The CARE of HEALTH in COMMUNITIES
Access for Outcasts

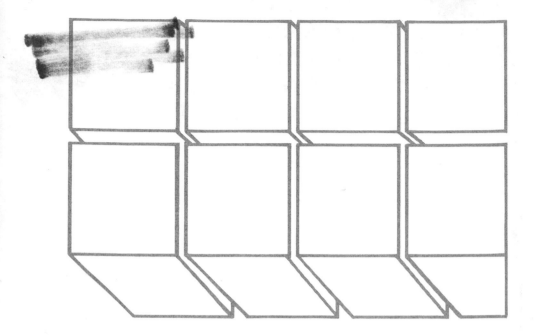

The CARE of

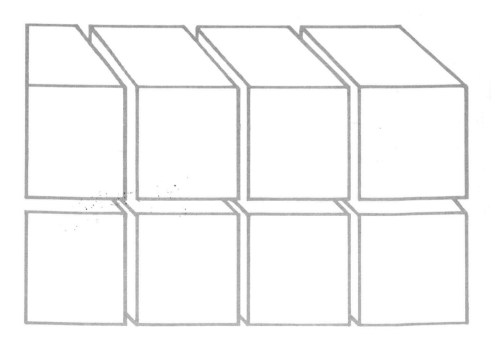

Nancy Milio

Boston University

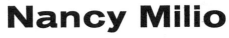

HEALTH
in
COMMUNITIES
Access for
Outcasts

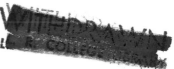

Macmillan Publishing Co., Inc.
New York

Collier Macmillan Publishers
London

Copyright © 1975, NANCY MILIO

Printed in the United States of America

MACMILLAN PUBLISHING CO., INC.
866 Third Avenue, New York, New York 10022

Collier-Macmillan Canada, Ltd.

Library of Congress Cataloging in Publication Data

Milio, Nancy.
    The care of health in communities.

    Includes bibliographical references and index.
    1. Medical care. 2. Medical care—United States.
3. Underdeveloped areas—Medical care. 4. Minorities—
Medical care. I. Title. [DNLM: 1. Community health
services. 2. Delivery of health care. WA546 M644c]
RA393.M5   362.1   74–6634
ISBN 0–02–381130–7

Printing: 1 2 3 4 5 6 7 8   Year: 5 6 7 8 9 0

To the memory of
MARGARET G. ARNSTEIN
who was not afraid to question
or to be questioned

Preface

It is easy to be concerned about health when it is lost. This book is for those who are concerned about health before it deteriorates. It is for those who are entering the health or health-related fields, and those who have worked in these fields but want a broader perspective of what they themselves are part of. It is also for those who think that the care-of-health must be significantly changed.

These pages are written recognizing certain realities: that no sector of a nation, and no nation, can any longer view its problems in isolation from the big picture—the national and international context, which increasingly limits or widens possibilities for action. And that efforts at the care-of-health and the rendering of health services can no longer be judged by the good *intentions* and purposes of the policy makers and practitioners. The painful job of looking at—and first of learning how to look at—the *effects* on people-in-communities of collective decisions and actions is now an essential instrument for repairing, revising, and reordering the environment and the health services, both of which can either support health or stifle it. If these things are not done, individual good intentions are wasted, nullified, and turned into frustration.

Recognition, the development of a critical consciousness, does not, of course, lead to answers, but without that questioning awareness we cannot even begin an effective search. Any acceptable answers must, at a minimum, not create more problems for those who are already outcast—whether nations or groups, minorities, the aged, women, the poor, and those geographically isolated. It is to this end—to further a critical consciousness in service of the search for acceptable answers—that this book is written.

Beginning with a global view, Chapters 1 and 2 attempt not so much to explain the intricacies of environment, health, and health services as to make the most important connections between people and their socio-political and ecological surroundings. This is done in the broadest context, comparing rich and poor nations and contrasting the rich and poor groups within these nations. Then, in Chapters 3–10, we change our focus to an affluent nation, the United States, and discuss its outcast groups and its system of health services. International comparisons are used as a reminder of other ways of seeing and dealing with the care of health. Placed between the major sections of the book are "Images of Access," vignettes of people and places in other countries, where reality illustrates the intertwining of the problems, dimensions, and clues to the solution of access for outcasts.

Following a general description in the second chapter of "outcasts, U.S.A.," who they are and how healthy they are, Chapter 3 shows where these outcasts are and their access to health services. The detailed material in the Appendix, contrasting differences among the states, may afford benchmarks for those who want to make further comparisons of the distribution of U.S. health services.

Chapters 4 and 5 go on to begin to explain the disparity in access to health services, revealing the sickness–inpatient–acute care focus of health care in its organization and financing patterns. Related to this is the specialist emphasis and personnel pyramids in the health occupations, taken up in Chapters 6 and 7, and the limited access that outcasts have to the health field. This comes through discussion of the makeup and direction of the health professions, using the new primary care practitioners as an illustrative focus. The section closes with an approach that can help increase access to the health field and to health services.

The foregoing ultimately are shaped, however, by the concerns of the final chapters (8–10) on various kinds of decision making—control, evaluation, and change making. They begin with a view of decision making as a bargaining—and therefore a political—process. Then follow detailed illustrations of this bargaining, concerning controls of various kinds, particularly planning, peer review, and the new professional standards review organizations (PSRO) and HMO (health maintenance organization) development.

Chapter 9 deals with questions of determining the effectiveness of decisions about health services and health. Chapter 10 deals with reshaping the alternatives for the care-of-health in the United States. It presents an analysis of nine major legislative proposals in terms of the types of provisions they set forth and their methods of approaching problems in health care. The effect that these provisions would have on outcasts is discussed also, as are missing alternatives. The chapter closes with the prospects for affecting changes in the decisions that provide for the care-of-health.

Wherever possible, the material was put into tables or graphs for those who may wish to use it in other ways. Appendix Table 18 summarizes the important facets of health services systems in a number of rich and poor countries. The notes provide an extended bibliography for those who want to pursue certain issues further.

The information concerning health care in other countries, in addition to the cited publications, was derived from my field research in Scandinavia, August 1967; in India, Hong Kong, Japan, the U.S.S.R., eastern and western Europe, January–December 1971; and in England, June–July 1973. For helping arrange these opportunities I am indebted to many people, especially to the late Margaret Arnstein, Yale University School of Nursing; Thelma Ingles, Rockefeller Foundation; Verne Robinson, U.S. Soviet-American Cultural Exchange Commission; the late Margaret Dolan, University of North Carolina School of Public Health; Dorothy Johnson, University of California at Los Angeles; Carl Taylor and Alice Forman, Johns Hopkins University School of Hygiene and Public Health; Lilo Hoelzel-Seipp, Wayne State University; Kusum Nair, Michigan State University; Myron Wegman, University of Michigan School of Public Health; Jeanne Carriere, Université La Val, Quebec; LeRoy Allen, Rockefeller Foundation; John Webb and Achyamma Thomas John, Christian Medical College and Hospital, Vellore, India; Miss A. Cherian, Indian Ministry of Health; Rama Rani Ray, Orissa State Ministry of Health; Shigeko Hayashi and Sachiko Ito, University of Tokyo; Erika von Amann, University of Heidelberg; Antonja Mol, University of Amsterdam; Jane Lowenstein, St. Christopher's Hospice, London; Muriel Skeet, British Red Cross; Kathleen Wilson and Lisbeth Hockey, University of Edinburgh. I am indebted to many of these individuals as well for helping me feel at home in their homelands, a debt that is unrepayable, as perhaps only those who have been "foreigners" can fully understand.

Others whom I can only thank for their reading of the manuscript in earlier forms, their helpful criticism, and other kinds of support and encouragement are Thelma Ingles, Ruth Hubbard Wald of Harvard University, Hans O. Mauksch of the University of Missouri Medical Center, Mary Catherine and Edward Conroy of England, Keith and Elma Hueftle of Detroit, Henry Silver and William Himelhoch of New York, Catherine Gutmann of Boston, and for bearing the typing, Elaine Blanchard.

N. M.

Contents

section I
The Global Context

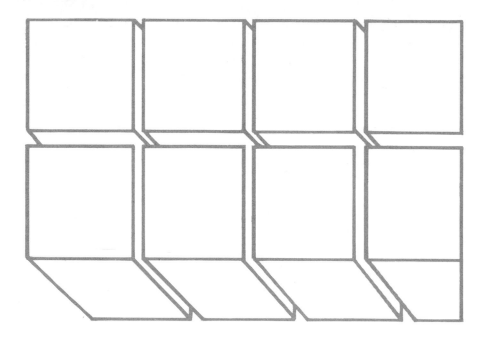

part one

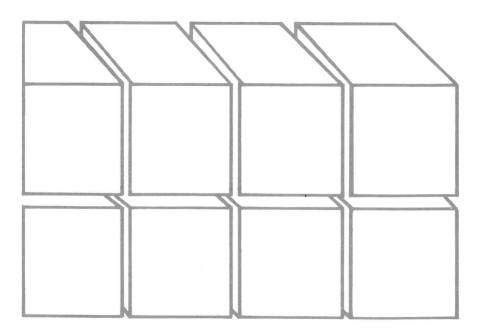

Environment, Health, and Health Care

The Lepers

"Ammal, Ammal.
Pasi . . . Pasi."

Fingerless hands
Upraised for daily bread.
Pleading. "Lady, Lady. Hungry . . . Hungry."

Formless stumps
raised to shelter
dust-reddened eyes from the searing sun.
Insensate skin
lifeless muscle,
pregnant only
with living death.

Brothers and sisters in torment,
outcasts through centuries of fear.
Rag-wrapped limbs
the only means allowed them
to keep their living parts alive.

N.M.
South India, 1971

chapter 1

Rich and Poor Nations: The Widening Gap

To view today's world environment as a system in which increasing demands are being made on finite resources in ways that do not allow the recycling of limited supplies—true as this is—is nevertheless to miss the more crucial aspect of global ecology. That is the question of distribution. It is the fact of a growing unevenness in what is available to meet the survival needs of more than two thirds of the world's people and what is available to the other 1 billion to meet their consumption needs. In general, the larger group is the poor, living primarily in developing countries in Asia, Africa, and Latin America. The more fortunate third live in the technologically advanced countries.

The reality of this increasingly discussed widening gap between poor and affluent nations, the causes and effects, constitutes the socioeconomic–physical environment in which 3.6 billion of us live. It sets the alternatives that may or may not allow persons to be born and live in health, to become aware of their options, to acquire the capacity to choose, to change, to expand the array of chances available to themselves and others.

What follows is an attempt to define the major aspects of this widening gap, in terms of available food, living space, jobs, income, education; to illustrate how the uneven distribution of these essentials for humane existence, between and within countries, affects chances for life and health and death, and in turn how these life chances affect the growth of populations, which again, depending on numbers, age groupings, and consumption styles, make variable demands on and contributions to the environment.

Demands On the global level, humankind demands increasingly more from its habitat through population growth (at about 2 per cent per year) and through a faster rate of increase in the young years (2.35 per cent among the 5–19 age group). This in turn augurs even higher growth rates for the future (1).

Consumption demands on water, petroleum, and marine protein are increasing at 3 to 4 per cent per year. And, in an effort to increase food

Table 1–1   The World Environment

Major Sources of Demand and Potential Regenerative Resources

	Major Sources of Demand		Potential Regenerative Resources[c]		
Data years					Data years
	Population increase		**Allocative decisions**		
1970	Total	3.632 billion	Redistribution of resources		
1963–1970	Rate of increase (annual average)	2%	Redirection of technology		
1960–1968	Rate of increase, 5–19 age group	2.35%	**Economic development of habitat** (% of annual increase)		
1960s	**Consumption, renewable and non-renewable resources** (% of annual increase)		GNP	4–5	1950–1972
			Income per person	4–5	1960s
			Food grain production[a] (ratio of increase to population increase)		
	Water	3			
	Marine protein	4	1950–1960	2:1	
1969	Petroleum	4	1960–1970	1.3:1	
est.[b]	Minerals and fuels	4.3–30	1971 and 1972	0.8:1	
	Other: land, timber				
	Pollution, air and water				
	Chemical fertilizers (% of annual increase) 7				
	Other: pesticides and other toxic elements, radiation, solid wastes, noise				

[a]FAO goal is 1.5–2% annual increase above annual rate of population increase.
[b]World demand as percent of 1969 world demand, producing 130–900% increases by the year 2000.
[c]The type and distribution of these would often place them on the "demand" rather than "regenerative" side of the balance.

Sources: International Planned Parenthood Federation, *Family Planning on Five Continents* (London: IPPF, 1972).
International Commission for the Development of Education, *Learning To Be* (Paris: UNESCO, 1972).
L. Brown, *World Without Borders* (New York: Random House, 1972).
FAO Report, *The Times* (London), June 7, 1973.
United States Council on Environmental Quality, *Environmental Quality–1972* (Washington, D. C.: Government Printing Office, 1972).

production, the use of chemical fertilizers is increasing at 7 per cent yearly, placing an additional burden on the environment by polluting water and threatening sea life (2).

World economic development, summarized as *gross global product* (GGP), the annual total monetary value of goods and services produced, itself produces deficits for the habitat. While on the credit side it can accelerate food production and human safety, it also depletes resources by using energy and mineral supplies without recycling them. Thus, although in the 1960s the GGP and the income per person worldwide was actually increasing 4–5 per cent annually, production and consumption styles were depleting world unrenewable supplies.

Of immediate impact was a 1 per cent drop in total food production instead of the 4 per cent increase that had been expected (3). The rate of food production, which was increasing twice as fast as the population was growing in the 1950s, slowed, relatively, to 1.3 in the 1960s, and was less than 1 per cent relative to population growth in 1971 and 1972 (Table 1–1).

World Distribution of Socioeconomic Resources   The advantages of world economic growth have been unevenly distributed however. About 40 per cent of the world's people are malnourished, and one third live in substandard housing. Over half the people received yearly incomes on the average of less than $100, while one fourth, the most affluent, received $1,000 or more (Table 1–2).

Table 1–2   World Distribution of Annual Income, 1970

Average per Capita ($)	% of Total Population
Under 100	51
100–1,000	24
1,000 or more	25

Source: L. Brown, *World Without Borders* (New York: Random House, 1972).

If the ability to read and write enhances people's capacity to use the advantages of economic development, then this capacity is also unevenly distributed throughout the world, increasingly so in terms of the numbers who are illiterate. Between 1960 and 1970, in spite of the fact that the proportion of illiteracy dropped 5 per cent worldwide, there were almost 50 million more illiterates, and the vast majority of these were women (Table 1–3).

Table 1–3   World Distribution of Illiteracy
Men and Women, 1960 and 1970

	1960		1970	
	%	N (millions)	%	N (millions)
World total (population over 15 years old)	39.3	735	34.2	783
Men	33.5	307	28.0	315
Women	44.9	428	40.3	468

Source: International Commission for the Development of Education, *Learning To Be*
(Paris: UNESCO, 1972).

People in Nations

Although numbers such as these suggest the increasing disparities between affluent and poor, they are nevertheless abstractions. The picture becomes more concrete, and more grave, when viewed as a comparison between developed[1] and less developed[2] countries.

Population   The industrialized countries of North America, Europe, and the Soviet Union hold less than one third of the world's people, including about one fifth of the world's children, and a small proportion of the world's women in child-bearing years (age 15–44). Most of these women, ranging from 4 to 8 out of 10, use methods of contraception. Most of the world's expenditures for direct fertility control, through contraception or abortion, are spent in these countries. This means that the affluent countries can look forward to slowing population growth, now only about 1 per cent per year; several countries already have or will soon achieve zero population growth—where the number of births equals the number of deaths.

The less industrialized world sectors of Asia, Africa, and Latin America are a virtual mirror image of this population profile. Already housing more than 70 per cent of the world's population, and 78 per cent of its children, they are growing by about 2.5 per cent per year. Further, they have most of the world's women of child-bearing age, fewer users of fertility control, and they spend the lesser amount, about 30 per cent, of all direct fertility control monies (Figure 1–1). The relationship of direct fertility control and other ways to deal with population growth will be discussed later.

Wealth   The share of the world's economic wealth as measured by

[1] Countries of North America, Europe, the U.S.S.R., and Oceania.
[2] Countries of Africa, Asia, and Latin America in the data cited unless otherwise noted.

Figure 1–1   Distribution Between Affluent and Poor World Sectors

Population and Direct Fertility Control

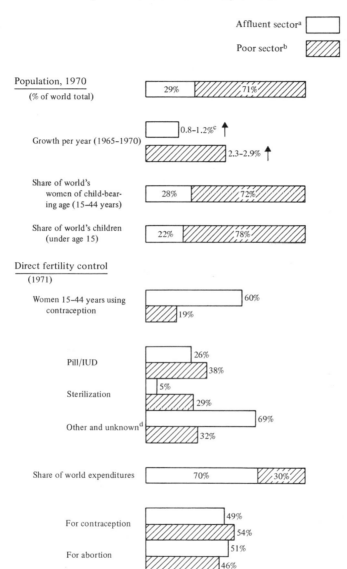

Affluent sector[a] ☐
Poor sector[b] ▨

Population, 1970
(% of world total)
29% 71%

Growth per year (1965–1970)
0.8–1.2%[c] ↑
2.3–2.9% ↑

Share of world's
women of child-bear-
ing age (15–44 years)
28% 72%

Share of world's children
(under age 15)
22% 78%

Direct fertility control
(1971)

Women 15–44 years using
contraception
60%
19%

Pill/IUD
26%
38%

Sterilization
5%
29%

Other and unknown[d]
69%
32%

Share of world expenditures
70% 30%

For contraception
49%
54%

For abortion
51%
46%

[a]North America, Europe, U.S.S.R., Oceania (Australia, New Zealand).
[b]Africa, Asia, Latin America.
[c]Range reflects differences between countries within each world sector.
[d]Includes 55 million abortions.

Data sources: International Commission for the Development of Education,
                Learning To Be (Paris. UNESCO, 1972).
            International Planned Parenthood Federation, *Family Planning
                on Five Continents* (London: IPPF, 1972).
            J. Robbins, "Unmet Needs in Family Planning: A World
                Survey," *Family Planning Perspectives,* 5:232-36 (Fall 1973).

9

gross national product (GNP) is even more unevenly divided. The developed sectors have more than 5 times the wealth of the less developed sectors. Both sectors grew at about the same rate during 1960–1968, roughly 5 per cent. But the gains per person differed because of differences in population increase. In the affluent countries, per capita gains averaged 3.9 per cent, while in the poorer countries, it was 2.7 per cent. Translated into dollars, this meant an average increase of $300 per person each year during the 1960s in the industrialized sector, and $10 in the less industrialized countries (4).

Jobs Growing populations and increasing numbers of children mean of course more people seeking jobs, a relatively more pressing need in the poorer countries. There, during 1960–1970, the labor force—persons registered as seeking work or having had some form of work, however temporary—grew 22 per cent and is expected to grow by 26 per cent in this decade. By contrast, the labor force grew by 12 per cent in the 1960s in the affluent countries and may increase by only 11 per cent in the 1970s (5).

The abundance of available jobs also is in contrast between affluent and poor nations. This translates into virtually no or low overall un- and underemployment figures in the rich nations, and high rates, estimated at 40 per cent, in the poor (Figure 1–2).

Urban Growth Although 70–80 per cent of the people in less developed nations have lived in rural areas, they are increasingly turning toward the cities for jobs and a better hope for survival. About 600 million are living in urban areas, which are now growing extremely rapidly, at over 15 per cent each year. Such growth far outdistances the capacity of urban services. Again this contrasts with industrialized countries, where urban concentrations are approaching 70–80 per cent of the population and seem to be stabilizing (6).

Available Food Given the growing differences in population, income, jobs, and living space, the gap in per capita food supplies becomes inevitable. The people of the poor countries have on the average fewer than two thirds the caloric and protein intake per day as those in the affluent countries (7) (Figure 1–3).

Education There is little question that formal education has had an important relationship to job getting and income, although its definition and efficacy are being critically examined nationally and internationally (8). Formal education is, then, in effect, a necessary resource for negotiating jobs, income, survival, or affluence. This is clearly so in the industrial areas of developed and less developed countries (9). This resource, too, reflects the widening gap in the world sectors.

Illiteracy In terms of illiteracy, the industrialized sector is reducing this problem by 1 per cent yearly for men, 50 per cent as fast for women;

Figure 1–2   Distribution Between Affluent and Poor World Sectors
Wealth and Employment

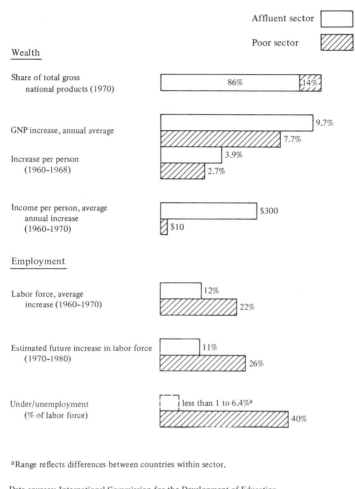

aRange reflects differences between countries within sector.

Data sources: International Commission for the Development of Education,
          Learning To Be (Paris: UNESCO, 1972).
          Committee for Economic Development, *Assisting Development in
          Low-income Countries: Priorities for U.S. Government Policies*
          (New York: CED, 1969).
          Great Britain Central Statistical Office, *Social Trends 1972*
          (London: Her Majesty's Stationery Office, 1973).

the less industrialized sector by about 5 per cent for men, but again, half
as fast for women. However, although the poor sector seems to be attack-
ing illiteracy at a faster rate, the paradox is that it had several million
more illiterates in 1970 than 1960 while the affluent sector had fewer
illiterates by several million. In other words, the growth in educational

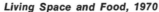

Figure 1–3 Distribution Between Affluent and Poor World Sectors

Living Space and Food, 1970

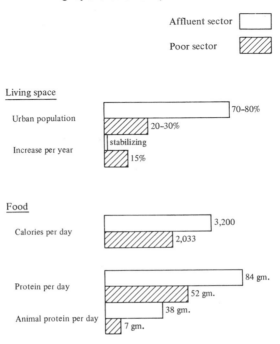

Affluent sector

Poor sector

Living space

Urban population — 70–80%

20–30%

Increase per year — stabilizing

15%

Food

Calories per day — 3,200

2,033

Protein per day — 84 gm.

52 gm.

Animal protein per day — 38 gm.

7 gm.

Data sources: L. Brown, *World Without Borders* (New York: Random House, 1972).
D. Jellife and E. Jellife, "The Urban Avalanche and Child Nutrition,"
J. Amer. Diet. Assoc., 57: 114 (1970).

resources was slower than population growth in the poor nations (10).

Prospects for narrowing this gap between the world sectors, under current conditions, are dim. The poor nations have a far smaller proportion of pupils enrolled in post-secondary education. However questionable the forms of higher education may be, its graduates will increasingly hold the higher-paying, decision-making positions in large-scale, computer-tied organizations. Even at the basic education level, the wastage ratio is considerably higher in terms of years of teaching per pupils graduated; overall public expenditure for education is lower (11) (Figure 1–4).

Perpetuating the Gap

Viewed in its various demographic and economic aspects, the widening gap in the distribution of world resources between affluent and poor sectors

Figure 1–4 Distribution Between Affluent and Poor World Sectors
Education

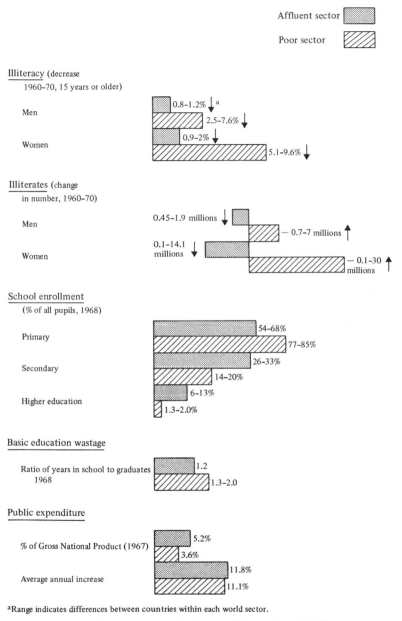

Affluent sector

Poor sector

Illiteracy (decrease
  1960-70, 15 years or older)

Men
  0.8-1.2% ↓ a
  2.5-7.6% ↓

Women
  0.9-2% ↓
  5.1-9.6% ↓

Illiterates (change
  in number, 1960-70)

Men
  0.45-1.9 millions ↓
  — 0.7-7 millions ↑

Women
  0.1-14.1 millions ↓
  — 0.1-30 millions ↑

School enrollment
  (% of all pupils, 1968)

Primary
  54-68%
  77-85%

Secondary
  26-33%
  14-20%

Higher education
  6-13%
  1.3-2.0%

Basic education wastage

Ratio of years in school to graduates
  1968
  1.2
  1.3-2.0

Public expenditure

% of Gross National Product (1967)
  5.2%
  3.6%

Average annual increase
  11.8%
  11.1%

aRange indicates differences between countries within each world sector.

Data source: International Commission for the Development of Education, *Learning To Be*
  (Paris: UNESCO, 1972).

is, in turn, a perpetuating cause in the further maldistribution of resources. Exchange on the global level increasingly favors the industrialized countries.

International Investment Multinational corporations admittedly regard the low development of the poor nations as an obstacle to investment; they therefore seek and often obtain home and host government protection, amounting to subsidies, for their investments (12). These multinational enterprises, the vast majority of which are headquartered in developed countries, are growing at about 8–10 per cent per year—twice as fast as global economic growth. An estimate is that by 1980, 75 per cent of world manufacturing assets will be concentrated in 300 corporations (13).

Technology Use The affluent world sector in 1964 produced virtually all the technological assets used in export. Well over 90 per cent of these resources were channelled through corporate enterprises between affluent nations. Thus the development and exchange of technology was oriented to the capital-intensive economies and profit-making ventures of the industrialized sector, and did little to benefit the labor-intensive economies or socioenvironmental problem solving of the poor sector (14).

Brain Drain Other means of exchanging technology, through the emigration of scientists, engineers, and physicians, have in the last decade shown a net gain for the affluent world. Highly educated professionals are coming to the affluent sector from the poor nations in increasing proportions (15).

Extractive Resources As the industrialized countries accelerate their needs for energy, they increasingly rely on the import of petroleum, from half to virtually all their needs, obtained for the most part from the poor sector. Likewise, they are importing more metallic ores, thereby becoming increasingly dependent for these on the less-developed countries (16).

Primary Products These primary products, nonmanufactured goods, still constitute 70–80 per cent of the exports of the poor countries, approximately the same as in the days of colonial empires (17). Even so, their primary agricultural products, such as sugar and cotton, have been allowed only restricted access to the world market as a result of protectionist trade policies by the affluent sector (18). As humanly irrational as it may seem, some countries, in Latin America, for example, are net exporters of agricultural products, although the quality of food eaten by their people has been slowly deteriorating during the last decade. Developed countries have 70 per cent of all world trade exchanged among themselves, and share only another 20 per cent with underdeveloped countries. Again, the proportions are diverging in favor of the rich nations (19).

Foreign Exchange Thus, the poor nations, able to sell and expand their trade only under terms and according to the needs of the industrialized world sector, find that their foreign exchange capabilities—needed to buy what they require for internal development—are severely limited. Almost 80 per cent of their foreign exchange came from exports in 1967 (and far less from foreign governmental aid or private investment) (20).

This is further illustrated by the fact that in the mid-1960s, the low-income countries that could expand their exports by only 2.6 per cent were able to develop their domestic economies by only 2.3 per cent. These countries contained more than half the people in the poor world sector (21). This economic growth did not keep pace with their population increase, much less the 11 per cent growth rate in GNP estimated to allow steady progress toward industrialization [This emphasis on GNP over people problems is now being reconsidered on the international level (22).]

Indebtedness The competitive position of the poor nations in international trade is thus deteriorating. This has been true since World War II and the situation continues to worsen. Under current world economic conditions, without the market capacity to earn foreign exchange for financing their internal development and without economic growth rates that will attract private foreign investment—except for certain kinds of manufacturing processes and petroleum extraction—the poor nations have been debtors. The nature and extent of that debt is now so grave that debt service and other payments to the industrial donor nations are now outstripping the foreign exchange inflow. In other words, the net outflow of currency from poor to affluent countries is now becoming greater than the net inflow. In spite of this increasing deficit, aid to the poor sector has been given proportionately more in loans than in grants, and public, non-profit aid has been diminishing (23).

To begin to remedy this aspect of the widening gap, the United Nations Conference on Trade and Development (UNCTAD) recommended in 1968 that the affluent nations make 1 per cent of their GNP as the net contribution in financial transfers between themselves and the less developed sector, with 0.70 of this amount deriving from public sources. In 1970, 0.34 of the total was coming from public sources. The 1 per cent goal had not been achieved, and was 0.78 per cent overall from both public and private sources. A few countries, such as the United Kingdom and The Netherlands, went over 1 per cent. The United States was about halfway to the goal, 0.55 per cent (24).

Health Status

As the disparity in population needs and the distribution of resources grows between the affluent and poor world sectors, a wide gap continues in health status, which the World Health Organization reports is not closing (25).

Table 1-4   Differences in Health Status Between Affluent and Poor Countries

Life Expectancy of Men and Women

	Affluent Countries				Poor Countries			
Data Years		Men	Women			Men	Women[a]	Data Years
1970	Sweden	71.8	76.5		Central Africa Republic	33.0	36.0	1963–1964
1968	Netherlands	71.0	76.4		Nigeria	37.2	36.7	
1966–1968	Federal Republic of Germany	67.6	73.6		India	41.9	40.6	1951–1960
					Pakistan	53.7	48.8	1962
1966–1967	Yugoslavia	67.7	69.0		Chile	54.4	60.0	1961–1962
1970 (preliminary)	United States	67.1	74.6		Egypt	51.6	53.8	1961–1962
					Ceylon	61.9	61.4	1961–1962

[a] See Chapter 2, Note 105.

Sources: United Nations, *Statistical Yearbook 1971* (New York: UN, 1972).

United Nations, *Demographic Yearbook 1970* (New York: UN, 1971).

U.S. Department of Health, Education, and Welfare, Washington, D.C., 1971.

U.S. Bureau of Census, *Statistical Abstract of the United States 1972* (Washington, D.C.: Government Printing Office, 1972).

Life Expectancy   It is tragically unsurprising to find that the life-span of people in the poor countries is often only half that of those in affluent nations. The children in some African countries, for example, can expect to live until they are about 35, while those in Sweden will live until they are over 70 (Table 1–4).

Death in the Early Years   This is in large part because a far greater proportion of deaths occurs in the youngest part of the population in poor countries. In Latin America 44 per cent of all deaths are among children under 5 years, while 7 per cent of deaths occurs in this age group in North America. The gap in deaths for children of 1–4 years is widening.

Even more pronounced is the difference in life chances for infants, the age group most vulnerable to an environment that does not guarantee adequate food and protection. Infant mortality rates in poor countries—deaths of children under 1 year per 1,000 live births—are often more than double those in affluent countries, ranging from less than 20 in the wealthiest to more than 100 in the poorest (Table 1–5).

Table 1–5   Differences in Health Status Between Affluent and Poor Countries

Deaths in Early Years

Data Years	Affluent Countries		Poor Countries		Data Years
1966	Deaths occurring under 5 years				
	(% of total deaths)				
	North America	7	Latin America	44	
	Infant deaths (per 1,000 live births)				
1970	Netherlands	12.7	Liberia	188	1960s
1970	Japan	13.1	Brazil	170	1960s
1968	Sweden	13.1	India	139	1971
1969	Denmark	14.8	United Arab Republic	118	1960s
1971	United Kingdom	18.6	Guatemala	94	1960s
1970	Canada	19.3	Chile	92	1960s
1970	United States	19.8	Colombia	78	1960s
1970	Federal Republic of Germany	23.3	Argentina	58	1960s
			Venezuela	46	1960s
1970	U.S.S.R.	25.7			

Sources: Pan American Health Organization, *Goals in the Charter of Punta del Este: Facts on Health Progress* (Washington, D.C.: World Health Organization, 1969).

United Nations, *Demographic Yearbook 1970* (New York: UN, 1971).

Great Britain Central Statistical Office, *Social Trends 1972* (London: Her Majesty's Stationery Office, 1973).

World Health Organization, *Health Hazards of the Human Environment* (Geneva: World Health Organization, 1972).

Child Growth and Development   Adequate nutrition affects the growth and development of children, of course. This is clear from a comparison of school-aged children in the United States (where the GNP per person was about $4,000 in 1968) with those in India and the United Arab Republic, which had GNP-per-person shares of $100 and $170, respectively. The average height of U.S. children was 9 per cent higher than India's, 4 per cent higher than that of the U.A.R. Their weight was almost one third more than India's, and 10–20 per cent more than U.A.R. children (26) (Figure 1–5).

Disease Patterns   The widely diverging socioeconomic environments of rich and poor world sectors produce, again, very different disease pat-

Figure 1–5   Differences in Health Status Between Affluent and Poor Countries
Child Growth and Development

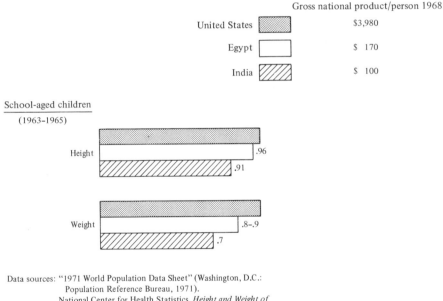

Data sources: "1971 World Population Data Sheet" (Washington, D.C.:
    Population Reference Bureau, 1971).
    National Center for Health Statistics, *Height and Weight of
    Children in the United States, India, and the U.A.R.*
    (Washington, D.C.: Department of Health, Education, and
    Welfare, 1970).

terns. The affluent nations are concerned about chronic disease, cancer, and accidental deaths. The poor name malnutrition, diarrhea, and certain communicable diseases as their major health concerns. In Latin American countries, for example, those with a lesser supply of animal protein and usable water had the highest death rates in young children dying from environmentally induced diseases. Over 90 per cent of these were considered preventable by sanitation and nutritional measures (27).

Applicable Technology Having diverging patterns of sickness, the medical technology of affluent countries has continued to develop in directions that make it less applicable in a variety of ways to the disease problems of the poor world, including the types of training needed for practitioners (28). This illustrates another aspect of the widening gap discussed above in relation to technology. The industrialized countries' technology is less and less applicable to the socioeconomic, as well as health care needs, of the underdeveloped nations.

In effect, the widening gap between rich and poor world sectors has become the most important characteristic in the world environment of the poor nations. That is, this growing gap sets the options under which they may or may not develop a survival threshold for the two thirds of the world population who live within their borders. This gap not only allows them diminishing proportions of world resources, but increasingly disallows them the chance to develop technologies, simple or complex, and other resources to solve their survival problems.

Population Growth

Viewed from the perspective of populations within poor countries, conditions which consistently, if not increasingly, threaten the availability of food and shelter, jobs, and other forms of security can only be seen as hostile. In this sense, a hostile, uncertain environment further encourages decisions that tend to aggravate the circumstances. Specifically, in the context of population growth, when the majority of people in poor countries experience deaths in their young, little paid work and low wages, and an uncertain future generally, they tend to bear more children. Their aim is, in effect, to ensure the survival of some who can earn at least some wages at low-skilled, labor-intensive jobs, and can care for them as they age. Until the means of survival are more assured—food; safe housing and surroundings; steady, paying jobs—there seems little motivation to limit births, even when effective modern methods are available, and even when fewer children might mean healthier mothers and fewer mouths to feed and persons to house.

Demographic Transition This illustrates the question of the demographic transition. Based on the experience of Western industrialized countries, the demographic transition refers to the initial increase in population growth, based both on longer life and fewer infant deaths, as industrial development made possible more stable living conditions for greater proportions of the population. As deaths decreased in the very young, births also began to decline, leading eventually to "aging" populations, which now exist in the affluent world sector (29).

Among the conditions necessary for this transition to occur—that is, to change from a pattern of short life-span, high infant death rates, high birth rates, and a young population to one of longer life, low infant death rates, low birth rates, and an aging population—has been what is called the socioeconomic threshold. This is the point at which the social distribution of resources allows an adequate food supply, living conditions that ensure the health and safety of infants and the aged, and literacy (30).

A very few developing areas, such as Taiwan, South Korea, and Hong Kong, have been able to slow down—but not contain—their rate of population increase in recent years. This they did through the effects of a 7–11 per cent annual economic growth rate, made possible in turn by the special economic attention given by industrialized nations (31).

Population Growth and Economic Development As implied above, growing populations can act as a deterrent to economic development. Through sheer numbers they make survival problems more difficult to solve and theoretically allow fewer social and economic resources per person. Since rapidly growing populations also mean more dependents, especially, young children, this further adds to the economic burden of the country. Further, under these conditions, workers are usually less healthy and therefore less efficient and consistent in production, another liability for economic growth (32).

Economic Development and Population Growth Conversely, when economic growth increases the survival resources in the environment of the population, in effect improving the health status of infants, mothers, workers, and the aged, the short-term effect is to have more resources available per person, more effective workers, and in the longer term, a slowly dropping birth rate (although the initial effect is a spurt in population growth). This, in turn, will have a positive effect on economic development (33) (Figure 1–6).

Population Growth and Family Planning It is at this point, the reaching of the socioeconomic threshold, that modern family planning programs have become effective in slowing population growth in the underdeveloped countries, as has occurred in Taiwan, South Korea, and Hong Kong (34). Without having attained the threshold which allows some assurance of survival, large-scale family planning programs have had little effect on hastening the demographic transition in the poor world sector (35).

India is a prime example. In spite of making family planning services a major emphasis in health care delivery since 1964, and expending more per person on this program than either South Korea or Taiwan, the population growth rate has remained basically unchanged, its 550 millions doubling every 28 years. Indications are now that the rate may even be increasing again (36). Rapid population growth is therefore a *result* of

Figure 1–6   Economic Development, Environment, Health, and Population Growth
Some Interrelationships

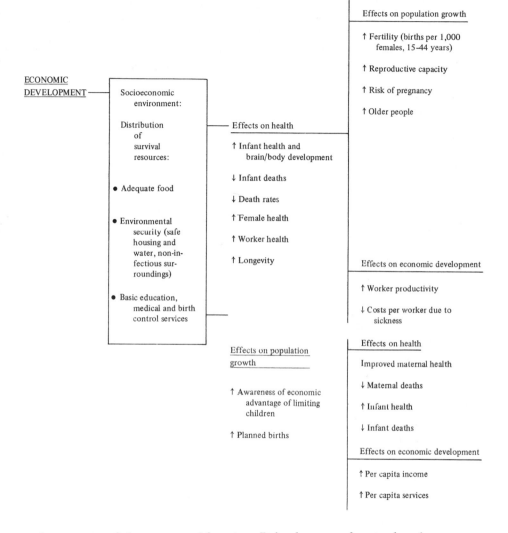

the poverty of the poor world sector. It is also one of several major perpetuating causes of that poverty and underdevelopment.

One way to summarize these relationships is to conclude that the reason underdeveloped countries are not following the demographic transition experienced by the industrialized countries is because they, the poor world, must contend with what eighteenth- and nineteenth-century nations did not have to face, namely, an affluent world sector.

A second major factor shaping the alternatives for the future of the poor world, and related to the emphases of the affluent world, is the criterion used to measure progress among the poor countries, the GNP. This figure, while it measures overall increase in production, says nothing about what kinds of goods and services are produced, or which groups are receiving what amount of benefits from economic growth. Even when divided by the population count, giving the per person GNP, this average tells nothing about the actual distribution of wealth and poverty within countries.

For this reason a number of groups with an international perspective have begun to advocate a refocusing of attention. From current emphasis on economic growth as measured by the GNP, they say a shift should be made to the immediate environment of poor populations, providing directly the steady supply of food, security in the form of housing, safe water, primary education and health care, and various means for increasing employment and income distribution (37). This approach is increasingly stressed (if not used), rather than awaiting the "trickle-down" effects of industrialization on the living conditions of the poor based on the former and, in part, current practices of affluent countries.

Summary

If on the global level a single pattern can be pointed to as denoting the critical aspect of environment that affects chances for the life and health of humankind, it is the widening gap growing between affluent and poor nations. The options of the poor world sector to meet merely their survival needs are severely limited by the increasing consumption of world resources by the affluent. In every essential for human life today—food, safe housing and living space, jobs, income, literacy—the smaller affluent sector continues to acquire larger shares. Further, its technologies tend not to be applied or applicable to the larger poor world's problems. Poverty brings rapid population growth and, so, more poverty. Thus the tragic irony: both the affluence of the rich world sector and the poverty of the poor world are making the poor poorer.

chapter 2

Rich and Poor Nations: Similarities

A further irony between the vastly different worlds of rich and poor nations is that when the distribution of resources is examined within their national environments, many of the problems of each seem strikingly similar. Recent reports by the World Health Organization and UNESCO have in fact pointed to the basic similarity of problems involving the delivery of health services and of education in both the developed and underdeveloped world sectors (1).

The fundamental difference underlying the similarities of course is that most of the people in the poor nations exist at a tenuous survival level, whereas most of the people in the affluent nations do not. Also, as earlier discussion suggests, the international widening-gap relationship between poor and wealthy world sectors has so far had a greater impact on the poor nations' internal affairs.

Disparities in Wealth and Income

In the Poor Countries

Reports now repeatedly show how patterns of world trade, increasingly determined by multinational corporations, as well as by forms of governmental foreign aid, are helping to widen the gap between rich and poor *within* underdeveloped countries. In India, 40–50 per cent of the population in 1970 lived below the official poverty level—the point at which malnutrition begins. Their income dropped, per person, in the last two decades, even though average income per person increased for the country as a whole (2). Thus while more than half the population were benefiting to some extent from economic growth, 200–250 million were becoming worse off (3).

Among those who prospered, some prospered far more than others. This was in part a result of the way the miracle-seed technology of the Green Revolution in wheat and rice crops was implemented. For example, the use of labor-saving, large-scale machinery, purchased from affluent nations, was encouraged, rather than developing new labor-intensive methods. Thus wealthier, large-acreage farmers—the 5 per cent who owned 20 or more acres—made the greatest profits while those owning less than 5 acres—75 per cent of all farm families—became, increasingly, debtors. This, among other things, further nullified the hoped-for redistribution of wealth through land reform (4).

Similar disparities resulted from farming and land reform programs in Latin America. As in India, also, manufacturing and export products, geared to the market demands of affluent countries and to the consumer demands of the affluent classes within their own borders, resulted in greater benefits to the tiny proportion of larger-scale entrepreneurs than to industrial or farm workers. In Brazil, for example, where the income of the wealthiest 1 per cent of the population was equal to that of the poorest 50 per cent, heavy industry grew at a yearly rate over 5 times that of wages (5).

URBAN–RURAL DISPARITIES

Urban Decay The economic patterns that we have been discussing have led to an increasing separation of affluent from poor in the underdeveloped countries, and to their isolation geographically. Accentuating the pattern of colonial times, the affluent live generally in the urban centers, the loci of international communication and trade and of national government. Most of the poor live in rural areas.

As already noted, they are coming to the cities in vast numbers seeking work, work that is being lost to them through the mechanization of farm labor and foreclosure on indebted small farms. But the cities cannot provide them all with work, both because they are arriving faster than industry is growing and because modern industry is not as labor intensive as in earlier eras. Thus are generated the slums and shantytowns of the large urban centers, now containing a third to one half of the urban residents in Latin American capitals (6).

Maldistribution of Area Resources This disparity between rich and poor, between urban and rural living, will almost certainly continue and increase, as attention and resources focus on cities. Even when national governments attempt to reverse this imbalance, their efforts may not be supported by foreign aid, which, in the cases of the largest nations, has tended to follow and support the interests of private business (7). The funds, for example, that were used to construct water supplies to rural areas in Latin America came from the national governments, with the U.S. Agency for International Development program furnishing but 2 per cent, many times less than was provided by it to urban areas (8) (Appendix Table 1).

Again, even when national governments undertake methods to re-distribute income within their countries, the methods used often either exclude the poorest segments of the population or are unenforceable on their behalf (9). Social security programs, for example, which insure against various risks of loss of income, are themselves a regressive form of taxation and tend to focus on the relatively small part of the popula-tion engaged in industrial work, located in urban centers; moreover, funds for these programs, in many African, Asian, and Latin American countries are under the control of the employer rather than the government, which legislated the program (10).

In the Affluent Countries

If in the underdeveloped countries, the poor are poorer than they are in industrialized countries, so also may the wealthy in affluent nations be richer and far more powerful in terms of the consequences of their de-cisions regarding the allocation of resources.

Disparities Between Affluent and Poor   In Japan and Great Britain, for example, the ratio of the wealthiest to the poorest fifths of the popula-tion is 9:1 in terms of their pretax income. This figure was 16:1 for indi-viduals in the United States (11).

Great Britain illustrates how wide affluent–poor disparities persist, even in a country favoring socialist principles. Going beyond the simple money-income measure of affluence to include all personal property, 5 per cent of Britain's population owns over 40 per cent of its wealth (Table 2–1). According to government accounts, efforts at redistribution of in-come, through social insurance programs and taxation, require a relatively larger share of the incomes of poorer households. Thus, after cash benefits are paid, through pensions, family allowances, and other means, the net redistribution of income is very small (12). Such programs are of course legislated by Parliament, whose Lords themselves own almost 10 per cent of the British Isles (13). However, a substantial redistribution of income does occur when all benefits of the programs are taken into account,

Table 2–1 Distribution of Resources Within Affluent Countries

Wealth and Money Income

| | Total Population | | |
	Most Affluent Group	Remainder or Poorest Group(s)	Country
Wealth[a]			
Ratio (richest to		9:1	United Kingdom
poorest fifths)[b]		9:1	Japan
		16:1	United States
Proportion (%) owned by	Richest 5%	Remaining 95%	
	41	59	Great Britain (1970)
Money income (%)[c]			United States
Share by families	Richest fifth	Poorest fifth	
1962	41.7	5.1	
1965	41.3	5.3	
1970	41.6	5.5	
Share by individuals	Richest 5%	Remaining 95%	
1965	20.2	79.8	
1970	20.5	79.5	
Share of wage and salary income (male workers)	Richest fifth	Poorest fifth	
1958	38.1	5.1	
1970	40.5	4.6	

[a] Wealth—includes monetary assets as well as property such as land, buildings, and equipment.
[b] Richest 20% of population in relation to poorest 20%.
[c] Money income—derived from wages, salaries, and earnings from holdings.

Sources: L. Brown, *World Without Borders* (New York: Random House, 1972).

Great Britain Central Statistical Office, *Social Trends 1972* (London: Her Majesty's Stationery Office, 1973).

U.S. Bureau of Census, *Statistical Abstract of the United States 1972* (Washington, D.C.: Government Printing Office, 1972).

U.S. Department of Labor report, *New York Times,* Dec. 31, 1972.

principally the comprehensive health, education, and social services available to the entire population. The narrowing income gap which thus results is still among the less wealthy 80 per cent of the people, the share of the wealthiest fifth remaining relatively untouched.

Most affluent countries have numerous and increasingly extensive post-income tax programs aimed at redistributing income. Some, such as Sweden's, are more effective than others. In recent years, many countries, such as West Germany, are broadening their social security programs, including wider health care coverage, channeling them more directly through central governments, relying less on indirect taxation—such as exemptions and other incentives—and less on employment-related benefits. This slowly shifts the focus to traditionally less favored segments of the population (14). The United States is least advanced in this respect.

U.S. Income Distribution   The distribution of income has not changed very much in the last 25 years in the United States. The poorest 20 per cent of American families have received about 5 per cent of the total money income while the wealthiest 20 per cent received over 40 per cent of all U.S. income. This income gap becomes more disparate when the income of *individuals* is measured separately, since average *family* earnings are appreciably higher (about 30 per cent) through the pooled efforts on two or more wage earners, principally wives. Thus the share of the wealthiest 5 per cent of all *individuals* has remained *more* than 20 per cent of all income (15) (Table 2–1).

There is some evidence that in certain respects the U.S. income gap may be widening. In terms of wage and salary income, the poorest workers were receiving a lesser share in 1970 than in 1958, while the most affluent earners increased their share of all earnings (16). As for nonearned income, the benefits of interest and dividends on 80 per cent of all U.S. stocks and bonds accrue to the wealthiest 1 per cent of shareholders. Thus, as profits increase faster than wages, the most affluent increase their wealth at a faster rate (17).

URBAN–RURAL DISPARITIES

Income Gaps   The disparities in income in the affluent nations are reflected, as in the poor nations, in urban–rural economic differences. In England, for example, earnings in the rural areas in 1971 were 25 per cent less than in urban areas, and unemployment was up to 3 times higher. A similar problem exists in other of the eight European Economic Community (EEC) countries, as well as the socialized countries of East Europe and, to a lesser extent, Japan (18).

In the United States, urban–rural gaps are reflected in such figures as the proportions of families in poverty in urban–metropolitan areas—7 per cent—and in nonmetropolitan areas—14 per cent in 1969. Families with incomes of over $15,000 composed 26 per cent of urban areas, and 15 per cent of nonurban areas in 1970.

Within nonmetropolitan areas, the disparities are further visible in the income of self-employed farmworkers, who earn only 80 per cent of what the average self-employed worker earns. A still greater gap exists between hired farmworkers and all wage-earners. The hired hands make less than one third the average wage (19). The generally rural and isolated section of Appalachia has had an increasingly widening gap between the income per person and that of the metropolitan areas of the country. Moreover, it is in the large urban centers that the gap—between Appalachian and other U.S. cities—is widening fastest (20).

Urban Decay The income-disparity situation illustrates a second aspect of the urban–rural problem which developed countries share with the underdeveloped nations. That is the deterioration of the large cities, whether by shantytown fringes or urban-core slums. Rapid population shifts, to the city by the poor, or from the city by the affluent, have aggravated the problems of resource distribution. Graphically, as one travels from the center to the suburbs of American cities, median income increases directly, so that it is 37 per cent higher at the suburban fringe than at the core (21). Twenty-eight per cent of urban residents were living in poverty areas in 1967, not far from the 33 per cent figure for Latin America (22).

Acknowledging this deterioration, several European countries and Japan have recently begun urban redevelopment programs. The EEC collectively is also planning to redistribute specially designated Common Market funds to poverty areas within its borders. However, this will be financed largely by a regressive 10 per cent tax on consumer goods (23).

Access to Education

Just as disparities in wealth are reflected in the quality of urban and rural living space, so also are they visible in the use of formal education in both affluent and poor nations. Education, in turn, as a resource that enhances the likelihood of higher earnings, has had the effect of bringing greater economic advantages to the affluent than to the poor, thereby widening the rich–poor gap (24).

Education and Social Class

Studies in recent years show that students from low-income, working class backgrounds and those from rural areas have been less represented at higher levels of education than those who come from higher-income professional families and from urban areas (Table 2–2). In Japan, for example, affluent families, which composed about 9 per cent of the total population in the 1960s, furnished over half of the students in higher education, while working class families (44 per cent of the population) furnished just 8 per cent of those students (25).

This general pattern of greater access to education for higher-status families has been found to exist in India and other underdeveloped countries, on the European continent, in Great Britain, the U.S.S.R., and the United States (26). This holds true even for students with the highest academic abilities—those who are bright and poor have less chance for advanced learning than the bright and affluent—in spite of research findings which show that intellectual potential is evenly distributed throughout all social classes (27) (Appendix Table 2).

Table 2–2   Distribution of Resources Within Affluent Countries

Occupation and Income Group Differences in Access to Higher Education

		Parents' Occupation		
		Professional and Managerial		*Working Class*	
Data Years		*% of Students Enrolled*	*% of Population*	*% of Students Enrolled*	*% of Population*
1960–1966					
	Japan	52.8	8.7	8.7	44.2
	England and Wales	62.9	21.5	27.2	71.5
	United States	52.4	22.9	26.6	57.4
	Yugoslavia	17.9	8.8	19.0	28.0
		Family Income			
1970		*$15,000 and over*	*$10,000– 15,000*	*$3,000– 5,000*	*Under $3,000*
	Families with members 18–24 years old (% with full-time college students), United States	61.0	45.8	19.9	13.9

Sources: International Commission for the Development of Education, *Learning To Be* (Paris: UNESCO, 1972).

U.S. Bureau of Census, *Current Population Reports, Special Studies,* Ser. P-23, 40 (Washington, D.C.: Government Printing Office, Jan. 1972).

Those with higher education have then had higher lifetime earnings than those without, a gap that tends to widen throughout most of adult life. Virtually everywhere it confers, to some extent, enhanced status, if not power (28).

Educational Growth   Given this situation, higher education, in terms of enrollment, teachers, and therefore expenditures, grew more rapidly in the 1960s in both rich and poor nations than any other form. It has expanded more than 2 or 3 times faster than preschool, primary, or adult education, which tend to have greater benefits for poorer and rural families (29). In effect, proportionately more public resources are being invested in the educational programs that give greatest advantage to the smaller, affluent groups within both rich and poor nations, an advantage that grows incrementally as the years pass.

Geographic Availability Beyond the question of preferential access by affluent groups to higher education, a second educational enigma common to both wealthy and poor world sectors is geographic access. Educational facilities are concentrated in prosperous urban areas rather than dispersed throughout urban poverty or rural areas (30). This is true in Latin America, where basic education is more than 10 times as available to urban as to rural children, in India, and in the United States (31). These conditions are again both a consequence of and a perpetuating cause of the sustained and sometimes increasing gap between wealthy and poor, urban and rural populations (Appendix Table 3).

Usable Education

The mushrooming of higher levels of education, fostered by hopes for enhanced status and economic mobility, has produced some anomalous outcomes. From the underdeveloped countries come reports that graduates are unwilling or unable to perform the practical tasks required in the world of work. They thus become under- or unemployed. Another way to view this is that the educational systems—and those determining the allocation of resources—are not preparing students for the work that needs to be done. They are overeducating them—in terms of concentrated time spans and specialized learning—and to that extent, at least, making them irrelevant to their country's needs (32). This has been done with the advice and aid of Western affluent nations, an approach recently coming under increasing criticism. Thus, because of uneven access and limited efficacy of education, the possibilities for effectively dealing with societal problems diminishes further.

Similar criticisms are made of academic education in the affluent countries, even though, relatively speaking, they can—perhaps—better afford the extravagance of irrelevent education, or miseducation. The charge of lack of efficacy has been made by those who show that job performance is not necessarily related to formal educational credentials (33).

Reform and Its Consequences At the same time, major educational reform, which is taking place in many countries, has focused, rather, on the second "universal" problem of education, that of providing access to all segments of the population. In such countries as England and the United States, some success in those reforms has not resulted in the expected narrowing of the affluent–poor income gap. Explanations suggested for this are that as educational opportunity increased, the higher-paying jobs became increasingly professionalized, and more formal degree requirements were emphasized, rather than secondary education or on-the-job-acquired skills (34). Differences have narrowed between high- and low-income students at the *secondary* level of education, in terms of providing more *years* of education to working class families, although not necessarily enhancing their income. The expansion of university education has given relatively more advantage to the higher-income groups (35).

An example of reform allowing improved educational access in the United States is black students, who, since 1967, are entering university and graduate programs faster than other social groups. At the same time, the education of low-income blacks is deteriorating. And, proportionately more blacks occupy the lowest economic levels in the country. Overall, significantly more have more education, but their unemployment rates have not diminished (36).

A related U.S. reform effort, the development of two-year community colleges, has had the effect of separating these students from the four-year college entrants on the basis of their high school track, not their ability. Further, since high school tracking (college preparatory or not) has been closely related to income and race, poor and minority students have more often entered community colleges (36a). In sum, education, as a resource with which to negotiate well-paying jobs, is more available to the affluent even after certain reforms have allowed access to broader segments of the population.

For this apparent impasse, a remedy has been suggested to the reformers who seek to use education as a means, through better job getting, to enhance the incomes of the poor. Given that social class is the most important determinant of educational success (graduation), a reversal of means and goals is advised. That is, reducing poverty through the direct provision of income to families may have the effect of improving the success of their children in education (37). This would not necessarily, of course, affect that other universal problem of education: that is, how to make it a lifelong, critical-consciousness-raising, participatory process.

Education and Employment

In the underdeveloped countries, enhanced access to education has meant primary and secondary education for greater proportions of the people. Ironically, however, unemployment—regardless of the type of job—is relatively higher among these, as compared to the very well educated and the illiterate (38). This is perhaps explainable by the types of work that need to be done. Since a vast proportion of jobs require low-skilled labor, employers, as they have done historically and in various countries, tend to hire those who will perform the task for the least wage, regardless of formal credentials (39).

Although employers in affluent countries have and do seek labor which can adequately perform the tasks at least wages, the job structure is virtually reversed (40). For example, in the United States the proportion of unskilled labor required now is less than 5 per cent of all jobs (41). The fastest growing occupations are professional, technical, and service (42). Thus skills—which, to repeat, are increasingly equated with formal educational credentials—become essential. And those who have been the subjects of the varieties of irrelevant education—whether maleducation (simply untaught), miseducation (taught untimely skills), or superfluous education—become the unemployed. In their greatest proportions, these are lower-income groups (a significant percentage of whom are excluded from unemployment statistics) (43). They thereby remain lower-income. All these interrelationships between education and jobs are important in looking at the problems in the health services occupations, to be discussed in later chapters.

Although formal education seems increasingly essential for employment, and well-paid employment, in the industrialized countries, it is not sufficient to assure such employment even when jobs are available. This is not only for the obvious reason that formal education does not necessarily guarantee competent job performance, but perhaps even more because of such considerations as ethnic identity and sex.

In England, for example, in the late 1960s job preference was given white over Asian Indians who were equally well prepared by education. The better educated the immigrants, the more was their experience with discrimination, even in communities considered "nonracist" (44). In a similar way, college-educated American Indians living away from the reservation had a higher rate of unemployment than those with high school education only (45). And, American women, having the *same* level of education as men were in jobs which paid them less than two-thirds what the men were receiving (46).

Outcasts East and West

These examples represent another commonality of both affluent and poor world sectors. This is the existence and persistence of groups in the population, growing in absolute numbers and sometimes proportionate to the whole, who receive less-favored treatment than those around them. They may be characterized by ethnic background, sex, and age, whether the very young or the very old. Whether their income level is affluent or poor, whether they live in urban or rural settings, their opportunities are fewer, their alternatives less, their choices narrower than those of their peers. These, with the poor and the isolates in rural districts or urban slums, are outcasts.

It is not too much to say that virtually anywhere in the world, to be poor and live in a rural area is harsh. And to be poor, rural, and an immigrant is worse. To be poor, rural, immigrant, and a woman is harsher still. But to be a poor, rural, immigrant, old woman is worst of all, in terms of one's options for life and health.

In the Poor Countries

In the poor world sector, outcast ethnic groups include refugee populations; linguistic, religious, and tribal minorities; and Untouchables, against whom less favored treatment is now illegal in India, but which exists, nevertheless (47).

Women in these countries are virtually excluded from administrative, major decision-making positions, and are represented only in small proportions in higher-paying jobs which are considered suitable for women (48).

Although official figures show some accelerated enrollment for girls at secondary schools, their actual attendance there and at the primary levels is far lower (49). In Asia, for example, where women enrolled in the 1960s at fastest rates in higher education, this rate also was slowing down —faster than the decrease for men—by 1967–1968. And, as pointed out earlier, there are increasing numbers of illiterates in the underdeveloped countries, 8 million more men, 40 million more women in 1970 than in 1960 (Table, 1–2; Figure 1–4). Thus, to the extent that education enhances status and income, these women will remain outcast (Appendix Table 4).

As for the aged, previous discussion of population changes and social security conditions suggests that those who are not fortunate enough to have family resources are likely to have their later years left to chance. The short life expectancies in the underdeveloped countries attests to their fates (Table 1–4).

In the Affluent Countries

The affluent countries, too, face the social fact of outcast groups. The elderly, a relatively dependent and traditionally poorer part of the age spectrum, now compose an increasingly large part of the population, from

6.9 per cent in Japan to 13.7 per cent in Sweden (50). Historical minorities persist, ranging from the linguistic groups within East European countries to Japan's lower-caste Buddhists and Koreans in urban slums or their indigenous Ainu population in the rural north—this in a country regarded as one of the most homogeneous in the world (51).

A new form of minority status which is, in a sense, the result of the super-affluence of many of the industrialized nations, has become visible in the last decade and is just beginning to gain official recognition in government statistics. This is their recruitment of workers from the relatively poorer nations for manual and service occupations. Workers, and often their families, have been going from the countries bordering the Mediterranean to central and northern Europe by the 100,000s (52).

In 1970 there were 2¼ million recruited workers in West Germany alone, adding not only to the nation's economic capacity, but to a perhaps less recognized demand on social resources which, for example, the almost half-million children of those immigrants require (53).

New immigrants make up about 20 per cent of the laborers in France —and a large proportion of the shantytown fringe of Paris. In Switzerland they compose almost one fourth of the entire labor force (54).

Another wave of immigrants derives from the former colonial empires. They seek new opportunities in the former mother countries, such as the Netherlands and Great Britain. In the period 1966–1970, while Great Britain lost 7,800 persons annually through emigration, it had a net increase of over 50,000 each year from its Commonwealth partners in the West Indies, South Asia, and Africa (55).

By 1972 the total of these new immigrants in Common Market countries was about 10 million (56). The United States is also gaining the new immigrant population. The 25 per cent increase in total immigration between 1965 and 1971 showed a drop in migrants from the most affluent countries, and increases from the Mediterranean, the Caribbean, and Asia, which had the greatest rise (57).

The figures suggest that not only the poor, but the poor from the underdeveloped countries, are increasingly seeking new chances in the affluent countries. Within the context of the affluent world, they become workers who are willing to labor for low wages (58). They are relatively less protected or unprotected by laws that regulate access to basic social resources such as housing and education (59). They are foreign to the sometimes-successful techniques for manipulating bureaucratic systems. Their presence creates resentment by low-income nationals, producing "social tension"

(60). They themselves may strike in protest to their less favored treatment
(61). They become outcasts.

The affluent countries share with the poor nations the practices that render
less favored treatment to women in terms of the distribution of social resources. Regardless of their income level, residence, or ethnic background,
women fare less well than their male peers, and men–women disparities are
wider among the poor.

Illustrative of this in Europe and the United States, men own greater
proportions of the wealth and have a far greater than half-share of the
resources which help them to attain and retain prestige, higher incomes,
and influence. Despite reforms that began in the 1950s, relatively smaller
proportions of women than men enter higher education, except at the
highest level of ability in the highest income group (Appendix Table 2).
Still fewer graduate, the least at the highest degree levels. They are under-
represented in the most prestigious occupations and in managerial and
administrative positions, whether in government, private business, or labor
unions (62). Even when in these more favored occupations, or in any other
job category, their full-time earnings are at best less than two thirds that
of their male counterparts (Table 2–6). These gaps did not narrow in the
1960s, and in some respects they may have increased. For example, the
proportion of U.S. women in the professions was less at the end of the
1960s than at the beginning (63) (Table 2–3).

THE BURDEN COMPOUNDED

It is clear that those who are outcast because they are poor or reside
in isolated living areas are even more unfavored in their access to resources
when they are also old and/or women and/or of ethnic membership. This
compounding of outcast statuses brings spiraling disadvantages, which in
turn tends to sustain their place as outcasts, in relative if not in absolute
terms.

Outcasts, U.S.A.

The compounding effects of outcast statuses is readily visible in the United
States. For example, in the already disadvantaged area of rural, non-
corporate farm life, further differences exist between the self-employed

Table 2-3 Distribution of Resources Within Affluent Countries

Wealth, Education, Employment, and Earnings by Sex

	Men	Women	Country	Data Years
Wealth				
Total, by individuals (billion pounds)	59.8	37.0	Great Britain	1970
University Education				
Students (% of sex)	n.a.	32	Great Britain	1963
	n.a.	25	West Germany	1968
	n.a.	35	Denmark	1963
	n.a.	29	France	1967
	40	29	United States	1970
Graduates (men–women ratio)	7:3		United Kingdom	1910–1960
Degrees				
B.A.	3:2		United States	1965–1969
M.A.	2:1		United States	1965–1969
Doctoral	9:1		United States	1965–1969
Employment (% of sex in labor force)				
Higher professions	42[a]	18[a]	France	1963
Managers, supervisors, foremen	13	5	Great Britain	1970
Managers and administrators	14.6	5	United States	1971
Engineers, scientists, and technologists	3	1	Great Britain	1970
Earnings (full time, per week)				
Median	$75	$43	Great Britain	1971
Manual occupation (ratio)				
1966	2:1		Great Britain	1971
1971	2:1		Great Britain	1971
Selected nonmanual (range)				
Health and welfare staff	$60–105	$35–67	Great Britain	1971
Academic and teaching staff	77–117	55–90		
Average income (annual ratio)				
1955	1.6:1		United States	1971
1970	1.75:1			

[a] As percentage of total labor force.

Sources: Great Britain Central Statistical Office, *Social Trends 1972* (London: Her Majesty's Stationery Office, 1973).

M. Craft (ed.), *Family, Class, and Education* (London: Longman, 1970).

U.S. Senate Committee on the Judiciary, *Report on the Equal Rights for Men and Women Amendment, Mar. 14, 1972.*

C. Silver, "Women and the Professions in France." *Amer. J. Sociol.* 78:836–51 (Jan. 1973).

Women's Bureau, report, *New York Times*, Dec. 31, 1972.

and the hired farmworkers, beyond their more than 2:1 disparity in average wages. Among hired workers were proportionately more women and more than 12 times as many from ethnic minorities; and about one third of them did not earn enough to qualify for social security coverage (64). Thus the disadvantages spiral into old age.

In a similar sense, those who are poor live also in poverty areas, and proportionately more blacks than whites live in the poor areas of the cities (65). Again, because women are poorer than men and have more difficulty obtaining work, they, like others who are of low-income, work more, and they work at lower-paying jobs and in less sought-after regions. As a final example, although more of the elders are poor, most blacks over 65 have poorer housing than their white counterparts, and old black women are poorer than old black men (66).

STATISTICAL PICTURE

A brief look now at a more systematic statistical picture of major outcast groups in the United States will give some perspective to later discussion of the problems in developing accessible health care services in the United States.

In terms of income levels and economically desirable living space, it is clear that families and unrelated individuals who are other than white— 90 per cent of whom are black—are less favored. They live in the South —more than half of all blacks live there—and in the poorer central cities and farm areas—where the black average income is below the official rural poverty level (67) (Figure 2–1; Table 2–4).

Income disparities have fluctuated, and among unrelated individuals may be widening (Figure 2–1). This perhaps reflects growing proportions of single women as well as of widowed elders, who are relatively poorer than others, as are the racial minorities (Figure 2–2).

Although women fare worse economically than men, minority women fare worse than women workers in general and compared with minority men as well, in fulltime earnings and as heads of families (Table 2–5), in employment in economically desirable occupations (Table 2–6) (67a) and in sustained employment (Figure 2–3). Their rate of unemployment (10.9 per cent) is even higher than that of women of Spanish origin (9.2), which is higher than that of minority men (9.1) or men of Spanish origin (8.9).

Similar patterns of favored treatment for white over minority races and those of Spanish origin, and of men over women, persist in general in education, for those completing 4 or more years of high school or of college (Table 2–7).

Figure 2–1   Distribution of Resources Within Affluent Countries

Income Differences by Race and Family Status, United States, 1970

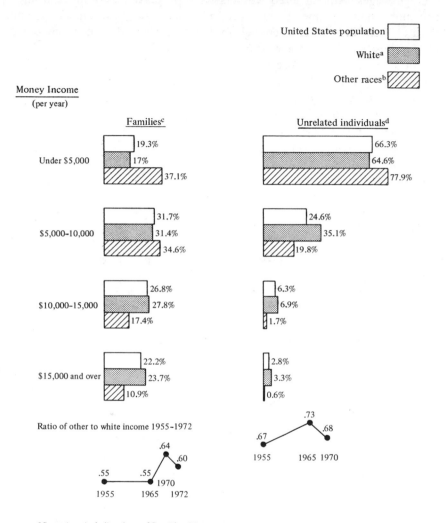

aCaucasians, including those of Spanish origin.

bNon-Caucasians, including Orientals, American Indians, and blacks who comprise 90% of "other races."

cBased on income of a four-member unit, 2 children, persons related by blood, marriage, or adoption; ratio includes all family sizes.

dPersons not living with others tied by marriage, blood, or adoption.

Data source: U.S. Bureau of Census, *Statistical Abstract of the United States* (Washington, D.C.: Department of Health, Education, and Welfare, 1972).

Table 2–4 Distribution of Resources Within Affluent Countries

Family Income Levels and Unemployment by Urban–Rural Residence and Race, United States, 1970

	White			Black		
	Under $5,000 (%)	Median Income	Unemployment (%, 1971)	Under $5,000 (%)	Median Income	Unemployment[a] (%, 1971)
United States[a]	17	$10,200	5.5	32.3	$6,300	9.9
Metropolitan[b] areas[c]	13.7	11,200	5.7	32.1	7,100	10.2
In central city	16.9	10,400	6.3	33.0	7,000	9.8
Outside central city	11.4	11,700		29.0	7,600	
Outside metropolitan areas[d]			5.0			8.8
Nonfarm	21.4	8,900	5.4	53.6	4,600	9.2
Farm	35.3	6,800	2.2	75.6	3,100	6.2

[a] Includes other races.
[b] Metropolitan area—a specific location composed of at least one county with at least one central city of 50,000 population or more.
[c] Urban family poverty level, $3,970.
[d] Rural family poverty level, $3,375.
("Poverty" is defined officially by the Social Security Administration each year as the amount required to meet the minimum annual food budget set up by the Department of Agriculture, multiplied by 3. Figures are set for various sizes of household and for urban or rural residence. Rural levels are now 85% of the urban poverty level.)

Source: U.S. Bureau of Census, *Statistical Abstract of the United States 1972* (Washington, D.C.: Government Printing Office, 1972).

Outcasts and Their Health

In the global context, earlier discussion showed how the uneven distribution of world resources is creating a widening gap between affluent and poor countries, producing, in effect, outcast nations. This has had dramatic consequences for the overall health levels of poor countries. Likewise, the skewed distribution of resources within countries makes certain groups outcast, within both affluent and poor nations. It also has effects for the health of outcast groups within nations.

Infant Mortality This becomes very clear from an analysis of infant mortality. Infant deaths, those occurring in the first year of life, in the United States were by 1960 almost twice as high for other-than-white[1] babies as for whites (Figure 2–4). In the mid-1960s a national study, the first of its kind, unraveled some of the causes for this disparity. It showed how socioeconomic status, measured by family income and parents' edu-

[1] Defined as all races that are not Caucasian; 90 per cent of these are blacks.

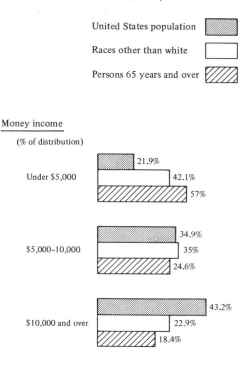

Figure 2–2   Distribution of Resources Within Affluent Countries

Annual Money Income by Minorities and Aged, United States, 1970

United States population

Races other than white

Persons 65 years and over

Money income

(% of distribution)

Under $5,000
21.9%
42.1%
57%

$5,000–10,000
34.9%
35%
24.6%

$10,000 and over
43.2%
22.9%
18.4%

Data source: National Center for Health Statistics, *Monthly Vital Stat. Rept.,* 22, April 2, 1973 (supplement).

cation, is the major determinant in a child's chance for life. And, in whatever income group, the higher the parents' education, the better a child's chance for life (68). This is consistent with the fact that higher education is closely related to affluent family background.

Other major life-reducing factors, such as very young or relatively older mothers, low birth weight, family residence, and disease or injury, pose a greater threat to the poor than to the affluent newborn. Regardless of race, deaths were 50–100 per cent lower in the highest social class than the lowest. However, a telling commentary is the fact that in this random sample there were not sufficient numbers of infants of other than white races in these highest social classes to compute mortality rates for them (69) (Figure 2–5).

In all income groups, infant deaths were higher in nonmetropolitan

Table 2–5 Distribution of Resources Within Affluent Countries

Median Income by Race and Sex, United States, 1970

	Total	White	Black
United States[a]	$9,870	$10,200	$6,300
Women (full time)	5,325	5,490	4,675
Men (full time)	8,965	9,375	6,600
Families (1972) with			
Women heads	5,115	5,840	3,645
Men heads (wife not working)	10,930	9,976	6,500

[a] Actual cost of urban living: family of 4, 1972, $11,446; on low budget, $8,106; on intermediate budget, $13,576.

Sources: U.S. Bureau of Census *Statistical Abstract of the United States 1972* (Washington, D.C.: Government Printing Office, 1972).

Women's Bureau, *Facts About Women Heads of Households and Heads of Families* (Washington, D.C.: Department of Labor, Apr. 1973).

areas and in the southern region of the United States, roughly approximating the more rural areas of the country. These are also the economically poorer areas, which makes for a cumulative threat to infants. In the south, for example, the deaths were not only higher for the poor than in other regions, but the gap between poor and affluent within that region was far

Table 2–6 Distribution of Resources Within Affluent Countries

Occupation and Income by Sex and Race, United States, 1971

Selected Occupations	Occupational Unemployment Rate	Labor Force					Total Minority (%)
		Men		Women			
		Median income 1970	%	Median income 1970	%	Minority (%)	
Professional and technical	2.9	$11,600	13.6	$6,700	13.3	10.6	9.0
Managerial and administrative	1.6	11,300	14.6	5,500	5.0	n.a.	4.1
Clerical	4.8	7,900	6.7	4,600	33.0	22.0	13.7
Service (excluding private household)	6.3	5,600	8.0	2,500	22.0	16.0	20.3

Sources: U.S. Bureau of Census, *Statistical Abstract of the United States 1972* (Washington, D.C.: Government Printing Office, 1972).

Women's Bureau, *Facts on Women Workers of Minority Races* (Washington, D.C.: Department of Labor, June 1972).

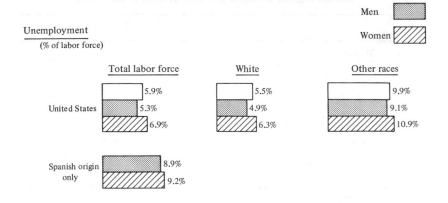

Figure 2–3 Distribution of Resources Within Affluent Countries

Unemployment by Sex and Race, United States, 1970

Unemployment
(% of labor force)

Men ▨
Women ▨

Total labor force   White   Other races

United States   5.9% / 5.3% / 6.9%   5.5% / 4.9% / 6.3%   9.9% / 9.1% / 10.9%

Spanish origin only   8.9% / 9.2%

Data sources: U. S. Bureau of Census, *Statistical Abstract of the United States 1972* (Washington, D.C.: Government Printing Office, 1972).
Women's Bureau, "Women Workers in Regional Areas, 1971" (Washington, D.C.: Department of Labor, June 1972).

Table 2–7 Distribution of Resources Within Affluent Countries

Secondary and Higher Education by Race, United States

	4 or More Years Completed[a] (% distribution)		
	High School (1971)	College 1960	1970
All races	56.4	7.7	11
White	58.6	8.1	11.6
Men	n.a.	10.3	15.0
Women	n.a.	6.0	8.6
Spanish origin	32.6	n.a.	n.a.
Black	34.7	3.1	4.5
Men	n.a.	2.8	4.6
Women	n.a.	3.3	4.4

[a] Persons 25 years and older.

Source: U.S. Bureau of Census, *Statistical Abstract of the United States 1972* (Washington, D.C.: Government Printing Office, 1972).

Figure 2–4   Differences in Health Status Within
Affluent Countries

Infant Mortality, United States, 1950–1972

Infant deaths
(per 1,000 live births)

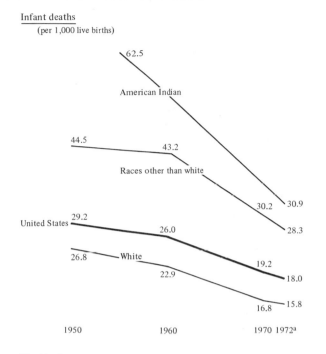

1950	1960	1970 1972[a]	

[a]Provisional.

Data sources: National Center for Health Statistics, *Facts of Life and
Death* (Rockville, Md.: Department of Health, Education,
and Welfare, 1970); and "Annual Summary for the United
States, 1972," *Monthly Vital Stat. Rept.*, 21, June 27,
1973 (provisional).

greater, a difference of 21.9 deaths per 1,000 live births, compared with a
2.6 difference in the more affluent Northeast (Figure 2–5).

This relationship of higher infant deaths in economically depressed
regions also exists in England (70). There, also, the life chances for infants was less for minority races (34.6) than for Britishers (26.8) in
1965–1969 (71).

A similar and widening gap between social classes was reported by
several European countries during the 1960s (72).

Low Birth Weight   Another important finding in the U.S. study was
that in babies of low birth weight, for whom the chances of death are
highest, there is a *small* difference in the chances for infants of poor or

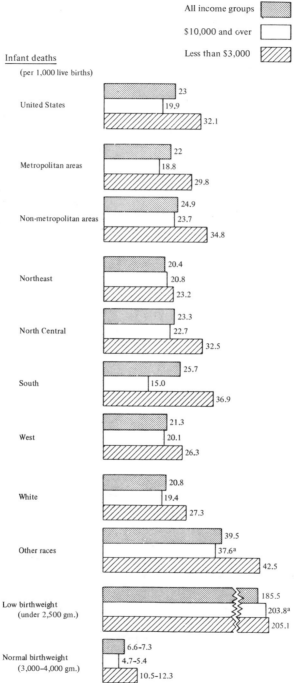

Figure 2–5 Differences in Health Status Within Affluent Countries
Infant Deaths and Income Group, United States, 1964–1966

All income groups

$10,000 and over

Less than $3,000

Infant deaths
(per 1,000 live births)

United States
23
19.9
32.1

Metropolitan areas
22
18.8
29.8

Non-metropolitan areas
24.9
23.7
34.8

Northeast
20.4
20.8
23.2

North Central
23.3
22.7
32.5

South
25.7
15.0
36.9

West
21.3
20.1
26.3

White
20.8
19.4
27.3

Other races
39.5
37.6[a]
42.5

Low birthweight
(under 2,500 gm.)
185.5
203.8[a]
205.1

Normal birthweight
(3,000–4,000 gm.)
6.6–7.3
4.7–5.4
10.5–12.3

44

[a]$7,000–10,000

Data source: National Center for Health Statistics, *Infant Mortality Rates:
Socioeconomic Factors, U.S.* (Washington, D.C.: Department
of Health, Education, and Welfare, 1972).

affluent families. In the normal birth-weight range, where life chances for the newborn are *best,* the poor have more than *twice* as many deaths as the affluent, and this difference increases after the first week of life (Figure 2–5). At this point, after the first week of life, poor babies die faster from respiratory and gastrointestinal disease and accidents (73). In other words, having left the technological environment of the hospital, the socio-economic environments of poor and affluent families then set the chances for life for the babies. Low-birth-weight babies remain longer within the hospital environment, of course.

The U.S. infant death rate is often compared unfavorably with those of other affluent countries. Higher U.S. mortality is thought to result in large part from the relatively higher and increasing proportion here of low-birth-weight babies (74). These babies have a higher risk of death than heavier infants, by 30 times, increasing the mortality rates (75).

A recent U.S. study of the increase in premature, low-birth-weight babies during 1950–1967 showed that 90 per cent occurred in other than white races (76). Moreover, more than 3 times as many low-birth-weight babies are born in the lower as in the higher-income groups, a relationship that occurs in England also (77). Thus, by separating out these babies of poor and nonwhite families, improvements in chances for life for babies of white families is similar to that in many affluent European countries (78).

Preventable Deaths Given this evidence, the U.S. study concludes that 47 per cent of infant deaths in this country are preventable (68 per cent is the comparable figure for Latin America), and most of the improvement can be made for babies in the normal-birth-weight range and after their first week of life (79). Clearly, this concerns those infants who do not come within the purview of specialized technology; nor are they, during this period of their lives, necessarily sought out by the system of health services. These babies are from poor families, from families other than white, and families who live in economically less desirable areas.

Nutrition It is comprehendable that the poor half of India's population is malnourished and that this is visible in the retarded growth and development of its children, as already noted. As unwelcome, but less easy to understand, is the evidence of malnutrition in the United States. In a recent national government survey, nutritional deficiencies were found most among blacks and persons of Spanish origin, more so in the lower-income groups, and were most prevalent among the poor in the lower-income states. In these same groups and regions child growth and development is more retarded than among the more affluent (80). This again represents the cumulative deficits of outcasts, and suggests how mounting deficits make them less able to throw off outcast constraints.

Disability Disability is another consequence for the health of outcasts, which in turn helps perpetuate their status as outcasts. The poor have more chronic disease, more limitation of activity from chronic disease, and more have severe types of limitation than the affluent, by 3–4 times; this makes them unable to perform major work, household, and school activities. Relatively fewer whites have such disability than those of other races; but among the poor, all races are roughly on a par, except for the severest forms of disability, when to be of other than white races is to have more disability (81).

Having more injury and illness also results in more days in bed and restricted activity for the poor, as well as for the aged, compared with the total population. As in other measures of health status, those who live in central city and rural areas, and in the South, experience more disabling effects from illness (82) (Figure 2–6).

Life Expectancy Given this picture of the poor, and of those who live in low-income areas, having fewer chances for healthful life and growth, their years of life can be expected to be shorter. Since greater proportions of other than white races are poor, including blacks and American Indians, life chances for the poor are suggested from life-expectancy tables arranged according to race. Although all Americans born in 1970 could expect to live on the average 70.9 years, whites would live 71.7 years, other races, 65.3 years. Further, where in the 1950s the higher death rates for other races were dropping substantially among persons 1 to 60 years, a steep rise occurred for those age groups in the 1960 decade, particularly in the young adult years (not including war deaths). This again widened the gap between the chances for life between other races and whites (82a) (Figure 2–7).

Population Growth This demographic pattern within the poorest segments of the population relative to the non-poor-white majority—of more infant deaths, and less chance for healthy and long life, and thus a younger average age—includes a higher birth rate, similar to that described in poor, underdeveloped nations and, in a broad sense, for comparable reasons. For example, the immigrant minority races in Great Britain have birth rates more than twice that of the home population (83). Similarly, in the United States, whites and the nonpoor have the lowest birth rates (84). What this means within affluent countries, however, is that the *main* source of population growth is nevertheless the number born to the majority (white) groups. This was recently officially recognized by a national U.S. Commission on Population and the American Future. It emphasized also that the problem of U.S. population growth could not be fully resolved until the issues of poverty and racism in America are resolved; and secondly that without controlling population growth, all other problems become more difficult (85).

Figure 2–6   Differences in Health Status Within Affluent Countries

Disability, United States, 1968 and 1969–1970

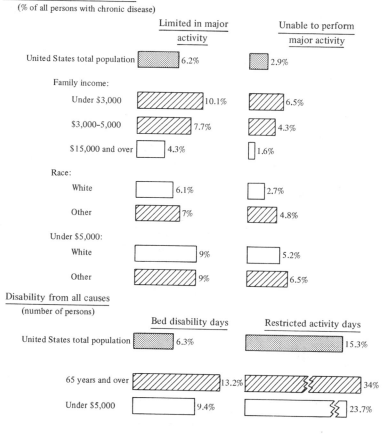

Limitation from chronic disease
(% of all persons with chronic disease)

	Limited in major activity	Unable to perform major activity
United States total population	6.2%	2.9%
Family income:		
Under $3,000	10.1%	6.5%
$3,000–5,000	7.7%	4.3%
$15,000 and over	4.3%	1.6%
Race:		
White	6.1%	2.7%
Other	7%	4.8%
Under $5,000:		
White	9%	5.2%
Other	9%	6.5%

Disability from all causes
(number of persons)

	Bed disability days	Restricted activity days
United States total population	6.3%	15.3%
65 years and over	13.2%	34%
Under $5,000	9.4%	23.7%

Data sources: National Center for Health Statistics, *Limitation of Activity Due to Chronic Conditions, U.S., 1969 and 1970* (Washington, D.C.: Department of Health, Education, and Welfare, Apr. 1973); *Current Estimates from the Health Interview Survey, U.S., 1971* (Washington, D.C.: Department of Health, Education, and Welfare, Feb. 1973); and *Health Characteristics of Low-income Persons* (Washington, D.C.: Department of Health, Education, and Welfare, July 1972).

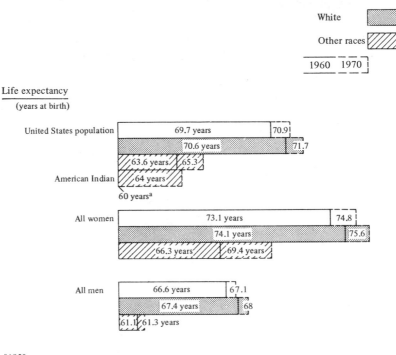

Figure 2–7 Differences in Health Status Within Affluent Countries

Life Expectancy, United States, 1960 and 1970

White

Other races

1960 1970

Life expectancy

(years at birth)

United States population 69.7 years 70.9
70.6 years 71.7
63.6 years 65.3
American Indian 64 years
60 years[a]

All women 73.1 years 74.8
74.1 years 75.6
66.3 years 69.4 years

All men 66.6 years 67.1
67.4 years 68
61.1 61.3 years

[a]1950.

Data sources: U.S. Bureau of Census, *Statistical Abstract of the United States
1972* (Washington, D.C.: Government Printing Office, 1972).
National Center for Health Statistics, "Final Mortality Statistics,
1970," *Monthly Vital Stat. Rept.,* 22, Nov. 14, 1973 (supplement).
M. Michal, et al., *Health of the American Indian* (Rockville, Md.:
Department of Health, Education, and Welfare, 1973).

Referring back to the socioeconomic threshold at which couples seek
to limit the numbers of children they bear, studies consistently show that
large proportions of the poor are ready to do this. [In fact, among blacks
in the United States, whose incomes are lower than whites, the fertility
rate (the births per 1,000 women 15–44 years of age) has diminished
since 1964, and that of whites has increased in 1968–1969 (86).] That is,
in affluent countries many of the poor have reached the "socioeconomic
threshold" for family planning. The next step, in terms of social planning,
is to provide safe and efficient technology for birth control to all men and
women who want it.

That the poor have fewer chances for life and health does not imply that the nonpoor are as healthy as they might be, or necessarily that they are becoming healthier.

Increasingly in recent years, concern is being expressed over the failure to control the rates of disease and death among nonpoor and affluent populations. Reports from Europe, Japan, and the United States show that death rates are no longer declining; they seem to be reaching a plateau or, in some instances, even increasing. Most of the lowest death rates in the age groups over 40, at least during the 1960s, occurred in less-affluent countries, such as Greece and Albania (86a).

Table 2–8   Differences in Health Status Within Affluent Countries

Death Rates, United States, 1950–1972

	Deaths (per 1,000 population)			
	1950	*1960*	*1971*	*1972*[a]
United States	9.6	9.5	9.3	9.4
White		9.5	9.3	9.4
Male	10.9	11.0	10.7	10.8
Female	8.0	8.0	8.1	8.2
Other		10.1	9.2	9.3
Male	12.5	11.5	10.8	11.1
Female	9.9	8.7	7.7	7.6

[a] Provisional.

Sources: National Center for Health Statistics, *Facts of Life and Death* (Washington, D.C.: Department of Health, Education, and Welfare, 1970).

National Center for Health Statistics, "Annual Summary for the United States, 1972," *Monthly Vital Stat. Rept.* 21, June 27, 1973 (provisional).

Death Trends   The U.S. death rate, for example, has changed little since the 1950s, reaching a low in 1954. Between 1971 and 1972 it rose slightly, from 9.3 to 9.4 per 1,000 population (Table 2–8). On closer analysis, the youngest and oldest, those under 5 and over 65, had relatively fewer deaths. Increased deaths were in the presumably most vigorous age groups, especially among those aged 15–65, following a pattern of the

1960s, where the largest increases in deaths occurred in the young adult years, especially among men. About two thirds of all deaths were caused by heart disease, cancer, and strokes, another 6 per cent by accidents, and 3 per cent by pneumonia and influenza, or 3 per 10,000 population. Younger adults died primarily from accidents, homicide, and suicide, older adults from the "diseases of aging"—or perhaps diseases of affluence—heart disease, cancer, and stroke, the three main causes of death (87).

A number of studies in various industrialized countries suggest that aging and affluent populations die from diseases described in a WHO report as having undetermined or indeterminate origin; from violence, self-inflicted or otherwise; and from certain infections no longer susceptible of treatment (88).

The death trends in pre– and post–World War II Czechoslovakia graphically illustrate the changes in life-span in a population that rapidly changed from a relatively poor to an increasingly industrialized nation, between 1930 and 1967. As urbanization, sanitation, medical technology, housing, and working conditions improved, death rates dropped and life-span increased. In the early 1960s, deaths slowly began to increase in the mature-age groups of a now-aging population. Deaths among infants continued to decrease, in a pattern comparable to those of other industrialized nations (89).

The obvious question, and the central problem for those concerned about promoting health, then, is what is it about "progress," urbanization, and industrial development that produces wider affluence, longer life, and better health but at the same time seems to threaten health and life?

Environmental Ties Just how environment affects health, particularly of affluent populations, is not clear. Perhaps answers will, in fact, be found, for the problem is now at the doorstep of the affluent world. Some interrelationships between health and modern life patterns are known, of course.

The urbanization of rural populations, for example, has been related to an increase in deaths from coronary heart disease in middle-aged men (90). One hypothesis offered for this kind of link is that urban life generates disease not only because polluted air, water, and food may have carcinogenic and traumatic effects on body tissues (91), but also because the intensity, aggressiveness, and sometimes overwhelming nature of city life may lower body defenses to infection, as well as to chronic disorders, in ways yet unknown. That is, those whose actions do not bring about what they aspire to are more likely to become ill than those who have sufficient control over their environment to reach their goals; or, lacking a degree of control, have some means, perhaps a buffering family group, to mitigate the impact of powerlessness (92).

Interpolating further, the powerless may not only be more susceptible to antigens and other potential pathogens, but they may also allow the awakening of internal "silent viruses" to work slow, degenerative processes (93). This concept is not the same as the older concept of psychosomatic illness, in which persons experience symptoms without physical signs of organic disease. Nor is it the anxiety component of illness which may result in heightened symptoms of physical signs of disease.

Living Patterns In a more direct relation to health, urban industrial life has allowed a wide choice of foods, especially for the affluent. A paradoxical result is that health-damaging obesity has now reached significant proportions, especially among adult Americans and adolescent boys. Further, the eating patterns of affluent populations, which emphasize high concentrations of refined sugars and starches, have been implicated in a wide range of diseases—from dental caries, constipation, and hemorrhoids to coronary thrombosis, diabetes mellitus, and gastric ulcers (94).

The forms of transportation and recreation, also associated with affluence, take high tolls in injury, disability, and death (95). Work environments have produced as many as 25 million injuries per year, increasing at about 3 per cent each year in the 1960 decade. Occupationally induced diseases kill 100,000 persons annually (96).

Consistent with these threats to health associated with urban life and affluence is the finding that in certain nonurban, nonpoor regions, death rates are below average and life-spans longer (97).

Mental Health Effects Environmental threats may be damaging of course in forms other than physical illness. The powerlessness hypothesis suggests an explanation for the increase in deaths by suicide and homicide in certain affluent countries (98). It may also help explain why adult women have had higher rates of severe mental illness than adult men (99).

Recently a common denominator for all forms of mental illness was offered. It is that of demoralization, or being unable to deal with situations which one and one's peers expect can be handled. It is the sense of losing control, and thus, of powerlessness. Offered in support are the findings that regardless of diagnosis or type of therapy, most psychotherapy patients show progressive improvement over time, particularly when the therapist, of whatever background or training, is genuinely concerned and supportive —a buffer to the powerless, perhaps. In this way the patients' fears and symptoms of powerlessness may subside and/or patients may become better able—or see themselves as better able—to control their environment, to attain what they want (or to want whatever they can attain) (100).

This latter outcome of treatment, acceptance of one's environment, suggests another way in which the environment in the form of mental health services may adversely affect health. If, in fact, the perception of relative powerlessness, particularly among certain groups, such as women or blacks, is realistic, then labeling the expressions of it as mental illness in some form would not be accurate. This is among the criticisms of applying mental illness labels, such as "paranoia," especially because "cure" then tends to mean learning to *accept* the environment rather than learning to change that environment (101).

This illustrates the question of the extent to which the environment fosters dis-ease as compared with whether the cause of dis-ease is within the patient (or victim, as some would say [102]). The answer determines the relative allocation of resources for "cure," whether to focus on environment or on the individual patient. This, then, is another crucial problem for those concerned about promoting health.

Health Services and Health   Psychiatric diagnosis is but one example of the therapeutic technology embedded in affluent living. As part of the environment, it affects "health" by defining those who are "unhealthy." Similarly, physical diagnosis may affect health by the mis-labeling of and therefore incorrect treatment of certain symptoms presented, for example, by women. Although clinical evidence in a recent study implicated disease based on organic causes, the origin of the symptoms were assumed by male obstetricians to be psychogenic, and thus women were ineffectively treated (103).

The technology for assessing the prevalence of illness may also adversely affect the perceived "health" of certain groups. For example, those in higher social status groups tend to know how to answer mental health questions in ways that suggest they are "mentally healthy." Lower status groups tend not to know how to do this. Thus those in lower statuses tend to be reported in surveys as having more mental illness than others (104).

In a more direct way, therapeutic technology may generate disease or injury, known as the iatrogenic effects of treatment. These include the damaging effects of x-rays, of prescribed drugs, and of hospital-induced infections. Superfluous surgery or other treatments are also counterproductive of health, of course, if only in the sense that they divert resources from those who are in real need of certain services (105). Likewise, over-investment of resources in prestigious but little-used diagnostic or treatment modalities inevitably deprives those who seek and require routine therapy (106).

Viewing health services from their intended, positive aspect—the prevention and treatment of disease, disability, and death—questions again arise. Little hard evidence in fact exists which can prove that many treatment regimens are efficacious (107). Only recently has the focus turned toward learning to evaluate health services (108). Some studies show that death rates for persons at various levels of health and illness were no different whether or not they received scheduled, complete physical examinations (109). Others show that those who obtain the regular "checkups" advocated by health professionals are persons in affluent social groups. But these people are not necessarily the ones who also engage in such health practices as not smoking, limiting cholesterol, avoiding overweight, getting exercise, and so on (110). In other words, contact with health professionals did not generate life patterns that could prevent or minimize the likelihood of disease.

On a broader scale, a national summary of studies shows that for persons who have the same level of education and medical care, death rates increased in the higher-income groups. In other words, as persons become increasingly affluent, the socioeconomic environment again becomes relatively more important in determining life chances than does medical care (111).

Health: Environment and Health Services

We have seen that for the affluent as for the poor, the socioeconomic environment is crucial for life and, by implication, health. For the poor this results from their limited access to basic needs, including medical care. For the affluent this results from their abundant access to their needs and wants in spite of medical care. For all groups, the physical surrounding takes its toll, and the evidence is that environmental degradation places a heavier burden on the poor (112).

Remedial Status Personal health services could become, of necessity, increasingly remedial in nature as industrialization and concommitant changes proceed. One can only conjecture about what will happen to the health and life-expectancy patterns of women, for example, given the changes in affluent countries culminating in women's liberation movements. Almost universally, women live longer than men and have lower death rates in every age group (Table 1–4). A major exception is in India and Pakistan—and not typical for underdeveloped countries—where female infant deaths are higher, and women's life-span shorter than men's (113). Recently, suicide among young women is increasing; in the United States, women's rates of limitation in major activity due to chronic illness increased over men for the first time in 1969–1970 (114); and the death rate for white women increased between 1960 and 1972 (Table 2–2).

These changes could mean, in part, that as women's environment shifts to what was traditionally a "man's world," increasingly more women will be under at least as many environmental assaults as men. This, then, may indeed mean more suicide, disability that limits occupational rather than household activity, and diseases that produce earlier deaths, such as coronary heart disease. Medical care will then alleviate the disease, but it cannot change the context, the societal patterns, which generate disease and prolong recovery.

Consumer Priorities   Health care "consumers" readily understand the relative importance of their environment over medical care. In a large urban concentration of American Indians, for example, those with incomes of less than $8,000 considered housing, clothing, and food as their priority problems. Those with more than an $8,000 income regarded clothing and medical care as priority problems (115). Similarly, surveys of the elderly consistently show that their first concern is income maintenance, and, as most have some illness, second is medical care (116).

Relative Efficacy   Recently an effort was made to test the relative efficacy of the environment and health services for the health of populations, measured by infant deaths and life expectancy, in 14 technologically advanced countries. Favorable levels of health were directly associated with the average income per person, but not with the number of available physicians or hospital beds. Further, the aspect of health care that was highly related to health was neither the amount of governmental expenditure on personal health services nor the type of governmental control over the delivery of services. It was, rather, the amount expended on nonpersonal, environmental public health care (117).

Dynamic Ties   This array of studies, disparate and tentative as they are, suggests a dynamic relationship in the relative importance of the environment and medical care to the health of populations. In a gross and admittedly oversimplified way, the relationships might look as shown in Figure 2–8. For groups in poverty, environmental resources such as food, housing, and sanitation are obviously more important to their life chances than medical care. As their socioeconomic conditions improve, they reach the survival threshold at which basic needs are more or less assured. At roughly that point, medical care may become relatively more important in sustaining health and life. As populations become more affluent and have a large excess income, they reach a point of "optimal opportunity," having a wide range of choices as to how to use their affluence. Their pattern of choices may enhance or damage their health in spite of the best medical treatment available to them. As already noted, affluent Americans, and perhaps affluent countries as a group, have tended to follow damaging patterns of choice. The poor have a narrower range of less desired choices.

The characterization in Figure 2–8 might in general terms be applied to countries in poverty or affluence themselves, or to groups that are poor or affluent within countries.

Shifts in Focus   As increasing recognition is given at national and international levels to the fundamental importance of the environment

Figure 2–8   Schema of Relative Importance of Environment and Medical Care for Poor and Affluent Populations

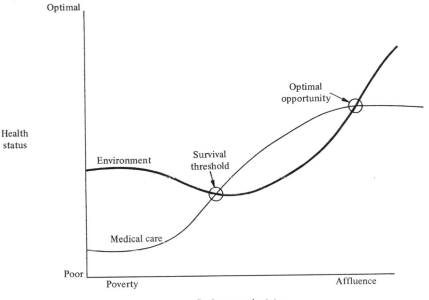

for health and for its further improvement, suggestions are being made to shift the focus of programs to environmental concerns, both to combat physical pollution and to provide social security through housing and income maintenance (118). Implicit here is the notion that the best hope for preventing disease, disability, and death lies in altering the environment in its ecological and socioeconomic aspects, and assuring individuals the resources to more effectively shape their own immediate environments.

Policy advisers, then, are proposing that major increases in governmental expenditures—and it is governments which are increasingly shaping health-related programs—give priority to changing environments over delivering personal health services. Thus health and other personal services would come, as they increasingly are, under closer scrutiny and would receive increased allocations only selectively (119).

This perceptible shift in emphasis, and the more selective, planned development of services, is also requiring a more total look at systems of personal health care and of the interrelationships and relative effectiveness of their components. WHO has recently recommended, as the best means for promoting the development of basic health services, that its assistance foster national health systems, rather than individual, isolated programs; that its experts provide long-term participatory, educative aid, rather than the short-term, advisory assistance of the past; and that the development of health systems be viewed for what they are in the national contexts of underdeveloped countries and in the perceptions of poor populations, namely an expression of popular demand for social welfare and social justice (120). These recommendations are virtually the same as those made by UNESCO regarding the development of education systems (121).

In the global context, then, health care systems have become not only a means intended to improve health but also to redistribute resources between affluent and poor, and therefore political entities. Within nations, too, as in the ghettos of New York, Edinburgh, or Kyoto, the demand for health services, as for education, is a call for the redistribution of resources between affluent and poor, majority and minorities (122).

Usable Perspectives Those concerned with health, regardless of what emphasis they choose and in what place and position they situate themselves at any given point in their lives, need a frame of reference based in the real world. In a literal as well as figurative sense, nothing less than a global view is now necessary for human health and development, if not human survival.

Any perspective that is to enhance an understanding of health care problems should include at least an awareness of the relative impact of the eco/socioeconomic environment and health services on health, and of the development and distribution of health services themselves as resources which those who "have-not," the outcasts, are now demanding.

Any major shifts in emphasis, whether between an environmental or health services focus, or within the system of health care, between types and loci of services, involve, of course, reallocations and new allocations of funds. The necessary decisions to be made, although they may include rational criteria, involve also the interpretations and perspectives of those whose interests lie in their control of current practices (123). Such decisions are political, in other words. In the sense used here, this means that they result from bargaining processes in which the groups involved seek to maintain or increase their resources, or to enhance their future bargaining capacity (124). This meaning takes on concreteness when one asks: What groups are receiving the advantages? What groups are paying? How are the allocation decisions made? In a perspective that offers a frame of reference for answering these questions there are also implicit criteria for evaluating outcomes, changes, and proposals for change.

The following chapters will now focus on the United States, a leading technologically advanced affluent nation, and its system of personal health services, a system at the crest of major changes, among a population peopled with outcast groups, a population demanding the redistribution of resources. The major questions in evaluating the current picture as well as the changes occurring and the proposals for change center on: Who has access to the advantages of health services and the health occupations? Who is paying? How are the decisions being made? Then, in evaluating the present, and possible future, is the question: Will the changes grant access for outcasts?

Summary

In the global setting the crucial fact is the widening gap between affluent and poor-world sectors. This gap is not merely the difference in the quality of consumption of the world's resources, consumption generated by growing populations among the poor and accelerating consumer economies among the affluent. It lies in the patterns of distribution of resources, which increasingly favor the affluent world, so perpetuating the gap. This has tragic effects on the chances for life and health in the poor world, further limiting their capabilities.

Despite these vast differences, rich and poor nations share certain common problems within their borders: wide disparities in wealth, both among income groups and between urban–rural areas; certain forms of urban deterioration; and the maldistribution of resources between urban and rural areas.

Education illustrates these disparities. Access favors the more affluent social groups and urban populations. Moreover, attempts at reform have favored the more advantaged groups. In these ways, given the links of family background to education, occupation, and income, the disparities between the affluent and the poor grow no less and sometimes widen. Beyond the question of access, the usefulness of current forms of education to enable persons to deal with the problems in their nations is called into question.

Among the most poor, and among those who more often live in the less desirable locations, are the ethnic and racial minorities, women, and the aged, to name some major groupings. Their numbers are growing in both affluent and poor nations, through immigration or by increasing proportions of the very young or very old. Not all outcasts are necessarily poor. What they have in common is the relative lack of access to social resources compared to those in the more dominant race, sex, age, income, or geographical groupings. Their less favored treatment tends also to limit their chances to overcome their outcast status, including the effects it has on their chances for life and health. Thus the deficit is cumulative. The burden is further compounded should they carry more than one outcast label.

As the environment thus weighs on outcasts, it also is having damaging effects on the life and health of the affluent. The affluents, both as nations and as groups within nations, are now beginning to attend to the eco/socio-economic environment, which in its physical assaults and the life patterns it fosters is becoming a threat to life and health for the advantaged—this in spite of their ready access to medical care.

In this new search for the environmental determinants of disease and the implied remedies that could be applied to the environment at various levels—international, national, regional, and local community—personal health services are coming under closer examination. To be most effective they will need to change in ways that will mesh with environmental patterns of solution. Their components will need to be viewed as part of a system of health care and as part of a community in which people have priorities based on their particular social character. A health services system will thus be evaluated along two dimensions: first, as a technological resource, in relation to its efficacy in solving one part of the problem of promoting health and life shared with other environmental efforts; and second, as a social and economic resource, in terms of whether it grants access for outcasts to its services, occupations, and decision-making processes. If instituted, this form of redistribution of resources would of course not eliminate outcast status in the United States. But at least the system of personal health services would no longer contribute to keeping outcasts outcast.

section II

The National Setting

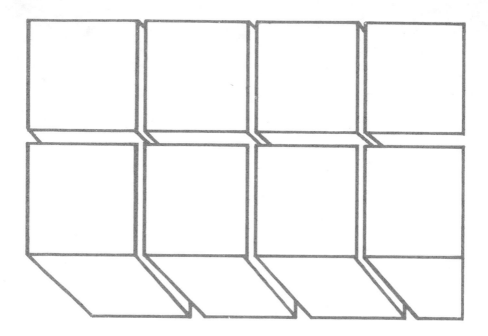

part two

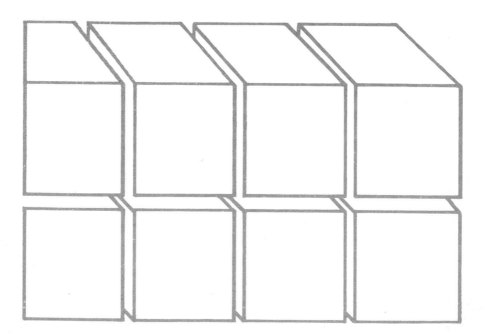

Access to
Health Services

The People Who Clean Up

Invisible people
weighted with linens
pails, brushes, and rags,
the pick-up brigade
smoothing our wrinkles
scrubbing our dirt
bringing freshness to staleness,
without choice,
or variation
or a nod.

Gaunt men of India
responding to "Boy!"
"Advanced" nations use women—
On the streets of Kyoto
dragging their brooms
flat-hatted, aging and round;
In Europe's once-elegant hostels,
harsh-sounding queens
in tiaras of white
with aprons to match
over black,
polishing wood and shining the glass.

So it's repeated all over the world
hauling and lifting
stooping and kneeling
        on Dutch tile
          German wood
            Italian marble
              British stone
                U.S. synthetics.
Bottom rungs feel the same.

N.M.
Glasgow, 1971

chapter 3

Distribution of People and Services

People have access to services in fact only when their resources consumed in time, travel, and fees are not more costly than the worth of those services in the contexts of their daily lives. When a full array of health services is not located where people are—the intended consumers—or when prices or other program characteristics intervene as barriers, people become outcasts of health care. As described earlier, certain social groupings are more likely to become the outcasts of services—namely those already outcast because of low income, poor living areas, old age, minority race, or majority sex.

What follows will first describe where the people are in the United States, giving a brief social and economic picture of the geographic regions; then, where the services are, the facilities, and the personnel; finally, the financial and programmatic aspects of access. Chapters 4 and 5 will then focus on the organization of delivery and payment for services, which will begin to explain why health services are distributed as they are.

Regional Distributions

Comparing the four census regions of the contiguous United States in relation to each other and to the country overall, a general pattern emerges. Roughly, the Northeast and South tend to be polar in most major characteristics, with the Northeast more similar to the West, and the South closer to the North Central states. For example, the Northeast and West are least populous, containing 24 and 17 per cent of the people; the South has the greatest proportion of the population, 31 per cent. The West and Northeast are most urban and most affluent, in terms of median family income; the South, least. The Northeast has highest density; the West, fewest persons per square mile (Figure 3–1; Table 3–1).

Such generalizations can be deceptive, of course, because of the variations within these large regions. The states of the mountain subregion of the West, for example, have the same per capita income as the South Atlantic states, $3,785, well below the national average (Table 3–1).

The regions, as would be expected, have unequal shares of some of the major outcast groups. Elders, those 65 and over, make up about 10 per cent of the U.S. population and are proportionately more white and female (Appendix Table 5). The Northeast has the most elders and fewest low-income families, relatively. The South has the most blacks and low-income families. [Black families are poorest in the South and most affluent in the West; white families are poorest in the South and most affluent in the Northeast (Appendix Tables 6–8)]. The West has the fewest blacks and the fewest elders (Table 3–2).

In sum, and with due regard to the danger of gross description, the people in the Northeast are oldest and most affluent, in the South least affluent and more black, in the West youngest, and in the North Central region somewhere between.

Contrasting Areas To make clearer the picture of health care available to these populations, and also because data often are not available on regional or subregional bases, we will draw a picture here, on the following basis. Eight States are selected, first on a geographic basis, two from each region, and then from contrasting subregions within each region. The intraregion contrasts are in incomes (per capita), urban–rural residence, and racial–ethnic composition.

There are four states, geographically dispersed, with high income, large urban populations, and a relatively high proportion of blacks and Hispanos: Connecticut, Illinois, Texas, and California. Their regional counterparts, with relatively low income, more rural populations, and smaller minorities (including American Indians), are Maine, South Dakota, West Virginia, and Montana. These last will be termed Less Affluent, and the others More Affluent States (Figure 3–1; Table 3–3). With one exception, the birth, death, and infant mortality rates were lower in the more affluent states in 1972. The exception was in the South, where Texas had a higher birth rate than West Virginia (Appendix Table 9).

Again, although generalizations about these contrasting states as more and less advantaged living areas are accurate in general, they do not imply advantage for every social group within them, particularly major outcast groups. It is true that the poor are relatively better off living in a more affluent than a less affluent state. But there are exceptions. For example,

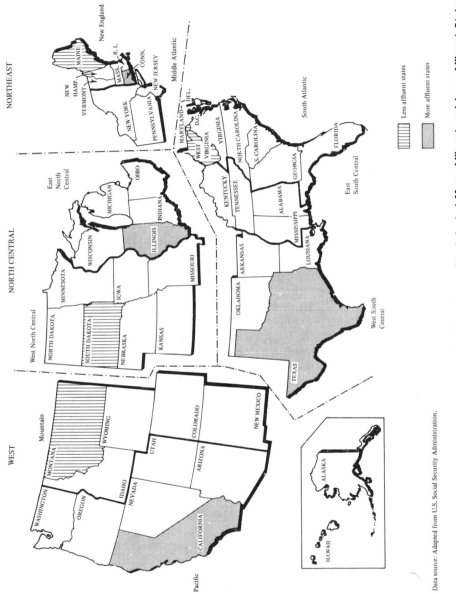
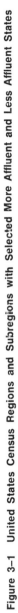

Data source: Adapted from U.S. Social Security Administration.

Figure 3–1   United States Census Regions and Subregions with Selected More Affluent and Less Affluent States

Table 3–1   Distribution of Population, United States

Income, Urban Residence, and Density by Region and Subregion, 1970

	Population (%)[a]	Median Family Income	Average per Capita Income (1971)	Urban Population (%)	Density (persons/mile²)
United States	100	$ 9,867	$4,138	73	58
Northeast	24	10,696		80	300
New England			4,469	76	191
Mid-Atlantic			4,701	82	374
North Central	28	10,327		72	75
East North Central			4,306	75	167
West North Central			3,904	64	33
South	31	8,552		65	72
South Atlantic			3,785	64	117
East South Central			3,146	55	72
West South Central			3,514	73	46
West	17	10,273		83	20
Mountain			3,785	73	10
Pacific			4,551	78	30

[a] Rounded.

Source: U.S. Bureau of Census, *Statistical Abstract of the United States 1972* (Washington, D.C.: Government Printing Office, 1972).

Table 3–2   Distribution of Population, United States

Elders, Blacks, and Low-Income Families by Geographic Region, 1970

	Total Population (1971)	65 Years and Over	Black	Family Income $—5,000	Families in Poverty (1969)
United States (%)	100	9.9	11	21.9	12
			% of regional population		
Northeast	24	10.7	9	15.4	8
North Central	28	9.1	8	16.9	8.5
South	31	9.1	19	25.0	15.0
West	17	8.7	5	17.6	8.0

Sources: U.S. Bureau of Census, *Statistical Abstract of the United States 1972* (Washington, D.C.: Government Printing Office, 1972).

National Center for Health Statistics, *Monthly Vital Stat. Rept.* 22, Apr. 2, 1973.

R. Morrill and E. Wohlenberg, *The Geography of Poverty in the United States* (New York: McGraw-Hill, 1971).

Table 3–3 Distribution of Population, United States

Elders, Blacks, and Low-Income Families by Geographic Region, 1970

	More Affluent States					Region		Less Affluent States				
	% U.S. Population	Per Capita Income (1971)	Persons Below Poverty 1969(%)	Urban Population (%)	Largest Minorities (%)			(%) U.S. Population	Per Capita Income (1971)	Persons Below Poverty 1969(%)	Urban Population (%)	Largest Minorities (%)
						Northeast						
Connecticut	1.5	$5,032	7.2	77	6 (Black)		Maine	0.5	$3,419	13.6	51	3 (Black)
						North Central						
Illinois	5.7	4,772	10.2	83	12.8 (Black)		South Dakota	0.3	3,446	18.7	45	5 (Indian) 0.2 (Black)
						South						
Texas	5.7	3,682	18.8	80	12.5 (Black) 6.4 (Mexican)		West Virginia	0.9	3,228	22.2	39	3.9 (Black)
						West						
California	9.9	4,677	11.1	91	7 (Black) 5.6 (Mexican)		Montana	0.3	3,479	13.6	53	3.9 (Indian)
Totals	22.8							2				

Source: U.S. Bureau of Census, *Statistical Abstract of the United States 1972* (Washington, D.C.: Government Printing Office, 1972).

67

hired farmworkers are economically worse off in absolute terms in affluent California than in less-affluent Montana (1).

Geographic Accessibility

Given now a sense of the relative advantages of people grounded in their living space across the spectrum of contiguous states, what access do they have to personal health services?

Health Care Facilities

Hospital inpatient services, measured in available beds per population units, are abundant in the less affluent states. Hospital general clinics, community mental health centers, and home health agencies are also proportionately more available in these states. Financing of these facilities has come from tax funds and has been allocated on a population formula that favors poor areas (Figure 3–2).

There is a clear difference in the distribution of facilities that are not publicly funded. Skilled nursing establishments, for example, are more available in the more affluent states. Even so, the two affluent subregions of New England and the Pacific illustrate how imbalanced combinations of services can limit access to certain groups, such as elders. The fact that the Pacific has almost twice as many Medicare enrollees, more than twice as many skilled nursing facility beds, but fewer than half as many home health agencies means that persons eligible for home services must be limited to the types of services available. Some, who might otherwise live at home, will be more likely to remain inpatients in the Pacific than in New England (Table 3–4).

The ambulatory services provided by medical groups are less available to the people of the less affluent states, except for nonspecialty groups. General practitioners in groups or solo practice are more available in those states (Figure 3–3; Appendix Tables 10–12).

Personnel

Generally, physicians and dentists, and specialists in particular, are more plentiful in the more affluent states and regions. Similarly, nurses and other health personnel are less available in the South (Table 3–5). An exception is the licensed practical nurse (LPN), used as a lower-cost nurse in the South (2). Texas, for example, categorized here as a more

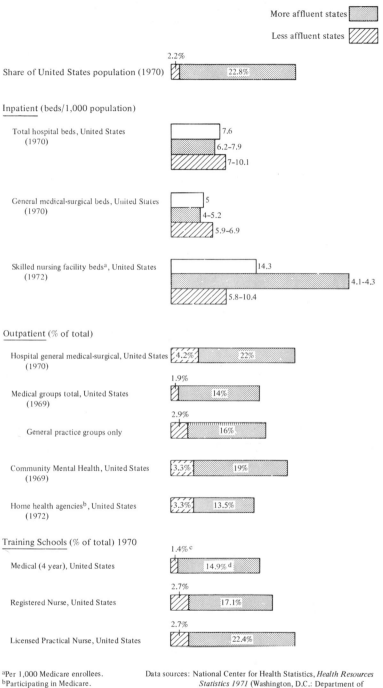

Figure 3–2 Distribution of Health Resources, United States

Service and Training Facilities in Selected More and Less Affluent States

More affluent states

Less affluent states

Share of United States population (1970)
2.2%
22.8%

Inpatient (beds/1,000 population)

Total hospital beds, United States (1970)
7.6
6.2–7.9
7–10.1

General medical-surgical beds, United States (1970)
5
4–5.2
5.9–6.9

Skilled nursing facility beds[a], United States (1972)
14.3
4.1–4.3
5.8–10.4

Outpatient (% of total)

Hospital general medical-surgical, United States (1970)
4.2%
22%

Medical groups total, United States (1969)
1.9%
14%

General practice groups only
2.9%
16%

Community Mental Health, United States (1969)
3.3%
19%

Home health agencies[b], United States (1972)
3.3%
13.5%

Training Schools (% of total) 1970

Medical (4 year), United States
1.4%[c]
14.9%[d]

Registered Nurse, United States
2.7%
17.1%

Licensed Practical Nurse, United States
2.7%
22.4%

[a] Per 1,000 Medicare enrollees.
[b] Participating in Medicare.
[c] All are private.
[d] 55% are private.

Data sources: National Center for Health Statistics, *Health Resources Statistics 1971* (Washington, D.C.: Department of Health, Education, and Welfare, 1972). Social Security Administration, "Medicare: Participating Health Facilities, 1972," *Health Insur. Stat.,* 48 (July 20, 1973).

Table 3–4   Distribution of Health Care Resources, United States

Medicare Enrollees, Certain Inpatient and Home Care Facilities in New England and Pacific States, 1972

		Participating Facilities	
	Medicare Enrollees (%)	Skilled Nursing (beds/1,000 enrollees)	Home Health Agencies (%)
United States	100.0		100.0
New England	6.3	16.1	15.6
Pacific	11.9	35.4	6.0

Source: Social Security Administration, "Medicare: Participating Health Facilities, July, 1972," *Health Insur. Stat.* 48 (July 20, 1973).

affluent state, had about as many LPNs as R.N.s per hospital bed, and more than 3 times as many per skilled nursing bed, depending far more on LPNs than any of the more affluent states (Appendix Tables 13 and 14).

Within the states themselves, there are again differences in access to physicians according to where people, and physicians, live. There are about 81 physicians (per 100,000 population) for those living in rural counties, and 132 for persons in metropolitan counties (3). Further, within the metropolitan areas, there are 4 times as many physicians for suburbanites as for central city residents (4).

In the cities, in the low-income areas of Chicago and New York, for example, where health is poorest, there are one half as many physicians and one fourth as many specialists as in the healthier and more affluent sections. These physicians, to whom the people of the poverty areas, mainly blacks and other minorities, do have access, often have no hospital staff privileges or opportunities for continuing education (one third of such physicians in New York) (5).

A recent analysis of where physicians choose to locate themselves shows that specialists are near medical schools, surgeons in particular near large hospitals, and other specialists near populations with higher education. General practitioners are likely to be near older populations, especially the elders (6).

Government Subsidies

Thus the federal dollars which built, or as some analysts say, overbuilt, the hospital facilities in the poorer and more rural states, did not serve to

Figure 3–3   Distribution of Health Care Resources, United States

Health Personnel in Selected More Affluent and Less Affluent States

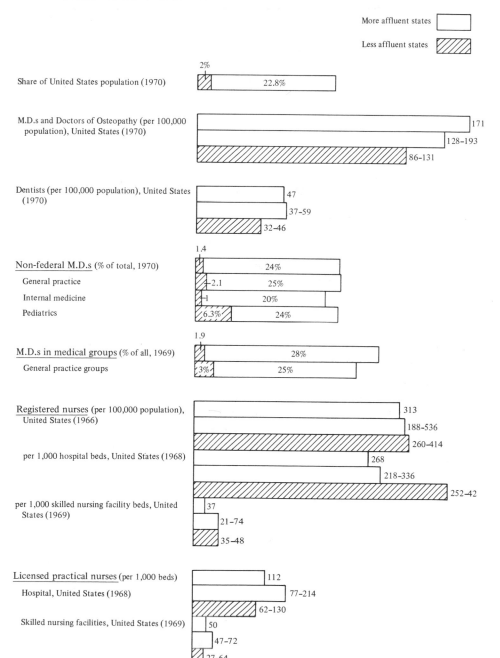

Data source: National Center for Health Statistics, *Health Resources Statistics 1971* (Washington, D.C.:
Department of Health, Education, and Welfare, 1972).

Table 3–5   Distribution of Health Care Resources, United States

Active Health Personnel by Region[a]

	United States	Personnel per 100,000 Population			
		North-east	North Central	South	West
M.D. and D.O.	148	181	133	114	161
M.D.s in group practice[b]	20	13.4	21.2	18.2	31.4
M.D.s in general practice groups[b]	1.3	0.3	2.0	1.3	1.9
D.D.S.	48	57	46	32	50
R.N.	310	417	307	217	325
Other professional and technical	258	298	260	205	294
LPN	137	181	109	138	115
Aides	346	385	413	281	298

[a] Estimated from 1960–1966 data.

[b] 1969.

Sources: S. Altman, *Present and Future Supply of Registered Nurses* (Washington, D.C.: Department of Health, Education, and Welfare, 1972).

National Center for Health Statistics, *Health Resources Statistics 1971* (Washington, D.C.: Department of Health, Education, and Welfare, 1972).

attract health personnel, particularly physicians, to staff them (7). Nor have nurses necessarily gone to the less affluent states, which have more hospital beds, although some movement has occurred among the traditionally lower-paid personnel with fewest job opportunities elsewhere (8).

These rural-poor communities received 62 per cent of federal funds for hospital facilities in 1965–1970. Other federal investments focusing on ambulatory care, with the exception of hospital-tied clinics, fell far short of what rural populations might expect is due them on a proportional basis. Nonmetropolitan areas comprised 35 per cent of the country's people in 1970 but received less than 25 per cent of funds to staff mental health centers, 15 per cent or less for health planning and development of regional medical care, and none for emergency care programs (Figure 3–4).

Training Facilities

Training facilities, as is the case with service organizations, might be thought of as an economic investment in a community and also as a means of attracting students who will eventually work in the locality. This latter

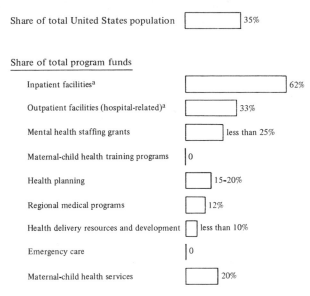

Figure 3–4   Distribution of Health Care Resources, United States

Federal Funds Allocated to Non-metropolitan Areas, 1970

Share of total United States population ____ 35%

Share of total program funds

Inpatient facilities[a] ____ 62%

Outpatient facilities (hospital-related)[a] ____ 33%

Mental health staffing grants ____ less than 25%

Maternal-child health training programs 0

Health planning ____ 15-20%

Regional medical programs ____ 12%

Health delivery resources and development ____ less than 10%

Emergency care 0

Maternal-child health services ____ 20%

[a] 1965-1970; communities of less than 50,000 population.

Data sources: Health Care Facilities Service, *Hill-Burton Program Progress Report 1947-1970* (Washington, D.C.: Department of Health, Education, and Welfare, Oct. 1971).
"Economic and Social Conditions of Rural America in the 1970's: Impact of Department of Health, Education, and Welfare Programs on Non-Metropolitan Areas in Fiscal Year 1970" (Washington, D.C.: Department of Health, Education, and Welfare, 1972).

strategy has apparently not been effective in the less affluent states. In the case of schools for registered and practical nurses, heavily financed by federal funds, the less affluent states have a larger share of facilities but relatively fewer students than the more affluent states, which have, for example, 17 per cent of R.N. programs and 20 per cent of R.N. students (Figure 3–2; Appendix Tables 15 and 16).

The less affluent states with no medical school within their borders have fewer students entering medical schools, diminishing a potential source of physicians. Those with a public medical school (they have no private schools) equal or exceed the student–population ratios of the more affluent states (Appendix Tables 16 and 17). Similar unevenness in training programs was also found by the Carnegie Commission's 50-state survey in 1969 (9).

This suggests that public investment in training may be necessary to generate health personnel in less affluent communities, but it is not sufficient to retain health workers. Again, this may vary with the type of personnel and their relative opportunities in more affluent regions, matters that will be discussed in Chapters 6 and 7.

As an economic investment, federal funds for Schools of Public Health have favored the more affluent Northeast in contrast to the South—in terms of support for both faculty and for students (Table 3–6).

Table 3–6   Distribution of Health Care Resources,
United States

Training Facilities and Public Funds, Schools of Public
Health, Contrasting Regions, 1972

	Total No.	Covered by Federal Grants (%)	
		Teaching Faculty	Students
United States	18	46	53
Northeast	5	44–77	41–73
South	4	15–49	20–61

Source: Association of Schools of Public Health, "Testimony Before U.S. House Subcommittee on Public Health and Environment," [Washington, D.C.: Mar. 28, 1973 (unpublished)].

Scarcity Areas

The question of health care shortage areas is summarized in the provisional government report of a national study. Of the more than 1,300 jurisdictions defining themselves as shortage areas, two thirds or more named personnel shortages and about one half or less named facilities deficits. The scarcest workers were physicians, dentists, and nurses, in that order. Most significant perhaps is that among the areas that specified the type of scarcity, virtually all listed inadequate, inaccessible, and/or ineffective use of services (10).

In other words, numbers of personnel do not necessarily translate into access to service by the people; nor do facilities necessarily guarantee that personnel will be available to staff them, or that either personnel or services are of a mix that allow effective and efficient use. This suggests that any health care strategies which seek to enhance access by increasing numbers of personnel or facilities without considering their types and interrelations in the context of communities cannot be, as they have not been, very successful. At a minimum, effective coordinating mechanisms have been absent. Another way to say it is that ways must be found such that the distribution of health services does not perpetuate, much less contribute to, the outcast status of communities.

Financial Availability

Health Insurance

The existence of nearby health services does not provide access to potential users who cannot pay the price of services of course. The most costly types, hospital and surgical, were covered to some extent for 78 per cent of Americans under age 65 in 1970. Of those with less than $3,000 income, just over 40 per cent had some insurance (Figure 3–5). The elders were covered by Medicare, and about half of them had additional private insurance (Table 3–7). About 20 per cent more white low-income families had some coverage compared to other races, but most higher income families of all races were at least minimally insured (Figure 3–6). These proportions vary regionally, smaller in the South, larger in the North Central and Northeast.

Out-of-Pocket Payments

A better estimate of the financial availability of health care than the insured is the direct measure of out-of-pocket medical expenses, which includes, but is not limited to, insurance premiums. Viewed in this way, 88 per cent of Americans had out-of-pocket medical expenses, but more of the elders, despite and because of Medicare, and more women than men, although women are somewhat better protected after age 65 than in their earlier years relative to men (Figure 3–5). Among low-income families, less than half of whom have any insurance, about 76 per cent had direct medical expenses, in spite of Medicaid (Figure 3–6).

Roughly half the people with private insurance, if they were under age 65, had some coverage for such out-of-hospital services as physician visits, medications, and visiting nurse. The elders had far less such coverage, and given their greater need, more of them had out-of-pocket expenses for these services (Table 3–7). The actual amount of these expenses will be discussed in Chapter 5.

Those with no out-of-pocket expenses, over 12 per cent of the population, are persons who had no medical care whatever, had services for which they were not charged, or whose insurance was paid by some other source and was sufficient to cover all the services they received.

Figure 3–5 Distribution of Health Care Resources, United States

Hospital and Surgical Insurance Coverage and Out-of-Pocket Expenses by Age, Sex, and Race, 1970

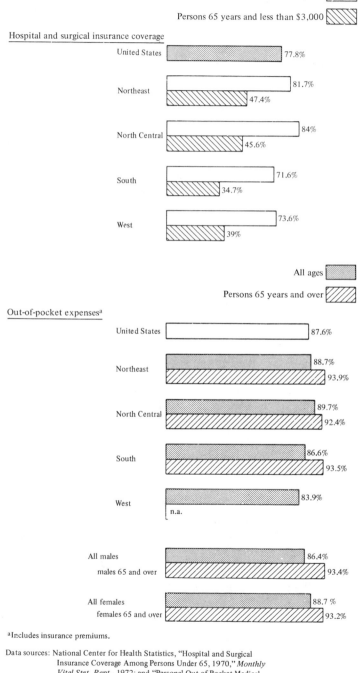

ᵃIncludes insurance premiums.

Data sources: National Center for Health Statistics, "Hospital and Surgical
Insurance Coverage Among Persons Under 65, 1970," *Monthly
Vital Stat. Rept.*, 1972; and "Personal Out-of-Pocket Medical
Expenses, 1970," *Monthly Vital Stat. Rept.*, 22, Apr, 2, 1973
(supplement).

Table 3–7 Distribution of Health Care Resources, United States

Private Insurance Coverage and Out-of-Pocket Expenses[a]
by Age and Type of Services, 1970

	Persons Under 65 (%)	Persons 65 and Over (%)		All Persons (%)	
	Private Insurance Coverage	Private Insurance Coverage	Out-of-Pocket Expenses	Private Insurance Coverage	Out-of-Pocket Expenses
United States					87.6
Hospital care	83.5	51.3	16.4	80.3	11.8
Out-of-hospital care					
M.D. office/home visits	48.0	19.5	n.a.	45.1	n.a.
Dental	6.6	0.6	25.2	6.0	40.0
Prescribing drugs	53.5	15.9	66.9	49.7	53.0
Visiting nurse	56.4	18.8 ⎫	14.4	52.6 ⎫	5.4
Home care	15.0	24.7 ⎭		16.0 ⎭	

[a] Includes insurance premiums.

Sources: Social Security Administration, *Social Security Bull.*, Feb. 1973.

    National Center for Health Statistics, *Monthly Vital. Stat. Rept.* 22 (Supplement), Apr. 2, 1973.

The important point is that major outcast groups have lesser access to services because of financial reasons. This is both because they do not have insurance protection that covers the extent and quantity of services they use, and because they have greater need for medical care.

Price, Need, and Use of Services

This relationship between medical need and the financial barriers to health services becomes clearer by looking at the actual use of services, measured in visits with the physician per year. (Physician visits is a better measure than hospital admissions since the consumers basically decide when they need to see a physician, whereas it is the physician who decides hospital use.)

The increase in physician visits by low-income persons between 1962 and 1968 (4.3–4.6), while visits by other income groups decreased (5.1 to 4.3), suggests an effect of the federal programs which funded health services and were initiated during that period (Figure 3–7). These figures do not indicate however the relative advantage of *new services started* in shortage areas compared with *payment for* services in already *existing* programs.

Figure 3–6   Distribution of Health Care Resources, United States

Hospital and Surgical Insurance Coverage and Out-of-Pocket Expenses by Income Group and Race, 1970

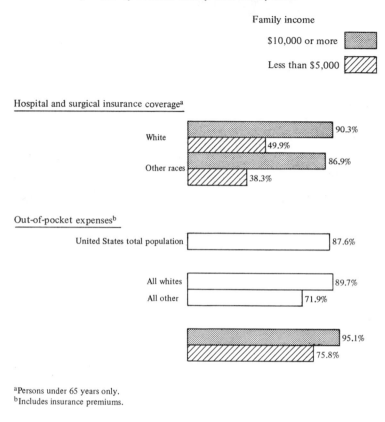

Family income

$10,000 or more

Less than $5,000

Hospital and surgical insurance coverage[a]

White — 90.3% / 49.9%

Other races — 86.9% / 38.3%

Out-of-pocket expenses[b]

United States total population — 87.6%

All whites — 89.7%
All other — 71.9%

95.1% / 75.8%

[a]Persons under 65 years only.
[b]Includes insurance premiums.

Data sources: National Center for Health Statistics, "Hospital and Surgical
Insurance Coverage Among Persons Under 65, 1970," *Monthly
Vital Stat. Rept.,* 1972; and "Personal Out-of-Pocket Medical
Expenses, 1970," *Monthly Vital Stat. Rept.,* 22, Apr. 2, 1973
(supplement).

A study in an eastern urban area showed that regardless of income,
having a regular source of health care is more important in affecting utilization of physician services. Then, for the poor, the other important factors
are whether they must pay for the service and how serious their health
problem is (11). As long as facilities are available on a regular basis,
guaranteed financial access for those who cannot pay will allow them to
increase their use of services.

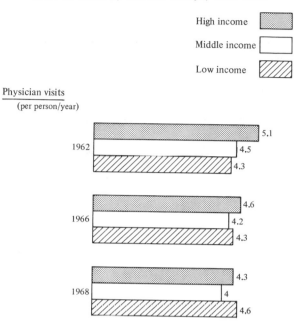

Figure 3–7 Distribution of Health Care Resources, United States

Physician Visits by Income Groups, 1962–1968

High income

Middle income

Low income

Physician visits
(per person/year)

1962
5.1
4.5
4.3

1966
4.6
4.2
4.3

1968
4.3
4
4.6

Data source: C. Schultz, et al. *Setting National Priorities: The 1973
Budget* (Washington, D.C.: The Brookings Institution, 1972).

This, however, is not the case for regular physical examinations or other preventive health services, for any income group. That is, a low price for these services does not increase their use, although those with more years of education use them more (12). However, this practice of obtaining regular physical examinations does not necessarily result in better health or more healthful living habits (13).

While certain federal programs have improved access to health services for the poor and the elderly, large deficits exist nevertheless. These depend upon where people live and whether or not they are white, especially among children. Children who live in urban areas, and children who are white, see physicians almost twice as often as others. The figures suggest that generally persons in the South and in rural areas have most limited access to physician services (Table 3–8).

Table 3–8 Distribution of Health Care Resources, United States

Physician Visits by
Income, Residence, Age, and Sex

	M.D. Visits (per person per year)			
	Total	Male	Female	Data year
United States	4.6	4.1	5.1	1970
Family income				1968
Low	4.6			
Middle	4.0			
High	4.3			
Residence				
Rural				
Adults[a]		3.0	3.7	
Children	2.0			1967
Urban				
Adults[a]		4.2	5.4	
Children	3.9			1967
Age				
Children (under 17)	3.6	3.7	3.5	1967
White	3.9			
Other races	2.0			
Region				
Northeast	4.1			
North Central	3.5			
South	3.1			
West	4.0			
Elders (65 and over)	6.4	6.0	6.7	1971

[a] In 10 most rural and most urban states.

Sources: Health Insurance Institute, *Sourcebook of Health Insurance Data* (New York: HII, 1972).

C. Schultz et al., *Setting National Priorities: The 1973 Budget* (Washington, D.C.: The Brookings Institution, 1972).

National Center for Health Statistics, *The Health of Children 1970* (Washington, D.C.: Department of Health, Education, and Welfare, 1970).

National Center for Health Statistics, *Current Estimates from the Health Interview Survey U.S. 1971* (Washington, D.C.: Department of Health, Education, and Welfare, 1972).

U.S. Congressional Record 118:H9679 (Oct. 11, 1972).

Program Access

Beyond geographic location and ability to pay, there are other program characteristics that limit services to certain groups. For example, certain medical treatments are excluded from coverage for women; or, because of the "experience rating" technique in the insurance industry, maternity benefits require higher premiums and are often optional to employer group plans, in effect penalizing the employer for providing a customary employment benefit and, further, for hiring women. The experience rating system has similar effects for elderly and handicapped workers (14).

Even when financing, facilities, and personnel are available, access may still be limited. Service programs, for example, may not extend themselves to those who need them most. In one Northeastern state where home health agencies are plentiful, only 2.4 per cent of the elders and 1.2 per cent of all disabled persons requiring home services did in fact receive them in 1971 (15).

Other studies show how the attitudes of health workers toward the aged, of upwardly mobile professionals toward the poor, of physicians toward women patients—in addition to the maternity-related practices already cited—affect the style and choice of treatment given. In effect, access to certain types of service is limited for reasons unrelated to health needs (16).

International Comparisons

The United States shares with other affluent, and with poor countries, the problem of uneven health services distribution. Rural areas as compared with cities have, almost universally, shortages of hospital beds, and far more severe shortages of physicians. Argentina, for example, with more than 50 per cent more physicians per unit of population than Japan, has more than three times as many physicians in its capitol as in the rest of the country. Similar or greater disparities exist in the urban–rural areas of such diverse nations as Denmark, the U.S.S.R., Japan, or Nigeria. There, in rural Nigeria, as perhaps an extreme, the physician–population ratio is 1 to 170,000 (Appendix Table 18a).

ENGLAND AND WALES

One of the most successful systems for distributing health care resources is in the United Kingdom (U.K.), England and Wales. Comparing certain contrasting regions, more and less affluent, rural and urban, hospital facilities, expenditures, and personnel are fairly evenly available in relation to population. The practitioners providing the greatest proportion of primary health services, the general physicians, are most evenly dispersed, 42 per 100,000 population in both rural and urban areas. Within regions, however, the average number of patients on a physician's "list" may vary substantially from the average 2,444. In some areas, such as the south-

Table 3–9   Distribution of Health Care Resources, England and Wales

Facilities and Personnel by
Contrasting Geographic Regions, 1971

	England and Wales	Selected Regions			
		South-west (rural)	North (rural–industrial)	North-west (urban–industrial)	South-east (including London) (urban)
Socioeconomic data					
Population (%)	100	7.8	6.8	14.0	35.5
Minorities (% population)	2.4	1.0	1.0	10.3	8.4
Median earnings (male, weekly)	$75	$70	$70	$75	$79
Unemployment (% 1972)	3.7	3.5	6.3	4.8	2.1
Infant Death rate	18	16	19	20	16
Hospital services					
Hospital expenditures (% 1970–1971)	100	7.2	5.5	9.1	24.7
Hospital beds (per 1,000 population 1970)	9.2	10.3	9.1	8.7	9.1–13
Personnel[a]					
Dentists (general) (%)	100	8.7	4.8	11.4	47.2
Gen. medical practioners (%)	100	8.5	6.3	13.0	36.8
Patients/M.D.	2,444	2,244	2,504	2,559	2,408
Specialists (per 100,000)	53	46.6	50.7	46.7	68.2
Hospital staff nursing (registered and midwives, per 100,000)	540	573.9	526.3	523.7	596.2
Training facilities (N)					
Teaching hospitals	36	1	1	1	26
District nurse training centers	32	2	1	2	7
Health visitor training centers	39	3	1	2	6

[a] Full-time equivalents, not individuals.

Sources: Great Britain Office of Population Census and Surveys, *Registrar General's Statistical Review of England and Wales 1971* (London: Her Majesty's Stationery Office, 1972).

Great Britain Central Statistical Office, *Social Trends 1972* (London: Her Majesty's Stationery Office, 1973).

Great Britain Department of Health and Social Security, *Health and Personal Social Services Statistics 1972* (London: Her Majesty's Stationery Office, 1973).

west, only 9 per cent of the GPs have more than 3,000 patients. In the less affluent north, 21 per cent have more than 3,000 patients (17). The people across the country have less access to specialists, who are up to 50 per cent more numerous in the London area, where the largest share of training facilities are also (Table 3–9).

Payment Systems

If most countries have not been able to assure geographic access to their populations, many have granted the financial availability of health services to all their citizens. This is increasingly the case for affluent nations. Through social insurance systems, virtually all the people of Scandanavia, the U.K., Canada, the U.S.S.R., and The Netherlands are assured that the health services they receive will be paid, as are over 90 per cent of the West Germans and Japanese. Most programs cover a full range of medical–surgical, maternity, dental, inpatient, and ambulatory services (18).

Most of the governments in the underdeveloped countries of Asia, Africa, and Latin America have established limited health insurance systems, thereby granting access to certain groups. The eligible persons are primarily workers in particular industries confined to urban areas, and covered for less than a comprehensive range of services (Appendix Table 18b).

Many of these governments, however, as is true for many affluent countries, are attempting to grant access to their total populations by providing health services directly under a system of governmental health services. Some have succeeded in this, but often only in the most favored regions of their countries.

Summary

Access to health services means being able to connect with the resources, places, and personnel that can render the needed care; it means assured payment for the services provided; it means services rendered in a manner and of a type suited to persons' requirements, not as a stereotyped response—all this done without undue effort, within the limits and priorities of those who need services.

Outcast groups—those in isolated and/or poor areas, the poor, elders, women—have more severe limits and therefore other urgent priorities, as well as greater need for health services, than their more favored counterparts. Yet they have least access to service because of geographic, financial, and program barriers. Training centers, private and tax dollars, service facilities, especially those for ambulatory care, and, most crucially, personnel, converge in most-favored areas among most-favored populations. This, in effect, places further burdens on outcast groups. It also has a wider environmental impact, adding to the pattern of unplanned metropolitan concentrations and the health deficits that process generates.

The obvious and urgent question is why such maldistribution of health services exists, a situation of which virtually no one approves. Some of the answer may be found by looking at how the provision of health services is organized and financed.

chapter 4

Organization—How Services Are Delivered

If the location and price of health care limit access to an array of needed services, what, in the patterns of health care delivery, contributes to maldistribution and high costs? What follows will portray the basic modes of providing health care in the United States, how they are changing, and, in part, why.

Hospital Care

To maintain a patient in an institutional bed in 1971 cost $36,000, not including the $50,000 entailed in construction costs per hospital bed. This fact, which summarizes the economic burden of inpatient services, led to a comprehensive study of health facilities costs authorized by the Congress. The study report, prepared by the General Accounting Office (GAO) recommended, in a word, deinstitutionalization, or, maintaining persons in as near to normal living in their community as possible. The intended effect is to reduce costs. From the viewpoint of the individual, community care means greater independence, wider choices, and a lesser likelihood of succumbing to the "sick" orientation that institutions tend to foster (1).

Ownership

Just over half the 7,600 U.S. hospitals were owned by private, not-for-profit organizations in 1970. More than one third were government-owned, and the rest were for-profit enterprises. Most government hospitals were under state and local jurisdiction, and about one fifth of the not-for-profit facilities were under church auspices. These proportions were about the same for the most common type, the general medical–surgical (non-specialty) hospital (Figure 4–1).

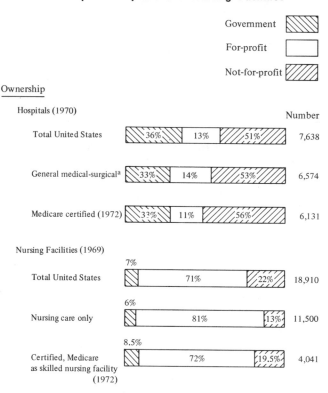

Figure 4–1   Organization of Personal Health Services, United States

Ownership of Hospitals and Nursing Facilities

Government

For-profit

Not-for-profit

Ownership

Hospitals (1970)   Number

Total United States   36%   13%   51%   7,638

General medical-surgical[a]   33%   14%   53%   6,574

Medicare certified (1972)   33%   11%   56%   6,131

Nursing Facilities (1969)

Total United States   7%   71%   22%   18,910

Nursing care only   6%   81%   13%   11,500

Certified, Medicare   8.5%   72%   19.5%   4,041
as skilled nursing facility
(1972)

[a]Federal, 5.5%; state and local government, 27.5%; church, 13%; other not-for-profit, 40%.

Data sources: National Center for Health Statistics, *Health Resources Statistics 1971* (Washington, D.C.: Department of Health, Education, and Welfare, 1972).
Social Security Administration, *Health Insur. Stat.,* 48 (July 20, 1973).

Nongovernment Hospitals

The changing picture of hospital care in the 1960s is evident in a comparison of the nongovernment hospitals before and after hospital insurance for elders became available under Medicare in 1966. The not-for-profit and for-profit hospitals certified to receive Medicare payments by 1972 were 56 and 11 per cent of the total, respectively, with government units making up the remainder (Figure 4–1).

Figure 4–2   Organization of Personal Health Services, United States

Not-for-Profit and For-Profit Hospitals: Changes in Revenue, 1961–1969

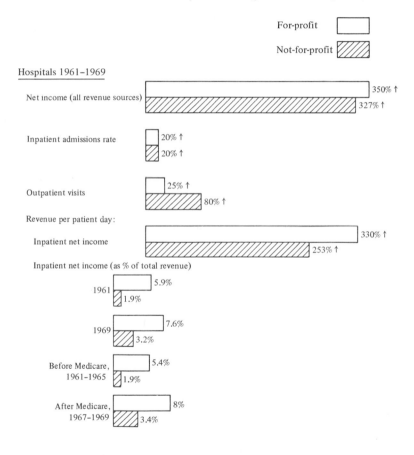

Data Source: Social Security Administration, *Net Income of Hospitals, 1961–1969*, Staff Rept. 6, Dec. 1970.

Through the 1960s the net income of nongovernment hospitals, their total revenue over expenses, increased by well over 300 per cent, the for-profits somewhat more than the not-for-profits. Each type had a 20 per cent increase in patients admitted, and the not-for-profits increased outpatient visits by more than 3 times the for-profits (Figure 4–2).

Most of their income increases came from inpatient care, a much higher rate of net income coming after Medicare was in effect. In other words, both not-for-profit and for-profit hospitals profited from Medicare payments.

According to a government study, the reasons that the financial position of all types of hospitals improved so considerably during Medicare's first year included (1) increases in bed occupancy (during the initial period only); (2) reimbursement for the cost of services to some elders, previously given at free or at reduced charges; (3) reduction of losses from uncollectible fees; (4) payment of an above-cost allowance of 2 per cent of allowable costs (that is, "cost-plus" reimbursement) (2).

FOR-PROFIT HOSPITALS

The for-profits may, in fact, have experienced a slowing of their earnings before Medicare; but by 1969 Medicare was responsible for 8 per cent of their net income, more than twice that for the not-for-profits (Figure 4–2).

Some of the reasons for the higher financial rate-of-return in the for-profit hospitals are their concentration on profitable services, such as laboratory, pharmaceutical, surgical, and medical supplies, and their avoidance of services that bring a net loss: room and board, emergency, maternity, no-charge clinics, longer-term illness, and special services that involve expensive equipment, such as intensive care (3). In other words, their focus is on a rapid turnover of patients, since the highest net income derives from the first three days of hospital care.

Since the late 1960s this focus has been complemented by organizational changes which allow other cost-saving measures, such as central purchasing and variations in personnel patterns. These changes also represent a shift in the type of ownership among for-profit hospitals. Initially begun in the 1950s by physicians, many have been bought and built in recent years by corporate enterprises, certain of them as extensions of the motel industry. Thirty such corporate chains now comprise about one third of the for-profit hospitals (4).

With this organizational background, the figures that describe the changes in the for-profit share of the nongovernmental hospital sector are more understandable. Between 1961 and 1969, their share of all hospitals decreased, but the number of beds remained the same; admissions and patient days increased, and outpatient visits decreased. The average length of stay remained less than in not-for-profit hospitals and increased at a slower rate. This is thus a profit-maximizing pattern of service (Table 4–1).

Given their profit-making emphasis, these hospitals are located expectedly in larger cities with higher per person incomes and where hospital insurance coverage is most extensive (5).

Changes Changes in the hospital component of personal health services which involve other than for-profit hospitals are more significant since they constitute about 95 per cent of inpatient, short-stay (less than 30

Table 4–1 Organization of Personal Health Services, United States

Share of For-Profit Hospitals in
Non-governmental Hospital Sector, 1961 and 1969

	% of Total	
For-Profit Hospitals	*1961*	*1969*
Hospitals	20.4	18.1
Beds	7.7	7.7
Admissions	8.4	8.5
Patient days	6.7	7.2
Outpatient visits	6.3	4.5
Length of stay (days)	5.8	7.0

Source: Social Security Administration, *Net Income of Hospitals, 1961–1969* Staff Rept. 6 (Washington, D.C.: Department of Health, Education, and Welfare, Dec. 1970).

days) hospital care (6). In the three-year period following Medicare, there was a continuing decrease in the total number of hospitals, almost 400 fewer, but an increase in government hospitals, 42. This decrease was almost all among small hospitals, those with fewer than 50 beds. Many of the for-profits of this size changed over to nursing homes.

Among the larger hospitals, of 100–500 beds, there was an increase in both governmental and not-for-profit hospitals. In the largest facilities, of 500 or more beds, there was a reversal in ownership through the closing of 29 government hospitals and the opening of 27 not-for-profit hospitals (7).

Thus the impetus of Medicare contributed to the closing of small hospitals which could not meet certification requirements for Medicare payments and to an increase in larger hospitals. The shift to not-for-profit ownership of very large facilities could, among other things, indicate the relative certainty of not-for-profit organizations for sustaining themselves through governmental health care payments.

Utilization

As described earlier, not-for-profit hospitals have received federal funds for construction and have garnered an increase in net income from Medicare payments. As nonprofit organizations, they were also eligible for other government funds; and, through affiliation with university medical centers, they received additional grants to develop specialized services.

The utilization of these services, the lack of use or misuse, has in turn contributed to the high costs of hospital care (8). For example, in some rural states which received construction grants, 35–40 per cent of hospital beds are unused. In the cities, this may be true for the majority of maternity and pediatric beds, as both physicians and patients move to the suburbs. Among all types of hospitals, bed-occupancy rates have steadily declined, from 83 in 1966 to 78 per cent in 1972 (9). Of the 360 hospitals with open-heart-surgery units, 71 per cent performed less than one per week in 1969, the minimum needed to maintain proficiency and justify costs; 37 performed no services at all (10). At the same time, the use of common surgical procedures, such as tonsillectomies, vary by 3–4 times in different areas of the country, and seem to be related to the number of hospital beds and surgeons in an area rather than medical need (11).

These practices of overbuilding/underuse of services, or the related overuse of facilities for payable services—whether paid by government or private insurers—implies cost increases. Such costs of course affect the users of health services through rising insurance premiums, taxes for government programs, and residual out-of-pocket payments—which may be billed even to low-income persons by some not-for-profit hospitals when Medicare payments do not cover the full costs (12).

Reversing the Primary Site of Care: Alternatives to Hospital Care

Nursing Facilities

Alternatives to hospitals for inpatient services are the extended care facilities (ECF), limited to an illness episode of 100 days, and skilled nursing facilities (SNF),[1] which provide nursing care and prescribed medical treatment. Other Personal Care Homes render some personal services beyond room and board; these were about 40 per cent of "nursing homes" in 1969. The average cost per patient in an ECF was less than one third that of hospital care in 1970 (13).

[1] The 1972 Social Security Amendments placed ECFs and nursing homes under joint Medicare–Medicaid standards, to be certified as Skilled Nursing Facilities.

Again, the advent of Medicare–Medicaid led to the closing of the smaller nursing homes, which could not qualify for payments. By 1972, of those certified as SNFs, the for-profit facilities made up about three-fourths; the not-for-profits, about one fifth (Figure 4–1). A fairly immediate effect of certification on nursing homes was an increase in the proportion having fulltime physicians (7.5 per cent) or having physicians on call (54 per cent) by 1968. Just over half had a full-time or part-time R.N. in charge; the others used other types of personnel (14).

Location As earlier noted, skilled nursing facilities are not distributed across the country in relation to home care programs. They also are not located in regions with high proportions of elders, but in more affluent areas (Appendix Table 13). California, for example, has 14 per cent of the SNFs but 3 per cent of the elders (15). Thus government insurance coverage for needed services (as Medicare), while it grants financial access, does not necessarily affect geographic distribution. This is because, in the case of nursing homes, which are predominantly for-profit facilities, construction funds have come from private sources and thus are focused on the best marketing areas. Also, as earlier discussed, where government construction funds were granted to not-for-profit hospitals in poor regions, a major problem of access to care was attracting personnel, principally physicians, to those regions (see Chapter 3).

Home Care

As an alternative to or progression from inpatient care, home care is often mentioned, primarily in terms of its cost-reducing potential. The cost of home care per patient was $8 per day in 1969. Estimates are that 5–50 per cent of days spent in acute care facilities could be saved through adequate home services; and possibly 20–30 per cent of patients who remain in the hospital after 30 days are there for nonmedical reasons, having few or no options for caring for themselves (16).

Changes Since 1966 when Medicare payments began to cover home after-care for hospitalized elders, more than 1,000 new home care agencies have been started. By 1971 there was a shift in auspices, with increases in official health department programs (now comprising the majority of all agencies), in hospital-based and in other programs, including the for-profit nursing facilities; there was a proportionate drop in the not-for-profit Visiting Nurse Associations (VNAs) and combined health department–VNA programs. Following the requirements for certification and/or pattern of payable services, these agencies increased their services beyond nursing care to include physical, occupational, and speech therapy, and, most markedly, home health aide services to provide personal care over an extended period of time. Such service nevertheless was available in less than 60 per cent of the agencies, and only one in five agencies offered more than one service beyond nursing care (17) (Table 4–2).

Apart from reducing the number of days in inpatient facilities, home care could conceivably prevent the necessity for hospital care, with maximum cost saving. It might also allow a wider range of choice to the 2.5–5.5 million nonaged adults who have severe functional limitations.

Table 4–2   Organization of Personal Health Services, United States

Home Health Agencies,
Change in Auspices and Services, 1966/67–1971

	Agencies	
	1966–1967	1971 (Medicare certified)
Total, United States (%)	100.0	100.0
	(N = 1,275)	(N = 2,333)
Auspices (%)		
Official (health department)	45.0	57
VNA	40.0	24
Combined health department/VNA	6.5	3
Hospital-based	6.5	9
Other	2.0	7
Services (% of agencies)		
Nursing	100.0	100.0
Physical Therapy	68.5	74.9
Occupational Therapy	13.9	19.9
Speech Therapy	20.6	27.0
Medical Social Service	22.8	21.1
Home health aide	34.3	57.6

Source: National Center for Health Statistics, *Health Resources Statistics 1971* (Washington, D.C.: Department of Health, Education, and Welfare, 1972).

These, along with 1.5 million elders, 40 per cent of whom have some limitation due to chronic disease, may need intermittent personal care or homemaker services in order to realize more of their potential (18). These services are not covered by government payments unless they are required following illness, even though experience in other countries suggests that such coverage lessens the need for institutional care (19). For various reasons to be discussed in later chapters, health care professionals in the nongovernmental sector have shown little or no initiative in this area or in home medical services, as the growing predominance of official government home care programs suggests. Further, Medicare payments for home care have steadily diminished while hospital payments increased between 1969 and 1972, and no public funds have been available to develop or expand inhome services or the array of personnel to provide them. Thus, for reasons related to both organization and financing, refocusing on home and community as the primary site for health-supporting, illness-preventing services is still far from a usable alternative* (20).

Ambulatory Care Arrangements

By 1972 allocation of federal construction funds shifted to ambulatory facilities. This came with the recognition that low-income states, after 26 years of hospital construction funding by the federal Hill–Burton program, had at least as many or more hospital beds relative to population as high-income states, and that alternatives to high-cost inhospital care were needed. Rural communities had long received a preponderance of inpatient facilities funds; of their ambulatory projects, most were public health centers rather than hospital outpatient facilities, perhaps reflecting the anticipated low rate of return to hospitals for those services. Early in 1972, half the federally supported facilities projects and almost 45 per cent of the funds were for ambulatory care (21).

Integrated Approaches

OUTPATIENT DEPARTMENTS

Although most hospitals (97 per cent) reported some outpatient, including emergency, services in 1970, 29 per cent actually had organized outpatient departments. Most of these are in the larger facilities. Most hospitals (82 per cent) had emergency rooms, but the majority of these (60 per cent) served only about one eighth of all emergency patients and were thus underutilized or overbuilt (22).

During the 1960s, people increasingly used these ambulatory facilities, about two thirds of the time for routine primary, episodic and emergency care, by 1971. The remainder of visits were made on referral to specialists. This latter type of visit can be an ambulatory alternative to what otherwise has been and often is done on an inpatient basis (23). More widespread use of this less costly alternative is of course realistic only if ambulatory facilities and necessary personnel are both geographically and financially available to those who need them.

* See Chapters 9 and 10 for further discussion.

One federal program intended to extend and regionalize specialist, that is, secondary and tertiary, services was the formation of Regional Medical Programs (RMPs) in the late 1960s. By 1973 the 56 RMPs were re-evaluating their emphasis on heart, cancer, stroke, and kidney disease management, and giving increasing attention to improving access to primary care, including emergency services (24). In effect, they were acknowledging the nonspecialist nature of most health care needs (25); that health services of any type are unusable without means of access by consumers; and that primary care may prevent the need for more costly specialized services. These changes followed changing emphases in federal funding (26).

TARGETED PROGRAMS

Other Federal programs to encourage the delivery of more or less comprehensive primary care are the neighborhood health centers, 60 per cent of the approximate 130 funded by the Office of Economic Opportunity. There were also 120 migrant health programs in 1971, as well as health services provided directly by the U.S. Indian Health Service on reservations (27) and to other special population groupings.

However, estimates are that but 0.5 per cent of Americans seek health services at neighborhood centers; about 11 per cent use hospital outpatient facilities; an equal number have no regular source of care; half as many use no services at all. Thus most Americans (65 per cent) go to private physicians, and another 8 per cent go to physicians in group practice (28).

MEDICAL GROUP PRACTICE

Medical group practice is simply a formally organized unit of three or more physicians who agree to jointly use equipment and personnel, although not necessarily practicing in the same facility; and who determine how costs and revenues will be distributed among themselves. The vast majority of these groups—which increased fourfold between 1959 and 1969—are partnerships or incorporated entities. In 1969 about 12 per cent were general practice groups, half provided a single specialty, and the remainder were multispecialty (two or more) organizations (29).

Thus the majority were not arranged to provide comprehensive services, which would include primary and secondary medical (specialist) and ideally, dental care, for all family members. About 16 per cent of non-federal active physicians worked in groups in 1969, or 21 per cent of all physicians in office practice—a very small proportion (7 per cent) of these were in general practice.

SOLO PRACTICE

Although the number of group physicians is increasing, solo practice is nevertheless the predominant mode. About 35 per cent of those in solo practice were general practitioners in 1970 (30). Again, solo practice does not afford, by definition, comprehensive care, although general practice is more likely to provide family primary care than can specialist solo practice, which most often focuses on a particular disease, age, or sex group (Table 4–3).

PREPAID GROUP PRACTICE

A relatively new form of medical practice organized specifically to provide comprehensive services to the array of persons represented by family is the prepaid group practice. It combines the group pattern of delivering services with an insurance method that provides coverage for services to well and to sick persons, thereby encouraging treatment in the early stages of disease and sometimes preventing illness. This is one way its intention to decrease the necessity for high-cost hospital services is carried out (31).

A second way is through the financing mechanism that makes the prepaid group practice, the providers of care, economically at risk for excess costs paid out in insurance for, for example, hospital care. This is possible because each consumer member, such as an employee and his or her family, pays a "prepaid" fixed monthly insurance premium and is, in turn, eligible for all basic services, regardless of quantity, in- or outpatient, during each year of coverage. The physicians in the group are paid then by the group on a salary basis or by capitation, that is, a fixed annual amount for each person for whose primary care they are responsible, whether or not that person requests services. Since physicians are reimbursed out of the same insurance fund which pays the group's overhead and all service costs, patients are not likely to receive unnecessary ambulatory or hospital care.

Curtailing of unneeded services is of course also in the interests of the consumer by keeping premiums low. In this sense, and because additional out-of-pocket expense can be relatively very small, the prepaid group practice improves the financial access to a full array of health services for the perhaps 5 million Americans enrolled in these programs (32).

The prepaid group practice (PPGP), as an organized means of fi-

Table 4–3   Organization of Personal Health Services, U.S.

Major Types of Ambulatory Care Arrangements. Integrated and Segmented Patterns[a]

Integrated			Segmented		
	N	% of total		N	% of total
General medical practitioners	55,000[b]	30	Specialist physicians	134,000[b]	70
Solo M.D.	52,300	35	Solo M.D.	96,600	65
Group M.D.	2,700	7	Group M.D.	37,400	93
Group medical practices[c]		12	Group medical practices[c]		88
General	784	12	Single specialty	3,114	50
PPGP	est. 140–350	(2–4)	Multispecialty	2,377	38
HMO	40		Ambulatory surgical facilities	est. 525	100
FMC	61		Maternal and Infant project	56	100
Hospital Ambulatory care			Child and youth health centers[d]	58	100
Outpatient department	2190	29	Family planning clinics	est. 3,500	100
Emergency Room	6,200	82	Federal funding	1,000	30
Neighborhood health centers[d]	129	100	Hospital sites	641	9
Migrant health program	120	100	Community mental health centers[d]	609	100
Regional medical program[d]	56	100	Freestanding psychiatric clinic[d]	1,109	100
			Government administration		55

[a] Figures are for various years, 1971–1973, unless noted.

[b] Nonhospital M.D.s, in office practice, 1970, excluding university and federal M.D.s.

[c] 1969.

[d] Primarily federally supported.

Sources: National Center for Health Statistics, *Health Resources Statistics 1971* (Washington, D.C.: Department of Health, Education, and Welfare, 1972).

Comptroller General of the United States, *Study of Health Facilities Construction Costs* (Washington, D.C.: Government Printing Office, 1972).

R. Egdahl, "Foundations for Medical Care." *N. Eng. J. Med.* 288:491–99 (Mar. 8, 1973).

M. Creditor and D. Nelson, "Regional Medical Programs and the OMB." *N. Eng. J. Med.* 289:239–42 (Aug. 2, 1973).

nancing and delivering health services, has many variegated forms and names. Perhaps 140 fall in this general category. Depending on the particular PPGP, the insurance premiums may be paid by individuals, by insurance companies on behalf of individuals or groups whom they insure, by employer–employee–union arrangements (with services in some plans delivered in labor union–owned group practices), or by a government–client combination, which has recently become possible for Medicare recipients and others. The PPGP can operate on a not-for-profit or for-profit basis, the profits accrued for physician–owners or other organized groups of investors (33).

Health Maintenance Organizations   When the enrolled membership of a PPGP, typically 30,000 people, is defined on a geographic basis (rather than an employee or other basis), confined to a particular neighborhood or district, it is known as a health maintenance organization (HMO) (34).

Foundations for Medical Care   There is a similar and newer organizational pattern, focusing on controlling costs and run by county or state medical societies. It is the foundation for medical care (FMC). There were 61 in 27 states in 1973. What has been called the key element in this pattern is the "incentive reimbursement system" for physicians. That is, it allows physicians, located typically in their office practices, to bill the FMC on a fee-for-service basis for services rendered to patients. The FMC then processes and/or approves these physician-generated claims and in turn sends them on to the insurance companies in which patients are enrolled, such as Blue Cross, or, as in California, Medicaid–Medicare.

Because the FMC is run by physicians, this process amounts to peer review of physician services, including their necessity. This form of cost control in its many aspects[2] has resulted in less overutilization of hospital care, thus lesser amounts paid out by insurers. For this service, then, the FMC charges the insuring agencies, including government programs, 2–5 per cent of the premiums paid (35).

Again, there are variations among FMCs. Some limit the fees that physicians may charge for each service rendered; sometimes this is on the basis of family income. Under this arrangement of traditional sickness insurance, patients may have significant out-of-pocket expenses (36).

A few FMCs are of the comprehensive type. That is, they not only furnish claims' approval and processing services, but also set up a package of health services and negotiate an agreement with an insurer to deliver these services for a given price per capita. In effect, the FMC resembles an HMO, except that physicians may practice out of their own offices; they would be likely to share some equipment, records, and personnel for cost saving and administrative simplicity; and although they may bill the FMC

[2] This will be discussed more fully in Chapter 8.

on a fee-for-service basis, their payment is, at least for certain insurers such as Medicare, guaranteed on a capitation basis, with perhaps additional fees divided among physicians from total revenues. This arrangement is then similar to a PPGP.

Another variation is that an FMC, as a financial entity, may sponsor an HMO, a delivery entity.

Probable Future The varieties of HMO legislation introduced into the 93rd Congress, 1973–1975, the final form uncertain at this writing, basically broaden the definition of HMO to include comprehensive FMCs, or any organized entity that provides directly, or by arrangement, comprehensive health services to a defined population (geographic or otherwise) on a prepaid capitation basis, with the HMO assuming some of the risk of higher costs.

Thus whatever the operational form, the HMO will be aimed at controlling costs, mainly by eliminating unneeded inpatient care. Current estimates are that there are likely to be not more than 100 HMOs developed or operating under federal funds by 1977. Fourteen federally-assisted HMOs were delivering services to 69,000 enrollees in 1973; this number is not likely to be more than 1.2 million by 1977 (37).

For purposes of clarity, HMO will here be used for the type of delivery housed in a common setting, with a consumer population defined by geographic limits. *FMC* will then refer to the dispersed form (sometimes called "individual practice") of physician services, which are limited to peer review activities; those which also provide a basic set of health services will be referred to as FMC(comp.) (Figure 4–3).

Current Effects The effectiveness of PPGPs for decreasing the number of hospital admissions of its enrollees, thereby avoiding expenditures for those services, is apparent from the evidence available (Table 4–4). More limited is the evidence that insurance premiums or out-of-pocket expenses are lower (38).

A wide range of PPGP types show fewer hospital days than fee-for-service delivery arrangements under Blue Cross or commercial insurers, by at least one third to one half as few. The HMOs have fewer than the FMC(comp.). Individuals seem to receive more total services under the PPGPs, most under HMO arrangements, and fewer hospital services. Moreover, inpatient surgery for such procedures as tonsillectomies and woman-related surgery are less than half the rates under typical not-for-profit (Blue Cross) or commercial plans. At the same time that PPGPs require only half the number of beds for their enrollees as other patterns of health care delivery, there is no evidence that members' health or mortality is any less than others' (39).

The question of whether persons enrolled in PPGPs, usually of middle-income families, are not healthier to begin with, and thus in less need of

Figure 4–3   Organization of Personal Health Services, United States

Comparison of Prepaid Delivery Systems: HMO and FMC Prototypes

	Health Maintenance Organization (HMO)	Foundation for Medical Care (FMC)
Sponsor	Any for-profit or not-for-profit organization, (including Foundation for Medical Care, labor union, hospital, medical center, community group, government, insurance company, bank, or other corporation)	State or local medical society
Patient population	Voluntarily enrolled, on a defined geographic (or other) basis	Insured persons accepted by M.D.
Services Type	Comprehensive (including M.D., laboratory, X-ray, nursing, drugs, ambulatory and in hospital)	Referred to needed services
Place	Group practice facility (free standing or attached to hospital, community center, and so on)	M.D. offices
Equipment, records	Shared	May be shared
Financing[a]	Fixed premium	Insurer-experience-rated; cost-sharing with insured
Out-of-pocket cost	Relatively low	Potentially high

Payment basis:
  To system
  To M.D.
	Capitation
	Salary; capitation
		Capitation; fee schedule
		Fee-for-service; capitation

M.D. personnel	Closed panel (hired by system)	Open panel (approved by medical society)
Cost control[b] Prospective budget	Yes	No, usually

Claims and other
  Types of peer review
  M.D. liability
	Yes
	Shares percent of risk
		Yes
		No, usually

[a]See Chapter 5.
[b]See Chapter 8.

Data sources: Comptroller General of the United States, *Study of Health Facilities Construction Costs* (Washington, D.C.: Government Printing Office, 1972).
R. Egdahl, "Foundations for Medical Care." *N. Eng. J. Med.* 288:491-99 (March 8, 1973).

medical treatment, is just beginning to be addressed. Two recent studies of low-income populations admitted under federal financing to HMOs show that visits to physicians increased initially and then diminished to the HMO average, which is less than the national average; hospital days decreased by one third and were similar to HMO rates; prescribed drugs also diminished (40). These low-income members were a small proportion of the five HMOs under study, and the actual cost of services to them was

Table 4–4 Organization of Personal Health Services, United States

Comparison of Delivery Arrangements,
Utilization Rates, 1968

Delivery Arrangement	Benefits Received[a] (% enrollees)		Hospital Days (per 1,000 persons/yr)	Inhospital Surgery (per 1,000 persons/yr)		
	Any Benefit	Inhospital		Total	Tonsillec- tomies	Gyneco- logical (Women's)
Fee-for-service[b]			534–1,167			
Blue Cross	33.2	9.9	924	75	6.9	9.2
Commercial insurers	26.1	9.0	987			
Prepaid Group Practice			410–744	34	2.4	4.8
FMC(comp.)	75.7	6.6	471			
HMO	80.6	4.9	422			

[a] Nonmaternity.

[b] Solo or group.

Sources: *Hearings,* House of Representatives Subcommittee on Public Health and the Environment, Mar. 6, 1973 (Federal Employees Health Benefits Program data), Ser. 93–26.

Comptroller General of the United States, *Study of Health Facilities Construction Costs* (Washington, D.C.: Government Printing Office, 1972).

higher than for others' because some additional care (up 15 per cent) was needed, and special "support" services such as transportation were added.

Limits to Access Thus the question remains whether PPGPs as they exist can be cost-saving for all segments of the American people, although they have shown improved financial access for the middle-income, privately insured population. If it is acknowledged that health services to the poor will cost more—if only because the initial quantity of needed care will be greater—the question is: Who will pay the added costs? A new pattern of health care *delivery* may control costs generally, but that fact will not be sufficient to grant financial access to lower-income people.

Nor will PPGPs necessarily locate in health-scarcity areas. Of the approximate 55 HMOs and FMCs(comp.) in operation in 1973, 47 were in urban areas. All but 2 states have laws which in some way restrict the development of HMOs, although 17 are considering somewhat looser requirements (41).

It is reasonable to expect that HMOs operating on a for-profit basis would locate in more affluent areas, as other for-profit health care providers have done (42). However, requiring HMOs to be not-for-profit in order, for example, to receive federal subsidy payments for low-income persons under Medicaid may not necessarily broaden access to health care. Where this was required in one state, there are now under litigation cases in which ostensibly not-for-profit HMOs contracted basic services with allegedly their own for-profit enterprises, and, as well, provided extremely low use of hospital services (43).

The problem of improving both geographic and financial access for all social groups to HMO delivery systems is, as the above suggests, not inherent in the HMO pattern itself but in the decisions over the allocation of resources—the amount, type, and controls—needed to develop HMOs. The HMOs' forms then follow from those decisions.

Similarly, the 1972 Social Security Amendments allow Medicare coverage for elders who choose to receive health services through an HMO. There was, however, no provision for coverage of health care they may need outside their particular HMO, no acknowledgment of transportation problems, no provision as to how elders might become aware of their options (44). Under such circumstances, choice is in reality highly limited. The result might then be that elders will little use HMOs, because they have little access.

Current efforts, then, to develop HMOs—the demonstration approach by the federal government, and the pilot projects of several insurance companies—and the limited number of operational private HMOs suggest that this delivery pattern will not make a numerically significant impact on health services during most of the 1970s (45). The prospects could change markedly, however, through the passage of certain kinds of national health legislation, of which the Professional Standards Review Organization, mandated in the 1972 social security amendments, is but a small example (see Chapter 8).

Potential Variants Future potential variants of the HMO delivery pattern include the transformation of neighborhood health centers, hospital satellite clinics and outpatient departments, local health department clinics, community mental health centers, and home health agencies. In other words, any of these, given the financial and other organizational resources, could expand their current service programs to include a basic set of comprehensive health services and provide them to a defined community population in such a way as to meet the delivery, financing, and control requirements that define the HMO pattern. These are not merely theoretical possibilities. Visiting Nurse Associations have, for example, initiated neighborhood health centers (46). Neighborhood health centers are being obliged to alter their financing methods (47). Recent legislation has been introduced in the Senate that would enable and encourage these kinds of transformations (48).

Whatever the realistic possibilities for such changes, the surgence of organized comprehensive ambulatory health services is some years away (although in the British experience, such programs increased very rapidly once the concept was accepted and institutionalized) (49).

Segmented Approaches

The more typical U.S. pattern of ambulatory care is a *segmented* approach rather than the *integrated* approach just described which focuses on persons, of varying ages, and both sexes. Segmented services, emphasizing particular diseases, health problems, forms of treatment, age or sex groups, include the specialist medical practices, maternal and child care facilities, and family planning and mental health centers (Table 4–3). These problem-oriented, categorical service programs may provide basic, primary care, as do Well-Child Clinics, or secondary care, as do medical specialist practices, or both, as in community mental health centers. They are all limited to particular health problems or certain social groups.

Limitations   This segmented "crash approach" may have an advantage in altering some aspects of problems affecting personal health, particularly when societal conditions allow or support improvements in health. For example, widespread new subsidized family planning clinics, and, increasingly, legally controlled abortion services, have contributed to declining birth rates and infant deaths; and government-supported Maternal and Infant Projects helped lower perinatal deaths (those occurring from the seventh month of pregnancy through the fourth week of life) (50). However, these programs report their limited capacity to change, for example, the rate of prematurity (51) or affect the timing of births (in terms of mothers' age and child spacing) (52), which would be far more effective for reducing infant mortality. These changes are of course closely bound to socioeconomic environments. Any contribution personal health services could make would require, at a minimum, sustained contact with the most vulnerable social groups—which the very organizational nature of segmented services mitigates against.

In other words, the more that service programs require individuals to arrange separate visits, with the personal logistical costs they entail, the less likelihood any service program has of a sustained relationship with individuals, much less a familiarity with the interrelationships of their immediate world to the particular health problem which the facility focuses on.

In addition, segmented programs are independently financed and administered. This tends to add to overhead costs, produce conflicting requirements, and encourage competition among programs for available dollars (53). Each type of program may then be insufficiently large to have an impact on its focal problem. For example, the Children and Youth

Projects were not expected to reach more than 17 per cent of the 2¼ million poor children for whom they were to provide health care (54).

These organizational patterns and others have the effect of limiting access to comprehensive health services to consumers, especially those with priorities mandated by the burden of being outcast, thus depriving them of the full benefit of what personal health services can do for health.

Mental Health Programs   In certain segmented services, consumers have, in fact, required attention to their more comprehensive concerns. A neighborhood mental health center in a low-income area in New York, for example, was providing clinical psychiatric treatment for 5 to 10 per cent of those who came for help—since only 6 per cent of their requests pertained to psychiatric or family problems. Their major problems were financial, housing, child care, and general community problems. Most services were therefore related to assistance, sometimes limited, in those areas. Most clients were satisfied, and 85 per cent "felt better," an essential in the health equation (55). However, the vast majority of these community mental health centers did not locate in poverty areas (56).

Like other health services, given the high costs of inhospital care and the less segmented approach that community-based ambulatory programs make possible, psychiatric services have been deinstitutionalizing. Between 1950 and 1970, there was a 40 per cent drop in hospitalized patients; in the 1960s, the number of psychiatric beds was reduced by more than one fourth, while the rate of patients admitted almost doubled. This rapid turnover of patients partly resulted then in the threefold increase in outpatient visits between 1962–1970 (57).

Child Care Programs   On a broader organizational level, the segmented, categorical approach to services has also tended to separate health care from child care, which "falls" into "social services" or "education." Yet, with about one fourth of all children under 14 years having mothers who work, and with a rising proportion of young mothers who work (58), child care centers and after-school programs pose obvious possibilities for relating comprehensive ambulatory health care delivery systems to children and to places of employment. This is another segmented service, "occupational health." Most industrialized countries have far closer links to both child care and work settings, and far more advanced systems of young child care (59). In this they adhere to WHO recommendations (60).

Federal Organization   Segmented services are reflected in the organization of federal agencies, which fund many, if not most, of them. Bureaus of the Department of Health, Education, and Welfare are categorical in focus, following the legislation which produced their programs; fund granting is often separate from financing and policy from program implementation and evaluation, policy making residing in short-term appointees, thereby minimizing a longer-range, comprehensive planning approach.

Thus new problem-focus programs may be quickly generated, on a small scale, without much relation to each other and with little or no integration at either policy-making or delivery levels (61). This may have the effect of limiting interbureau conflict (62), but it also places costly demands, in time, effort, and taxes, on consumers. In return, consumers receive numerous, circumscribed, tenuous, and *ad hoc* programs.

Figure 4–4   Organization of Personal Health Services, United States

Department of Health, Education, and Welfare, Selected Agencies, 1973 Organization

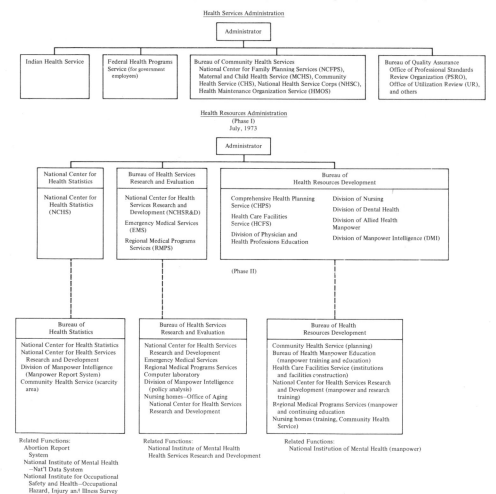

Source: Department of Health, Education, and Welfare, *Health Planning Memorandum* 48 (Aug. 16, 1973).

The organizational chart for the health care aspects of HEW has frequently been reorganized in recent years. Two of its components most directly related to the direct provision of personal health services or the funding of services delivery are the Health Services Administration and the Health Resources Administration, following a 1973 directive in its phased steps (Figure 4–4). Other components are the Food and Drug Administration; Alcohol, Drug Abuse, and Mental Health Administration; Center for Disease Control; and National Institutes of Health. The organization of payment for services is in the Social Security Administration, Social Rehabilitation Services.

Consequences for Access Thus the segmented nature of health services is importantly a result of the federal organization, which provides services and funds for health care, in turn a result of decisions as to how much and what types of resources should be allocated in what ways (see Chapter 8). Patterns of services are also heavily influenced by the health occupations (see Chapter 7).

The delivery of health services is, in effect, not a result of policy planning and coordination, but the consequence of almost chance convergence of a variety of facilities offering numerous types of services under several kinds of ownership and financing, initiated and located to ensure fiscal integrity and adhere to legal mandates, if not to uphold the spirit of the law. In any given setting, the available mix of services and the ways they are used, emphasizing inpatient or outpatient care; comprehensive, specialized, or primary care; integrated or segmented arrangements are closely related to what those services cost and ultimately to financial access for potential users.

Deinstitutionalizing Strategies

Organizational Changes

Some approaches then to lowering or containing costs, recommended by the 1972 study for Congress, were (1) providing care in the appropriate facility, deemphasizing inpatient care when medically possible; (2) developing new and in effect more usable forms of delivery, the comprehensive ambulatory care facilities; (3) sharing underused or overbuilt services within confined geographic areas, such as certain emergency rooms and pediatric or maternity beds; and (4) regionalization of specialized, therefore less needed and more costly, facilities (63).

The use of appropriate facilities assumes of course the existence of an array that emphasizes noninstitutional care. As already described, this is not the case in most communities; even when the programs exist, that does not assure their "appropriate use." Among the reasons cited for the slowness of changes that would allow full access to an optimum mix of services are the unwillingness of major providers to risk losing control over current patterns; lack of integration between hospital and nonhospital inpatient facilities; lack of consumer awareness of alternative arrangements; less than vigorous enforcement of current controls; and financial incentives for keeping hospital beds filled (64). Other changes, then, in financing and control—that is, ensuring the development, distribution, and necessary use of noninpatient, comprehensive services—have become increasingly discussed and to an extent initiated (Chapters 5 and 8).

Preventive Measures

Without doubt the best way to reduce the demand on costly health facilities is to prevent the need for their use. One obvious way is to control technologically controllable communicable diseases, which accounted for 2 per cent of inpatient days in 1970. In addition, hospital-induced infections added 2–4 days' stay to a significant proportion of inpatients in nonteaching (2 per cent) and teaching hospitals (5 per cent); 7 per cent of surgical patients incurred infections, adding $7,000 per person to the costs of their care (65).

The selective use of full physical examinations and screening for certain groups, tied to immediate and guaranteed treatment, would also prevent the later necessity of more extensive medical care. The control and prevention of chronic disease, which takes about 28 per cent of all inpatient days of care, depends, of course, as does the continuing problem of communicable disease, on what resource committments are made to changing the environment in the broad sense (66).

Finally, organized changes and preventive approaches are needed for another effect of industrialized society, the first cause of death in the younger years—accidents. Since two thirds of these victims die even before reaching a medical facility, emergency services must move into communities in various ways. This would not only save lives, but might also limit disability and shorten dependence on specialized care. The best "treatment" resides in prevention, through allocative decisions, which, for example, might make motor vehicles unnecessary (67).

International Comparisons

As countries attempt to make personal health services accessible to their populations, certain general patterns emerge. Concerning systems for delivering health services, virtually all countries are moving away from inhospital care, particularly industrialized countries, which historically have been hospital-oriented.

Examples of national health service systems in which the government owns the most or all health facilities and employs the most personnel are Sweden, the U.S.S.R., and Great Britain. These systems, although varied in organization, have the capability for refocusing health services. In Sweden, hospitals are owned by local, county government, with 50 per cent of ambulatory care given through outpatient departments. About 14 per cent of physicians are in private practice; although they are nonsalaried and work from their own premises, virtually all are affected by national health insurance fee schedules (68). About 35–50 per cent of physicians in many industrialized countries engage in general practice (see Appendix Table 18c).

While in Sweden local government has the ownership of hospitals, in the U.S.S.R. and Great Britain ownership resides at the national level. In 1974 Britain implemented a plan that will more closely relate national policy planning through regional coordination of graded services and local delivery of integrated services. This is in contrast to former patterns of regional hospital administration by quasi-autonomous boards and separate local delivery of segmented (for example, maternal–child) services (69). This has become possible in part because of the tenfold increase, between 1965 and 1971, of integrated primary care centers, health centers owned and staffed by local government support, out of which general practitioners agree to work—6 times as many GPs did so in 1971 as in 1965, roughly 10 per cent of all GPs. About two thirds work in some group practice arrangement, and they provide 90 per cent of necessary medical services (70). These changes have made separate maternal and child welfare facilities unnecessary, and these facilities are gradually being closed. With family planning methods newly payable under the national health insurance system, these programs as separate entities may eventually not be needed (71).

Further steps toward deemphasizing inhospital care have been the development of new options, such as one-day maternity facilities run by midwives and related to the GP, hospital, local health, and home care network; "open institutions" for the mentally ill; and rapidly expanding home care programs. Home care provides both temporary and permanent personal and/or health services to the elders, sick, disabled, or for maternity services in Britain, Sweden, Denmark, and other countries. Payment for these government services is based on ability to pay or may be without charge to groups such as the elders (72).

Canada, which has a national hospital and medical insurance program, is now considering a plan that is similar to other national health service systems and to systems now operative in certain of its provinces, as in

Quebec. The plan calls for high-level policy planning and resource allocation, regional coordination of services, and local program development of integrated services, emphasizing noninpatient options (73).

The industrialized countries with health services delivery systems that tie national-level policy planning to local programs seem able to implement on a relatively even basis such otherwise *ad hoc* services as emergency medical, ambulance, industrial, and selected screening and aftercare, throughout the population and regardless of ability to pay (74) (see Appendix Table 18c).

The delivery of health services in Japan is similar in ways to the U.S. pattern, emphasizing a categorical approach at the national level, and separating certain services, such as maternal and child, for prefectural and municipal health department provision to those who do not have access to private practitioners. Such care is given through MCH centers, which are mainly in rural areas. Most physicians, over 90 per cent, are not employed by government (75).

Certain less industrialized countries, such as India and China, have fairly well developed planned systems for delivering health services. In India, following a national plan, personal health care is, except for family planning services, the responsibility of the states. The plan, implemented in part, calls for community development blocks, with regional specialized facilities and district comprehensive health centers and related subcenters for maternal and child services. Now, the formerly segmented family planning subcenters are being integrated into the district network (76).

Several of the newly independent African countries are attempting to develop national health service systems, tying in remnants of their colonial inheritance. In Nigeria, Senegal, and Tanzania, for example, free government health services are available but only in limited ways (77).

With the major exception of Cuba, which has a fairly extensive national health service, most Latin American countries follow what is sometimes called a "pluralist" pattern of health services. That is, care is provided under a wide range of auspices which own or control varying proportions of facilities and services, and include the national and local governments; certain social security programs; special occupational groups, such as the military or police; and private for-profit and not-for-profit organizations. As already noted, these services are not evenly available (78).

Summary

In the United States, access to health services for all social groups has been limited in part because of the way health services are organized. The primary necessity of meeting budget, if not profit, requirements, has strongly influenced the development and location of certain types of facilities and services, following the most favorable private or federal-supported "markets," markets that have emphasized payments for high-cost inhospital care. Budgetary risks are, in turn and in part, based on the fact that health care organizations are dependent on profits or on attracting nongovernment support through development of prestigious images. Prestigious services, most prevalent in the largest sector of health care, the not-for-profit hospitals, are most often of the least needed and most expensive types. This adds to the total costs of care and in turn limits the financial access of certain groups of consumers.

When government support has been granted to mitigate costs, it has been done without benefit of national policy guidelines or regional planning; it therefore has been in the form of *ad hoc* funds for construction and/or services of categorical types. This in turn almost ensures the lack of comprehensive, integrated arrangements of most needed types of services in geographic areas of greatest need.

However, the resulting limits to access are also attributable to forms of financing, of servicing, and of control over health services, as the next chapters will show.

chapter 5

Paying for Health Care

As earlier pages suggest, financial incentives alone may change the number, types, and distribution of personal health services but do not necessarily produce the best and most economic combinations of most needed services in regions of greatest need. These pages will look more closely at how health care is paid for, by whom, to whom, and with what indirect as well as direct effects.

The Growing Problem

Health had become the second largest "industry" in the United States by 1971 measured by its share of national income.[1] It had grown by 87 per cent since 1966 (1).

National Health Expenditures and Personal Health Care Costs

Total national health expenditures amounted to $83.4 billion, representing 7.6 per cent of the GNP. These expenditures include governmental public health activities, medical research, medical facilities construction, and principally (91.2 per cent) personal health services. National figures do not include funds spent for the education and training of health workers

[1] Total earnings of labor and property arising in the current production of goods and services.

nor for pollution control.[2] Expenses for personal health care per person nearly doubled between 1965 and 1972 (Table 5–1).

Table 5–1   Financing of Health Services, United States

Total National Health Expenditures, Including Personal Health Services, Changes, 1950–1972

	Fiscal Years			
	1950	*1965*	*1971*	*1972*
Total health expenditures[a]	$12.1	$38.9	$75.0	$83.4
% GNP	4.6	5.9	7.5	7.6
Personal health expenditures[b]				
% of total	89.4	89.3	89.9	91.2
Per capita	$79	$198	$358	$394

[a] In billions; does not include expenditures for health care training and education, or air and water pollution control and treatment.

[b] Does not include government public health expenditures, medical research, or medical facilities construction; includes administrative overhead.

Sources: B. Cooper and N. Worthington, "National Health Expenditures, 1929–72." *Social Security Bull.,* Jan. 1973.

Social Security Administration, *Res. Stat. Note* 19:3 (Nov. 29, 1972).

Committee for Economic Development, *Building a National Health Care System* (New York: CED, 1973), p. 41.

I. S. Falk, "Financing for the Reorganization of Health Care" (mimeo), July 2, 1972. Paper presented at Sun Valley Forum on National Health, Idaho.

SOURCES OF PAYMENTS

The picture of who paid these accelerating expenditures has changed considerably. In 1950 government sources were paying for about one fifth of all personal health care; the federal share was just under half. Private sources paid the remainder, two-thirds coming directly from consumers of services, and about 10 per cent through insurance plans.

Twenty years later, 1970, the direct payments by consumers decreased by almost half (36 per cent), private insurance payments increased by about two and one half, and government sources covered 36 per cent of all expenses, the federal arm now the predominant source (Figure 5–1).

Current Trends   These trends continued for 1972, with direct consumer, insurance, and nonfederal government sources each paying lesser

[2] To be discussed below.

Figure 5–1   Financing of Health Services, United States

Sources of Funds for Personal Health Expenditures

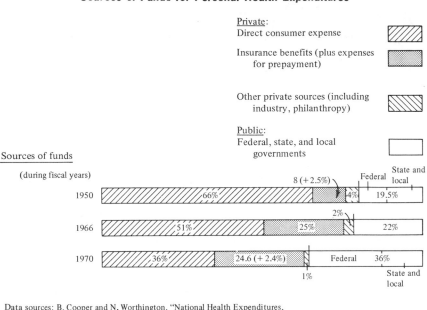

Private:
Direct consumer expense

Insurance benefits (plus expenses for prepayment)

Other private sources (including industry, philanthropy)

Public:
Federal, state, and local governments

Sources of funds

(during fiscal years)

1950   66%   8 (+2.5%)   Federal 4%   State and local 19.5%

1966   51%   25%   2%   22%

1970   36%   24.6 (+2.4%)   1%   Federal 36%   State and local

Data sources: B. Cooper and N. Worthington, "National Health Expenditures,
1929-1972," *Social Security Bull.*, Jan. 1973.
I.S. Falk, "Financing for the Reorganization of Health
Care," July 1972 (mimeo).
Social Security Administration, *Medical Care Expenditures,
Prices, and Costs: Background Book* (Washington, D.C.:
Government Printing Office, 1973).

shares and the federal government share rising concommitantly (2). Most of these funds went to hospitals (45 per cent), physicians (22 per cent), and for drug costs (11 per cent) (Figure 5–2).

These figures, then, show increasing expenditures for health services, increasingly paid through indirect private and governmental, especially federal, sources. These, of course, derive their income from insurance premiums or general taxes and social insurance payroll taxes. The federal government, further, grants an annual tax subsidy of $3 billion through income tax policies for individuals who buy health insurance and for employers and employees. Individuals may deduct about one half of their insurance premiums. A larger subsidy is given to employers and employees by excluding all employer health insurance payments from the taxable income of either group (3).

Toward an Accurate View   Unfortunately it is not possible to get an accurate view of *total* national health expenditures, the sources of payment, and the recipients of funds. This is because of the omissions noted above

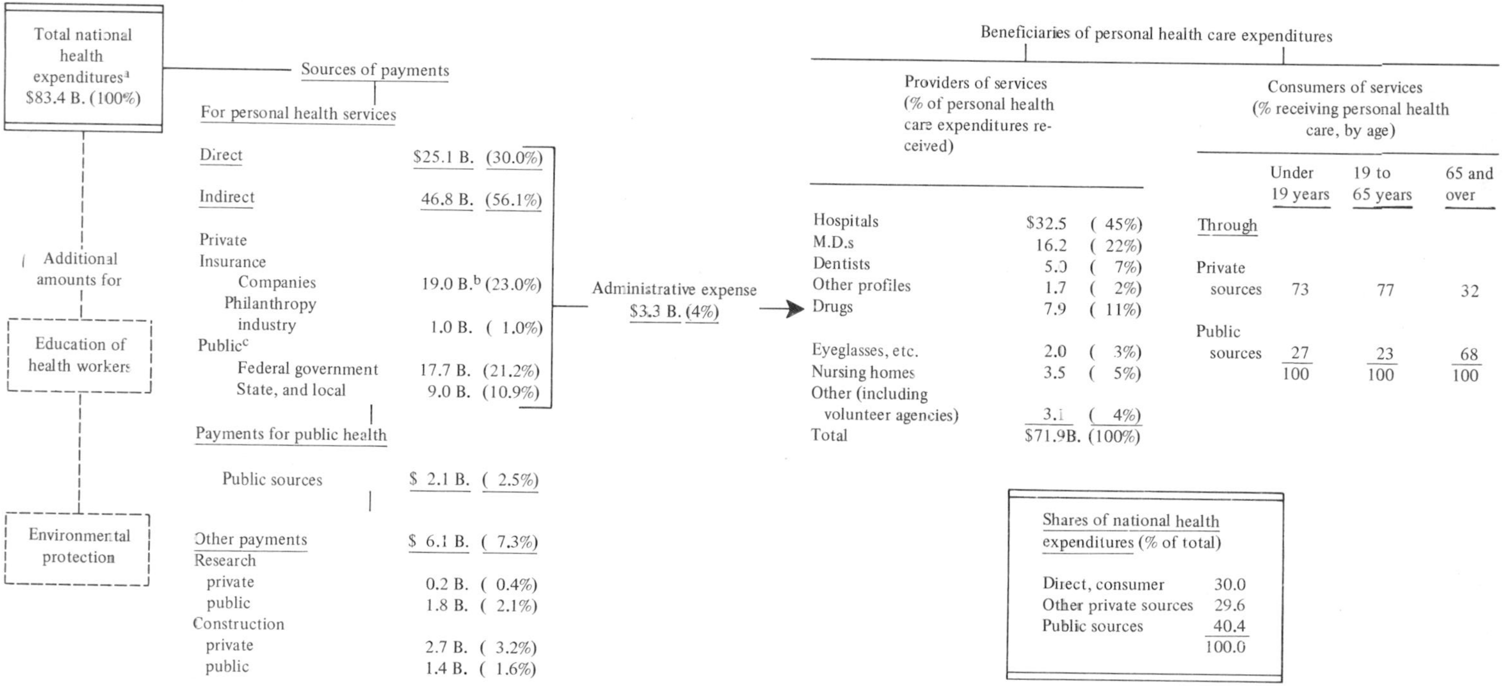

Figure content:

Total national health expenditures[a] $83.4 B. (100%)

Sources of payments

For personal health services

Direct	$25.1 B. (30.0%)
Indirect	46.8 B. (56.1%)

Private Insurance Companies — 19.0 B.[b] (23.0%)
Philanthropy industry — 1.0 B. (1.0%)
Public[c]
Federal government — 17.7 B. (21.2%)
State, and local — 9.0 B. (10.9%)

Payments for public health
Public sources — $ 2.1 B. (2.5%)

Other payments — $ 6.1 B. (7.3%)
Research
 private — 0.2 B. (0.4%)
 public — 1.8 B. (2.1%)
Construction
 private — 2.7 B. (3.2%)
 public — 1.4 B. (1.6%)

Additional amounts for
Education of health workers
Environmental protection

Administrative expense $3.3 B. (4%)

Beneficiaries of personal health care expenditures

Providers of services (% of personal health care expenditures received)

Hospitals	$32.5	(45%)
M.D.s	16.2	(22%)
Dentists	5.0	(7%)
Other profiles	1.7	(2%)
Drugs	7.9	(11%)
Eyeglasses, etc.	2.0	(3%)
Nursing homes	3.5	(5%)
Other (including volunteer agencies)	3.1	(4%)
Total	$71.9B.	(100%)

Consumers of services (% receiving personal health care, by age)

	Under 19 years	19 to 65 years	65 and over
Through Private sources	73	77	32
Through Public sources	27	23	68
	100	100	100

Shares of national health expenditures (% of total)

Direct, consumer	30.0
Other private sources	29.6
Public sources	40.4
	100.0

a Does not include expenses for air and water pollution control and treatment, nor private and public costs of education and training in health occupations.

b Includes about $1 B. for prepaid group practice plans.

c Includes Medicare ($8.4 B.), Medicaid ($7.3 B.), and $11.1 B. for other programs such as workmen's compensation medical benefits, military and veterans medical and hospital care, temporary disability insurance, school health, and so on.

Data sources: Social Security Administration, *Res. and Stat. Note*, 19:3 (Nov. 29, 1972).
Committee for Economic Development, *Building a National Health Care System* (New York: CED, 1973).
Hearings, House of Representatives, Subcommittee on Public Health and the Environment, March 6, 1973 (Federal Employees Health Benefits Program data), Ser. 93–26.

Figure 5–2 Financing of Health Care, United States Allocation of Total National Health Expenditures by Payors and Purpose, 1972

regarding health care training and pollution control. These omissions reflect the segmentation of the health care education sector and the environmental sector from health services. A true picture of U.S. health care, its directions and potential redirection, is not possible until these omissions are overcome.

Shares of National Health Expenditures   In an effort to view national financing of health care within the current definition of national health expenditures, Figure 5–2 shows the sources of payments, the payors, as proportions of the national total (rather than of personal health expenditures only, as is customary). Thus, excluding direct consumer payments, private intermediaries and sources account for less than 30 per cent of all health expenditures, including a tiny amount for research (0.4 per cent)[3] and the larger share of construction of medical facilities. This leaves about 40 per cent to government sources, and does not include the tax subsidy for insurance premiums.

Additional Educational Costs   However, a very conservative estimate of additional public funds spent for the education and training of health workers in 1972 would include over $700 million in nonresearch funds from the Department of Health, Education, and Welfare (HEW), plus funds from federal non-HEW agencies for 83,500 health trainees, and other—state and local—governmental funds which support the 892 publically owned health professional schools.[4]

Added Antipollution Costs   These amounts, along with public funds[5] used for air and water pollution control, sanitation, sewage treatment, and water supplies (at least $41 billion) represent well over half of *all* health expenditures. This, then, could cast a different shape to the presumed "private enterprise" model of health care in the United States (4).

PERSONAL HEALTH CARE EXPENDITURES

Focusing again on personal health care expenditures, some important questions are: Why are they accelerating? Why is the shape of payment changing? (See Figure 5–1.) The answers are intertwined.

Some of the increase in expenditures, about 10 per cent between 1965 and 1972, was due simply to population increase; another 38 per cent was a result of the increased use and scope of health services; the rest, 52 per cent, has been attributed to price increases (5).

---

[3] This does not include drug company product research, about $0.5 billion.
[4] This is 51 per cent of all (1,742) such schools.
[5] Private expenditures were under $10 billion in 1971.

Price Increases   Looking at price changes in the 1960s, it is clear that medical care prices rose faster than the overall Consumer Price Index,[6] and have grown at accelerating rates since 1965. Prices of certain components, such as hospital rooms and physician fees, led the increases, and drug prices moved from a position of decline to increase, almost doubling between 1965 and 1970 (6) (Figure 5–3).

Figure 5–3 Financing of Health Services, United States

Medical Care Components of Consumer Price Index, 1960–1970

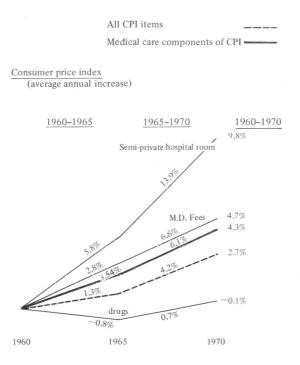

Data source: Bureau of Labor Statistics, Consumer Price Index.

[6] The CPI measures changes in average prices of goods and services purchased by urban wage earners and clerical workers and their families. It is the most generally accepted measure of price changes, and its medical care components are the most widely used indicators of health care prices.

Out-of-Pocket Expense These price increases meant that by 1970, of all Americans who paid for any health care, their average out-of-pocket cost, including insurance premiums not paid by employers, was $209 per person. It was $320 for persons over 65 (7). These amounts were higher for whites than for other races, higher for women than men, for the affluent than the poor, higher in the South and West, and higher for elders in every category (Table 5–2). These variations, as discussed in Chapter 3, reflect differences in prices, health care needs, and ability to pay.

Table 5–2 Financing of Health Care, United States

Personal Out-of-Pocket[a] Costs for Personal Health Services for All Persons and Selected Groups with Such Expenses, 1970

	All Persons	Persons 65 and Older
United States	$209	$320
Race		
White	212	327
Other	185	219
Sex		
Male	190	311
Female	227	327
Income		
Under $5,000	217	299
$10,000 or more	223	376
Region		
Northeast	206	293
North Central	188	326
South	210	321
West	253	365

[a] Includes insurance premiums.

Source: National Center for Health Statistics, "Personal Out-of-Pocket Medical Expenses, 1970." *Monthly Vital Stat. Rept.* 22, Apr. 2, 1973.

Family Budget Amounts Another way to see the impact of rising health care prices is to look at the proportion they require of family budgets. According to Department of Labor estimates of the actual costs of two-adult, two-children families living at lower, intermediate, and higher standard budgets, medical care required diminishing proportions at the higher levels. This meant in 1972, 7.6, 4.6, and 3.2 per cent for urban families living on $8,100, $13,600, and $20,210 per year, respectively, the lower standard bearing more than twice the burden of the higher standard of living (8). Understandably, such budget requirements have been rising (9).

Elders' Expenses   Increasing cost is particularly a problem for elders, 60–65 per cent of whom depend primarily on retirement benefits for their living expenses. About half of the single retirees in 1970 had neither pensions nor earnings to supplement social security benefits. This meant that their median income was $1,500 per year (10).

Examples of Financing

Social Insurance Financing: Medicare

To assist elders in meeting the costs of their medical care, Medicare was enacted in 1965. Under the social insurance principle of the social security program, financed by federal revenues (11 per cent) and employee contributions through payroll taxes (86 per cent), it pays elders' medical expenses, including hospital, nursing home, and certain home sick-care services.

Under Part B of the plan, physician and other medical services and supplies are covered; these are available for an ongoing monthly insurance premium. Both Parts A and B have deductible clauses which require the enrollee to pay up to $72 for the initial services. There are also co-insurance payments, under which the enrollee pays a flat rate or percentage of ongoing medical charges, such as the 20 per cent copayment for medical services in a given year after the initial $60 annual deductible has also been paid by the patient. Certain services are not covered at all by Medicare insurance. These include dental and eye care, hearing examinations and aids, general physical examinations, immunizations, orthopedic aids, and outpatient drugs (which cost $74 per user in 1971). (11).

Some Effects   This form of health insurance has thus insured a part of the financial risks of getting sick for elders and has subsidized most heavily the most costly forms of medical care. In so doing, it in effect encouraged more expensive forms of care by, for example, requiring hospital treatment for an illness prior to the enrollee's transfer to a skilled nursing facility. It also tends to encourage elders to avoid seeking a health, eye, hearing, or dental examination until they feel the symptoms of illness, since the insurance plan does not cover these costs (12).

Recent Changes   Changes in Medicare under the Social Security Amendments of 1972 ease somewhat the effects of its hospital-oriented sickness focus. For example, the 20 per cent copayment for home health services was eliminated, although the annual $60 deductible remains. Services to elders may now be paid when they receive medical care through HMO-type arrangements, including foundations for medical care or neighborhood health centers, when these groups meet certain quality standards. Such standards may be waived, however, if the HMO has fewer than 25,000 enrolled members. This is the case for most federally assisted HMOs, which are relatively small. Only about 2.5 per cent of elders are in areas in which HMO delivery systems exist, however. Other limitations of this provision were pointed out in Chapter 4 (13).

The early experience with HMO services was reported by the Social Security Administration to show 10–15 per cent lower payments for Medicare enrollees than for comparable elders who received their medical care under typical fee-for-service practice arrangements (14).

The 1972 Amendments also automatically placed under Medicare disabled persons who are not yet 65. They also allowed enrollment by elders who have been excluded from the social security system, including many never-employed women and sporadically employed workers, which includes a large proportion of farm laborers. These new enrollees would have to pay monthly premiums for Part A services ($33) as well as Part B, which were increased to $6.30 in mid-1973 (15). Thus the out-of-pocket costs per person for these elders would be over $470, in addition to the deductible and copayments required for medical care each year, unquestionably a deterrent to many of them if they sought no financial help.

Other Payers　This governmental–consumer social insurance program paid 42 per cent of the costs of health care for elders in 1971. Other government funds paid an additional 26 per cent of the costs; individuals directly paid another 26 per cent (amounting to $250 per elder), and private insurance plans paid about 6 per cent (16). In effect, elders, large proportions of whom have low incomes and chronic diseases, have paid through their work life and in ongoing insurance and direct payments a large proportion of their health care costs, which tend to be rendered under high-cost arrangements (Figure 5–4).

These, then, are the financing mechanisms underlying the sources of payment for the personal health care expenditures for elders. As earlier noted, public sources pay for 36 per cent of the expenditures for all age groups. For elders, all public sources account for over 67 per cent of payments, although the actual financing for those dollars is derived in large part from elders themselves (17) (Figure 5–2).

Public Revenue Financing: Medicaid

The Medicaid program represents another method of public financing for personal health services. It is intended to pay the costs of health care for

Figure 5–4   Financing of Health Services, United States

National Programs for the Aged and Poor: Medicare and Medicaid, 1973

	Medicare	Medicaid
Eligible beneficiaries	1. Social Security retirees and other aged. 2. Chronically disabled; certain others.	1. Recipients of categorical aid programs (e.g., Aid to Families with Dependent Children). 2. Medically indigent, determined by each state: 23 states limit their programs to (1); 28 states cover both (1) and (2).
Coverage Basic services	Part A: Hospital care; skilled nursing facility care; Home health services (with time limits).	Mandatory: states must provide physician services, in- and out-patient hospital services, skilled nursing facility, and home health care; family planning.
Supplementary	Part B: Physician, home care; physical therapy, and out-patient hospital services.	Optional: state may provide drug, dental, and eye services.
Financing	Social insurance, plus 1. Individual premiums (Part B). 2. Deductibles (Parts A and B). 3. Copayments (Parts A and B).	Government revenues (federal and state) matched by 1. Monthly premiums from medically indigent. 2. Copayments may be imposed by states.
Proportion of personal health care covered for eligible groups	42%	26%

Sources: Social Security Amendments of 1972 (P. L. 92–603).
Perspective (4th Q, 1972).
Health Law Newsletter, 25 (May 1972).

the "categorically needy"—those already receiving public assistance, such as under the federal Aid to Families with Dependent Children (AFDC) program—and the "medically indigent"—those too poor to pay for health care, including elders; "indigent" is determined by each state. The states are required to make available certain health services to these eligible persons, including hospital, physician, nursing home, home care, and family planning services. In addition, they may provide such optional services as drugs, dental, and eye care. Federal funds have then paid from one half to over three fourths of the costs, and the states finance the remainder of covered services. (Figure 5–4). However, because many services are not covered, low-income families must pay for over one third of their health services directly out-of-pocket. This amounted to $77 per person in 1970. (18)

Under the 1972 Social Security Amendments, medically indigent people must now pay monthly insurance premiums; states now have the option to impose copayments as well (19). A large proportion (38 per cent) of Medicaid funds were used in 1971 to pay the deductible and coinsurance costs for elders who were too poor to pay for their Part B Medicare services (20).

Toward Consolidation

For the first time, the Medicare and Medicaid programs were joined legislatively in the 1972 Amendments. This was a beginning effort to untangle the sometimes contradictory definitions and requirements which confuse recipients and impede administration. For example, the "extended care facility" under Medicare and "skilled nursing home" under Medicaid became the Skilled Nursing Facility, with a single set of certification standards. Unlike Medicare, however, Medicaid does not require hospital care prior to SNF care (21).

FISCAL CONTROLS OVER UTILIZATION

Consumer Cost Sharing   Under both programs, the HMO option is now allowable, and in both, cost sharing—the deductible and copayment provisions—has become prominent. This is, of course, an attempt to control health care expenditures by discouraging the use of services or, more accurately, the unnecessary or overuse of services.

Studies of the effects of the cost-sharing strategy show that the imposition of copayments does discourage the use of physician services and reduces the costs of care per person (22). Or, to put it conversely, whenever consumers no longer pay directly for a particular service, such as physicians' services, they tend to increase their use of that service. These "induced services" or "induced demands" result in "induced costs" and higher total expenditures (by about 2.5–4.5 per cent, depending on the type of service) (23).

Effects of Copayments   However, *low* copayments do not deter the overuse of services; and copayments that are high enough to deter use also unduly burden the poor, who become the first to forego health care. Recent experience with Medicare showed that the deductible and copayments for ambulatory care had greatest impact on persons in low-to moderate-income families. Almost one third of these failed to use services compared with smaller numbers in more affluent families or among those who had other governmental or private insurance to cover most of the deductible and copayments. The low- to moderate-income group also had higher proportions of other races than white, of lesser educated persons, and more of those who needed, but could not afford, to see a doctor (24). Thus those in greatest medical need may become the first to avoid even publically supported insurance programs—intended for the indigent—when copayments are required.

In any case, cost-sharing strategies are likely to have greatest impact on first-contact health services, where the consumer has the major choice of initiating health care. This is usually some form of ambulatory care, and so is the relatively less expensive type. It is the physician who primarily determines utilization of high-cost care, that is, inpatient services. At that point of decision making, the fact that a patient must pay the now proportionately small share of hospital charges is not likely to deter a decision to use in-hospital services—particularly if a patient has delayed needed medical care to avoid the copayments.

Insured Services   Here the relationship of hospital utilization and increasing costs is more closely tied to the types of services insured. As suggested in Chapter 3, those insurance plans which more heavily cover inhospital services show perhaps 20 per cent greater use of hospital care than the plans which emphasize other-than-hospital care (25). Again, under experience with Medicare, the inpatient facilities that were eligible to receive payments for care increased their patient care in the before and after periods of Medicare (26).

In sum, fiscal means to control health expenditures are likely to have greater impact by focusing on the types and amount of benefits covered which can *discourage*—through physician decision making and consumer encouragement—use of the *high-cost* (inpatient) types. To use copayment requirements to deter consumers from coming for health care can prevent the poor from using the services which the tax-supported programs, at least, were intended to induce them to use.

Limited Eligibility: Experience Rating   Another means, also focusing on the consumer, used to control the use of health services is to limit the types of persons eligible for insurance. This is done in private insurance plans, for example, through the use of "experience rating." This technique sets the rates for monthly premiums based on the company's experience with a particular category of enrollees. Thus women or handicapped persons or elders, who use more health services, are charged higher premiums. This has the effect of detering them (or their employers) from seeking any, or all but minimal, health insurance. For the insurance companies, the consequence is relief from higher-risk, medically needy enrollees (27).

An alternative to this is the "community-rating" technique used by some of the larger HMOs. Here, premiums may be based on family size in the eligible population or community, but not on individuals' past or projected medical care requirements. In effect this does not penalize those who need more services, although it may mean on the average slightly higher premiums for the more healthy enrollees. This result has been offset in some instances, as described in Chapter 4, by federal subsidy payments for elders, the disabled, and the poor (28).

Provider Risk Sharing: Capitation A mechanism used by HMOs to control the unnecessary use of services, as noted earlier, is to tie the provider's income to the cost of services. This is done through the capitation method, which guarantees full care on a yearly basis to the consumer for a fixed, prepaid monthly payment. With the qualifications pointed out in Chapter 4, this method of reimbursing providers has been successful in encouraging lower-cost ambulatory health care.

Salary Another method of reimbursement that attempts to control expenditures directly and focuses on the providers is salaried income. This obviously allows budgetary planning on a more predictable basis than the more open-ended fee-for-service method. A crucial minority of health personnel in the United States—the physicians, dentists, as well as optometrists and podiatrists—are usually paid under fee-for-service methods. The vast majority of health workers, of course, are salaried.

A recent survey of physicians showed that payment on a capitation basis over fee-for-service methods was preferred by a minority of AMA members (30 per cent) and by 47 per cent of non-AMA members (29).

In sum, these and other fiscal techniques—which focus on either consumers or providers—to control health expenditures directly or indirectly have gained prominence in recent years, along with other nonmonetary attempts at cost control.

INDIRECT AND UNINTENDED EFFECTS

Rising Costs Accelerating costs are in part an unintended consequence of public financing of health services for the poor and aged. This result is principally from the emphasis on most expensive types of care—inhospital coverage paid on an open-ended cost-reimbursement basis—and from the open-ended fee-for-service reimbursement method for physician services (30).

Institutional Relief Another indirect effect of Medicare and Medicaid has been, by paying for services in medical centers and teaching hospitals, to increase the salaries of resident physicians and their supervisory medical school faculty. This thereby relieved hospitals and medical schools of a portion of their personnel budgetary costs (31).

Profits An additional consequence of public financing for the higher-medically-at-risk poor and elderly is an apparent improvement in profits for commercial insurers. Although they were reporting losses in the health components of their insurance plans in the 1960s, the 20 largest companies, which have 75 per cent of the private health insurance business, reported a profit by 1972 (32).

OTHER PUBLIC PROGRAMS

Although Medicare/Medicaid under the Social Security Act are the largest publically financed programs for personal health care, there are numerous others.[7] These include financing and/or delivery in varying mixes with other public or private groups, principally Department of Defense health services, the Veteran's Administration programs, and programs administered under the health or social security agencies of HEW and authorized under welfare and employment sections of the Social Security Act; or under other legislation, such as the Public Health Service Act, Economic Opportunity Act, or Mental Health and Mental Retardation Act (33).

ADMINISTRATIVE COSTS, PUBLIC AND PRIVATE

At a minimum, authorities that overlap add to health expenditures through their aggregate administrative costs. This amounted to 7 per cent of the benefits paid for the public insurance programs. This figure, however, compares favorably with the 10 per cent rate in employer–employee group insurance programs, and the 30 per cent administrative cost among individual health insurance plans and comparable high service charges in the not-for-profit Blue Cross–Blue Shield plans (34). For the total administration of this variety of health insurance programs, U.S. consumers paid in 1972 $3.3 billion, 4.6 per cent of all personal health expenditures (35).

Financing of Health Training

The administration of funds for the training of health personnel has the same kinds of problems as does the services programs. As earlier noted, these dollars, possibly several billion and increasingly paid through public sources, are not included in the official national health expenditures total. In 1970 there were almost 150 federal training programs, authorized by over 40 pieces of legislation and administered by almost 50 units of the

[7] $8.4 billion for Medicare; $7.3 billion for Medicaid; $11.1 billion for all others.

federal government, the majority within the Department of Health, Education, and Welfare (36).

Problems

Among the problems cited in the cost study of the education of health professionals, mandated by Congress, were the lack of coordination of financing policies for various types of programs and little coordination between sources of federal funds—such as research grants, training programs, and Medicare–Medicaid payments. This segmented approach was found to foster special claims by special interests, and it provided no mechanism to assess or balance those claims (37).

Moreover, there is no means for developing long-range policy for health personnel training and supply, nor for relating such a policy to the provision of health services. Under these circumstances, federal support for health personnel training has been increasing rapidly through the 1960s, but with little means to assess its effects. No sources of consistent financial data for all health schools exist (38).

Some Effects

As has been the case for health services delivery programs, health schools, too, have changed as a result of federal financing. Medical schools alone, receiving a 52 per cent increase in federal research grants between 1965 and 1969, increased their full-time faculty by 59 per cent, while student enrollment grew by 16 per cent only. In effect, the educational institutions changed because of the availability of certain types of federal funds, not because of the demands of student enrollment (39).

Similarly, by a federal policy decision in 1950, university resources were chosen (rather than federal facilities) for furthering basic research. This rapidly accelerated the research focus of medical schools. In 1947 a small part of medical school income (11 per cent) derived from federal research and research training funds; by 1968 this had grown to 42 per cent, paying one third of the total faculty budget and shared by 40 per cent of the full-time faculty members (40).

Thus although public funds, especially since the 1960s, have increasingly been used to pay for all facets of personal health services, including the training of personnel, relatively little attention has been given to developing mechanisms to monitor and assess the direct or indirect effects of such funding.

Potential Effects

With continued public funding, health schools are likely to have their expenditures more closely scrutinized. Taxpayers and legislators are likely to view "productivity" and "results" in terms of the numbers of students admitted and graduated. This, in turn, may mean not only changes in fiscal accounting by the schools, but also a renewed emphasis on basic rather than graduate programs, as recent experiences suggest (41).

Further, former "charity" patients, who traditionally provided clinical experience for health students, now have the buying power under Medicaid to go to other than medical center facilities. Health schools may need to refocus attention on the community aspects of health services delivery and somewhat less on academic concerns in order to reclaim their patient clientele. As one result, faculty may be increasingly spending more time in the direct delivery of health care (42).

International Comparisons

Affluent Countries: National Health Insurance

Most affluent countries have a national, statutory health insurance system, whether or not they also provide health services directly through a government-owned health care system. Most of these national health insurance programs pay both cash benefits as well as for health services needed during maternity and sickness. Cash benefits are paid to patients in lieu of missed work. Payments for health care may be made to either government-owned or to private facilities and individual providers. In the U.S.S.R. and other similar socialist countries of eastern Europe, the governments own all facilities and employ all health personnel. Thus in those countries insurance payments to providers are not the method used for financing health care (43).

PAYMENTS TO PHYSICIANS

In many countries, payments to physicians who are not employed by the governments are made on a capitation basis. A potential uneconomic effect of this method is that busy physicians may not spend enough time with time-consuming patients such as the aged and others who require much medical care. Thus they might overly refer patients to specialists while still retaining their capitation fee (44).

In recent years the British system has sought to offset this by paying a larger capitation to GPs for each aged patient. British GPs refer 12–14 per cent of their patients to specialists, which compares favorably with the 10 per cent referral rate of salaried district medical officers in Sweden (45).

The Netherlands uses another means of assuring full care under the capitation method. The full capitation rate is paid the physician for each of the first 1,400 patients accepted in his or her practice; a lesser rate is paid for the next 1,400; thereafter, no capitation payment is made (46). Thus there is no economic incentive for building a large practice.

Most specialists in these systems are hospital-based and salaried. One problem for assuring health care delivery which the salary method offers is that physicians may emphasize their private or nonsalaried practice over the salaried practice. Sweden recently attempted to resolve this by no longer allowing specialists to collect separate outpatient payments in addition to their salaries; a straight salary method is now used (47).

QUEING

In countries where direct payments by consumers are very nominal, such as Great Britain, patient visit rates to physicians are similar to those in the United States. Inhospital *elective* surgery, however, has placed a demand on these facilities which has resulted in waiting lists (although the lines are shorter now than in the past). This, in effect, represents another means for controlling the use of certain services, queing. This amounts to an alternative to the copayment method for limiting the use of health services. Presumably most people are willing to wait for nonurgent care.

In these and other ways, national health insurance systems can use fiscal controls to bring about planned effects in health care delivery, such as emphasizing most-needed services and most-economical forms of care for various population groups.

OTHER FISCAL PROGRAMS

Other fiscal measures that can enhance health care services by preventing or easing the effects of illness, are the economic-support programs that most affluent countries have. These are the old-age, disability, and survivors' pensions; work injury and unemployment insurance; and family allowances for the total population (Appendix Table 18b).

In many of the poor countries of Asia, Africa, and Latin America, national health insurance programs, where they exist, are limited. They usually cover only certain worker groups. Small proportions of government revenues, if any, supplement the employer–employee payroll tax fund out of which benefits are paid. Benefits are often limited to cash and/or specific services, such as maternity or hospital care. Services in Latin America are often obtainable only in facilities owned by the national health insurance agency. India's program resembles those of the Western countries in form, although it covers lower-paid workers in certain urban firms only. Physicians who receive patient care payments under these systems are usually based in inpatient facilities and are salaried.

A few countries, among the poorest, use an alternative to the social insurance approach. Nigeria and Tanzania, for example, have provident funds. Certain groups of employers and employees are required to jointly build up a fund that employees may have in cash benefits for sickness or other grave needs. The benefit is limited to the amount a worker contributes. It is, in effect, an enforced savings. Moreover, it is difficult to assure that the fund will be justly administered (48) (Appendix Table 18b).

Summary

Although the picture of U.S. health care expenditures is not precise—because financing programs are not sufficiently coordinated to allow or require full and consistent reporting—what is clear is that the size of health expenditures is rapidly growing, with the greatest share of services increasingly paid out of federal government funds for those with the highest risk of medical need. In addition, there is growing prominence of government funding for the education of health personnel, as has been true in biomedical research and environmental protection. Public financing has thus allowed lower-risk health activities to be shaped by private interests.

The consequences of these segmented programs, as well as the open-ended payment methods and sporadic methods of control over services covered and service utilization, have included spiraling costs. This has placed added burdens not only on the users of services in outcast groups (who often encounter direct-payment requirements), but also the working-class taxpayers, themselves an already burdened group. Institutional budgetary relief and profits have been the consequences for many service, educational, and financing organizations.

Thus the attempt to enhance financial access to health care for the poor has had inequitable effects in terms of redistributed resources. This has resulted from the choices over the sources of financing, the services covered, the methods of payment, and fiscal control. These program strategies have had planned or unforeseen consequences, directly or indirectly affecting the distribution of facilities and personnel, the arrangements for the delivery of services, and the shape of the education of health personnel. Chapter 6 will examine the latter effect more closely, particularly as it relates to the access of individuals to the health care occupations.

Images of Access

In the day-to-day world people in communities go on living and dying, aware to a limited extent or totally unaware of far-removed systems which shape their options for humane living. In everyday life, within the big picture, efforts continue, aimed at granting access to services necessary for humane living.
The vignettes that follow portray three such efforts, in settings that limit or broaden the likelihood of the wider impact of those efforts. All, however, aim toward making certain services accessible to outcast groups in New Delhi, Holland, and London, making personnel and facilities available where and when they are needed, without financial barriers to the users.

i For Farmer Migrants, New Delhi

In the chill of midwinter mornings in New Delhi, the choking smell of smoke fills the air and creates a layer of haze over the city. It comes from the mud-stove fires of 60,000 workers, men and women, who make their homes on the construction sites where they work. They live in housing, made by them of brick supplied by the construction bosses, a few feet square and roofed with vine or scrap boards and metal, located on the fringes of as many as twenty to thirty building sites.

These workers are farmer migrants from Rajasthan, the large desert state to the west, who came to Delhi seeking to lessen the burden of survival in their rural area. Today, more of India's people are rural, 4 out of 5, than in the mid-nineteenth century—before Britain effectively transformed its economy to her own purposes, according to the late Prime Minister Nehru.

In the capitol's construction work, these wives and husbands can earn a relatively good income for their six days of heavy labor. Wages vary from about 150 to 700 rupees per month, about $20–100. Economically, they are low- to low-middle-income families. Socially, as immigrants and Muslims, they are often regarded by the Hindu majority as money-hungry and backward.

They, in fact, do have less formal education, particularly the women, who are kept subservient to men. Literacy among women is about 6 per cent in Rajasthan, about 42 per cent in urban Delhi, and about 15 per cent in India overall. Women are allowed to learn little or no English— the second language of the country; sometimes they are still required by their families to observe *purdah,* the veiling of their faces in public. They earn greatest approval—even more than for their Hindu counter-parts—by bearing many sons for their husbands.

The children of the Rajasthanis, perhaps 30,000 of them, grow up as transients as their parents move from site to site following work. They do not usually enter school, which is compulsory for six-year-olds, for they have no birth certificates. Besides, they are more useful caring for younger brothers and sisters. So all are left to live and play in the slush of mud and dung and human excreta that surrounds their tightly packed dwellings. Or they run outside the wire walls of the site into heavy motor scooter–animal traffic, one of the most accident-laden environments in the world.

By law, building contractors must provide crèches, group nursery care, for the workers' preschool children. But this law is virtually un-enforceable, according to Meera Mahadevan, founder of Mobile Crèches for Working Mothers. A member of the more comfortable class of Indian society, Mrs. Mahadevan says that she could no longer overlook these children, who are doomed by their beginnings to remain outcasts, as are their urban-nomad parents. With a young teacher, Mrs. Singh, daughter of a "poor Prince" and British-educated, they began the first construc-tion-site crèche in 1969.

The aim of Mobile Crèches is to take care of workers' children, re-gardless of their age, eventually on all New Delhi's building sites. Thus the crèches move with the workers.

Through bargaining, pressuring, and cajoling contractors, these women were given minimal crèche facilities. Forming alliances with voluntary relief organizations such as Brothers to All Men, they got food and other supplies, and a cash grant from the Canadian High Com-mission. Mobile Crèches had seven programs in operation by 1971.

One crèche is in Chanakyapuri, near New Delhi's "Embassy Row."

As we drove there in one of the common three-wheel canvas-topped scooters, Meera Mahadevan had to badger the big, turbanned driver to go beyond the Pakistani High Commission, where Indian troops were newly quartered on the lawn to quell protests over a plane hijacking. This was two months before the Bangla Desh secession.

At the shanty-town fringe of the Chanakyapuri construction site, after engaging in the necessary bargaining over the driver's fee, Meera Mahadevan was greeted with shouts from the children as we walked toward the crèche.

Sitting Indian-fashion on the ground, one group of six- to eight-year-olds was being taught to write Hindi on small slates by the head teacher, a young woman and university student. Another older group was learning about Indian leaders of the past by the assistant teacher, who had two years of formal education beyond the compulsory ten years.

Preschoolers were playing and singing nearby, unperturbed by incessant flies. And inside the three-foot brick wall under a partial sheet metal roof—the crèche facility—mothers were breastfeeding their infants, having been allowed to leave their building work. *Ayahs,* helpers (known as servants in the past) attended to the physical needs of the infants, cradled in tiny hammocks.

After their first year, twenty-five of the crèche's thirty preschoolers (three- to six-year-olds) could count to at least 50 and knew some of the alphabet. Seven of the thirty-three older children could do math, read, and write, and the rest could count to 100 and had learned the alphabet.

In the crèche the sexes are mixed, contrary to the ordinary pattern of separation, and male preference, in the public school system. Indian preference for males also shows up in the larger number of girl babies left for adoption; the giving of health examinations to groups of boys before groups of girls; the greater frequency with which parents bring male infants for medical treatment; the higher death rate for girl babies; and, unlike most countries in the world, the lower life expectancy for women.

At Mobile Crèches all the children share the essentials for their bodily well-being—clothing and blankets, health examinations and immunizations given by volunteer physicians, vitamins, and breakfast and lunch. Of necessity, the food is simple and based on combinations of milk, sugar, and gram wheats—the protein-rich pulses, or husked peas, beans, and legumes—ground into a versitile wheat that can be made into flatbread; filled, rolled, fried, or steamed as meat-cheese or vegetable cakes; or added to an array of sweets.

Because parents live so close to the crèche, family planning information, nutrition exhibits, and other education propaganda activity is brought to the construction site by other organizations, governmental and voluntary. Given the isolation of these families, such information seems more an entertainment than an intrusion.

The workers at the seven crèches, fifty in all, almost one third of whom are volunteers, were trained by Mrs. Mahadevan. She is reluctant to allow foreign women, Americans and British, to work in the crèches, although they are willing. But, she says her "Indian sisters," although they are free of the cultural and language barriers of foreigners, are often unwilling to get involved in "dirty work."

The paid workers, currently all women, get $20–30 per month, typical of the low incomes of preschool teachers, except for those who work in expensive English-language preschools, formerly the only kind available. They attribute the female-teacher pattern to the example set by the West, which some of them are now beginning to question.

Formal training for preschool teachers is done in privately run Nursery Training Colleges, in one- or two-year programs led by those who qualify as primary school teachers (with Bachelor of Education degrees); graduates are then licensed by the state Departments of Education.

The organizers of Mobile Crèches do not regard formal qualifications or femaleness as essential to do the job. The rigidities of formal education may, in fact, limit the imagination of the workers, and the emphasis on women limits the experiences of the children. So, as the program expands, hopefully to all thirty construction sites, Mrs. Mahadevan plans to train the enlarging child care staff, drawing on university students and others of both sexes, with a team of three professional workers "of the *right* kind"—those who are adaptable and can "laugh with the children." The three, a nurse, nursery teacher, and primary teacher, would initially do a week of demonstration teaching with the staff at each site, and then individually continue to rotate, supplementing the basics in child care and education.

Funds for this will, Mrs. Mahadevan hopes, come from voluntary sources. She hesitates to seek government monies for fear that political considerations might interrupt funds once granted. However, she thinks that building contractors in time ought to be required by law to pay for the Mobile Crèches (1).

ii For Urban Villagers, southern Holland

The birthplace of the painter Van Gogh, who produced a revolution in art, has itself undergone revolutionary changes, most of them in the last twenty years. The quiet village of Etten-Leur, not far from the Belgian border, is undergoing industrialization. In less than two decades its population has increased by over 4 times its original 5,000 members. Most of the new people came from southern Europe to find work. Work they found, and difficulties, but not the degradation that workers have historically endured in the large industrializing cities. These immigrants were entitled to certain social prerogatives legislated after World War II, thanks to the clear thinking of such people as Dr. Mol of Etten-Leur, who served as a Member of Parliament.

Still tall and straight at eighty years, with thick, wavy gray hair and wearing a dapper wool suit, Dr. Mol is obviously a revered citizen of the village. In many ways he is the picture of the family physician, a picture now fading in the memories of people in much of the modern world. For almost a half-century, Dr. Mol was the only physician for Etten-Leur. He literally knew every person. He was present, in spite of long distances and bad weather, at the beginnings and endings of generations. In the traditions of Catholic southern Netherlands, he and Mrs. Mol bore nine children, seven sons—four are physicians, one a veterinarian, one a dentist, one a psychologist.

But Dr. Mol saw the world, and The Netherlands, changing, and he recognized that the private practice of medicine had to change, too. So, as a legislator, he helped draft what is now the national health insurance program, among the most efficient and effective in the world.

His sons say that they wish everyone were required to use the national health insurance instead of only those whose income is less than 18,800 Dutch guilders (about $6,000), although these are the vast majority. As general practitioners they are paid quarterly by the government on a capitation basis: $1.20 per person per year for the first 1,800 patients who choose them as their personal doctor, and about $0.75 for each additional person, up to 2,800 people. This basic prepaid fee allows the patients as many office visits as they need. Because they are family doctors, the Mols also make house calls, eight or ten or twelve, each afternoon following the work at their office–clinics, located in their homes in the southern Netherlands. Like most physicians, they also treat a number of quite affluent "private patients," who are willing to pay high fees rather than use the national health insurance system.

For all its members, the Dutch system provides not only health care but also medical care—the treatment of illness—medication, dental care, and hospital care. The costs of childbirth in a hospital are not included for women who are expected to have a normal, uncomplicated delivery— only those with potential complications are hospitalized, about one third. Most women are safely delivered at home, attended by midwives or doctors.

The health and social security system provides many nonhospital benefits to mothers and babies and is responsible for their being among the healthiest in the world. For example, working women continue to receive their full salary for three months while on maternity leave, six weeks before and after delivery. Then, during the delivery at home, the services of a general practitioner or midwife are paid by the health insurance. Half of the mothers who bear their children at home use an additional form of maternity care, unique to The Netherlands in its extent, the *kraamverzorgster,* a woman who provides care during and related to childbirth—the "mother-keeper," or home help.

Dr. Mol's personal experiences attested to the need for this kind of service, especially as a village like Etten-Leur was beginning to burgeon with new workers and their growing families. He explained how many new mothers, especially those from southern Europe, who were isolated from their next-of-kin, welcomed the mother-keeper, whose services are covered to a great extent by the national health insurance.

The Kraamcentrum, the headquarters for Etten-Leur's mother-keepers' services, is a new, low, window-fronted building that is part of a large shopping center, a recent addition to the urbanizing village, which more closely resembles its U.S. counterparts than commerce in Amsterdam. However, unlike comparable buying areas in the United States, the local health center, primary school, and community center radiate from this natural crossroads.

The Kraamcentrum, which has an almost home-like rather than business-like atmosphere, is both a service and a training center. It is one of nineteen government-funded, nonprofit organizations, evenly distributed among Holland's twelve administrative regions. Etten-Leur's center covers 60,000 people in thirteen surrounding villages. The registered nurse in charge—in ordinary street clothes, but without the flare of women in Amsterdam—says she supervises the forty mother-keepers with two other nurses. The RNs' jobs also encompass the practical training of eight to ten student mother-keepers. Some of the students temporarily live at Kraamcentrum, which has comfortable dormitory quarters, when their homes are too great a distance from their working places.

The students, who may be as old as forty, but are usually close to the minimum age of eighteen, are given a year's training, including six months of practical experience at a kraamcentrum. To enroll they need only a primary education, six years, plus two years of house-keeping training in a kind of vocational school. The first three months of classroom teaching is done at a regional center by instructors in nursing, social medicine, housekeeping, and group work. Their diploma allows them to work at any of the kraamcentrums throughout Holland (not as private practitioners) at a wage of about $167 per month for twenty working days per month.

As an incentive to older women, Dr. Mol says, they may retire when they are sixty and receive their social security pension, now over $120 per month. He points out how, over the years, certain aspects of mother-keeper training have been especially conducive to young immigrant women and their families—the limited amount of formal education required and the fact that during the six months of practical work the trainees receive a salary of $137, plus room and board, in addition to $0.90 per day which is paid to their parents.

These conditions are clearly inviting to young girls from low-income families. Just as clearly, however, given such low wages, the job of mother-keeper is not intended to be liberating but rather a way to make more tolerable the straits of poorer families and the women in them. A further disadvantage from the perspective of the workers is that they cannot get advanced training in nursing schools if they do not have a secondary education, and they are not given certified, academic recognition for their experience as mother-keepers.

A consequence of all this, according to the nurse–supervisor, is the high rate of job turnover—most of the girls get married within four years and stop working. The numbers of workers seems adequate for the present, however. This is perhaps partly because modern birth control practices have become more common—the Catholic Church in The Netherlands is no longer an opponent. Another changing practice is that more affluent women seem to be choosing the hospital, at their own expense, for a normal childbirth—not because of medical necessity, but for the allure of "being modern" that hospital care seems to have, in spite of the fact that this may indeed not be the healthiest environment for normal new babies—the chances of infection are increased.

With the increase in childbearing women, some hospitals are beginning to hire mother-keepers to take care of maternity patients. Also projected is the possibility that mother-keepers may go with pregnant women to the hospital, attend to their comfort during childbirth, and help them at home following discharge from the hospital. These prospective changes in patterns of maternity care will be greatly affected by what services the national health insurance decides to subsidize—a clear example of how patterns of social and health behavior, of what "is done" or "not done," are shaped (2).

iii For the Dying, London

Great preparation is made for the great events in human lifetimes—birth, education, marriage, career, inheritance, perhaps also for an afterlife. But such concern is rarely paid that second most important event in every life—its end.

We do not think about, plan, or choose the way in which we would like to die. We somehow assume that the inevitability of death means also that we have no choice about how we shall die—where, with whom, in command of how many of our faculties, supported by how much medical technology. We learn little or nothing by any organized means in our lifetimes as to whether, indeed, we could command such options, much less what those options may be.

As part of society, health personnel are also imbued with the general avoidance-of-death mentality, usually supported by their formal education and work settings. They therefore become unable to offer a different perspective to terminally ill patients. In a few places people are working toward setting up the conditions that would make it possible for sick persons to determine their own way of dying; to not let the dying be isolated, outcast. One such place is in London.

The screeching of buzz-bombs, a terrifying momentary silence, and then the explosion. That was what the office girls in London lived with day after day during the Nazi Blitz, Angela told me. Then one day a bomb hit her office. She thought she was dead, but a beam had fallen, protecting her head. That was her first experience of being hospitalized.

Over the years, changes occurred in Angela's body, difficulties in seeing, moving, talking. Finally, unable to move except one arm, isolated and lonely, she took twenty sleeping pills, but she did not die. That was her second experience in a hospital.

From there she came here to St. Christopher's Hospice. She was expected to die months ago. Now she is writing her autobiography. She says she feels alive, and so no longer fears and dreads this time of waiting for the end of her life.

The Hospice is meant to be a humanizing respite before death. It is a place for feeling alive for those who know they must soon die. It is a kind of halfway house between the world of the living and the inevitability of death; but a house set in light and beauty, comfort and freedom from pain; a crossroads for the terminally ill, the busy world, the caring world, the world of nature, the realm of the contemplative. In other words, it is a place where the dying can choose how they will die. They are no longer outcasts, the objects of whispers, subjected to stilted conversation, deprived of information about themselves, acted upon solely in terms of what others decide is "best" for them, powerless recipients of drugs and procedures that totally divorce them from what they have known as human living.

The Hospice is set in a hilly, quiet residential area in southeast London, easily accessible by the red double-decked buses that go back and forth along the road outside its front door. It is otherwise surrounded by lawn, trees, and gardens. The windowspace, which forms a broad ribbon around this low modern building, is at a height that allows people in wheelchairs and those confined to bed to see the outdoors. A court surrounded by openable glass walls, connecting the outside with the inside, allows those who are able to be wheeled outside in bed or chair. Sometimes meals are cooked and eaten in the court. The use of the grounds and the building is very much left to the imagination and capacities of patients and workers. Chapel, the kitchenettes, and the art and craft equipment are available to patients and to their families. Lounges, carpeted and comfortably furnished, are conducive to afternoon tea for patient and family and, sometimes, workers.

Schedules and rules are kept at a minimum. Family members are welcome at any hour of the day or night. They may remain, or leave, may give much or little physical assistance to their dying one, may discuss or not discuss the approaching end of life, as they and the one who is dying agree.

For those like Angela, without family, others become a substitute family—among them, the elderly people, who occupy a housing unit which is part of the Hospice. It was originally intended as low-cost apartments to be offered as an inducement to workers. However, staffing is no problem at the Hospice, and so the apartments, pleasantly designed and decorated, are rented to the elders. They in turn have become interested companions to Hospice occupants, and at the same time have found for themselves a special reason for being.

The workers at the Hospice are also a kind of family for the patients. They use comfortable forms of address, mostly first names. They, and the patients, wear informal, noninstitutional clothing. Areas and ideas that are "off-limits" are rare.

But for workers to be comfortable in the presence of death, in something other than the outright denial of emotion that often exists in places where people have terminal illness, they must face their own feelings about death. For workers to be a kind of family, the usual barriers between various types of workers must dissolve. To work toward this kind of openness and melding, the Hospice staff meets weekly in small groups, including nurses, aides, volunteers, students, social worker, and chaplain.

Subjects for their discussions range from particular feelings related to a patient, to general social concerns such as abortion, delinquency, war, and the mass media. Topics and leadership come from the group, rotating among the members. Points of view cover a wide range, from radical to conservative. But the common denominator seems to be each person's right to his or her own views and to the expression of those views—exactly the kind of attitude that is also necessary to help terminal patients find their own way of dying.

To be comfortable in the face of death means in part for most terminally ill patients, especially those who have cancer, to be free of pain. Most of the patients at the Hospice have cancer. With the environment that the Hospice provides, far smaller amounts of drugs seem effective, the result being that the people who are dying are also much more alert and alive, able to make decisions about what they will do, how they will die. Patients are not subjected to experiments with anticancer drugs or other "heroic" surgical or medical treatments. They are given only treatment that will keep them as comfortable as possible.

Of the first 500 patients who came to the Hospice since its opening in 1967, 2½ per cent were able to return home because disease symptoms disappeared or because their pain was so well controlled that they could live a somewhat normal life at home for awhile.

Of the second 500 patients, 12 per cent went home. Now the Hospice has an outpatient service for those who return home, advising them on the best combination of pain medications, allowing them to talk about the fears and anxieties that arise, and helping them and their families to take steps to deal with some of the reasons for their worries, such as the economic ones. However, the British National Health Service covers virtually all health costs, and the social security system for disabled, retired, or widowed people covers basic living expenses, remedy for many anxieties.

Recently, the Hospice has made three of its staff nurses available to visit the homes of the patients. Under this home service, a nurse will call on a family once before the patient comes to the Hospice, so that they will know what to expect. Should the patient return home, the nurse will visit to help maintain the balance of medications or deal with other concerns, including when and whether to return to the Hospice.

Some people choose to die at home. Others want to go home for a weekend or a few days. Another alternative that the Hospice will offer to families in the future is that they will be able to remain overnight or for a number of days or weeks in studio-like apartments that will be attached to the patient unit in a new section of the Hospice.

Another facility that is being built is living quarters for physicians, nurses, clergy, and social workers who come to work for several months at the Hospice to learn to be comfortable themselves with dying and to help others to be comfortable (3).

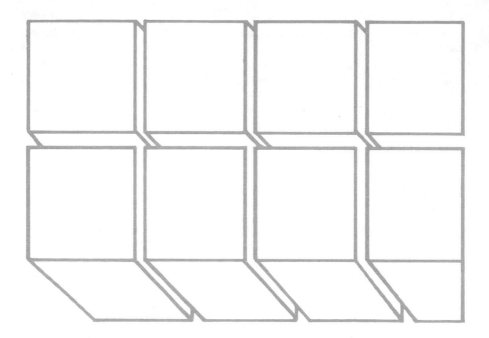

part three

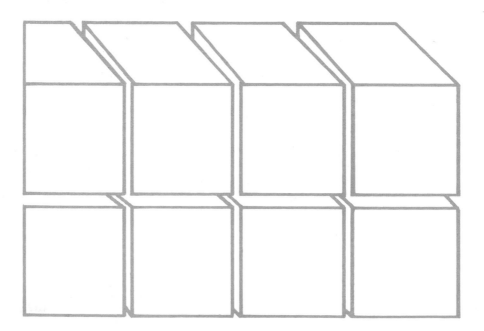

Access to the Health Occupations

chapter 6

From Student to Practitioner: Patterns and Effects

The predominant outcast groups in our country, known by their income, residence, sex, race, or age, have had at best limited access to personal health care facilities, services, and personnel. Changes in the organization and financing of health care have so far only served to accentuate the uneven distribution of resources.

Certain social groups have also had restricted access to the health care occupations. This chapter attempts to draw a picture of the occupations, their composition—which groups enter, where they go, what their rewards are—and the consequences of these patterns. Chapter 7 deals with the changes going on in the occupations and their effects both on health services and on outcast groups.

Occupations in Outline

In Environmental and Personal Health Services

Health, as the second largest U.S. "industry," is so, in large part, because it is labor-intensive, a service system requiring many people-oriented personnel and skills. By 1971 health-related services were rendered by about 4¼ million people. Only about 7 per cent of these provided environmental and food and drug protective services. [This does not include newer pollution control personnel; there were 7,000 air and water quality workers, the largest of these categories (1).] The other 4 million gave personal health care, mostly within inpatient facilities (Figure 6–1).

Figure 6–1   The Health Occupations, United States

Personnel in Environmental and Personal Health Services, Inpatient and Ambulatory Care

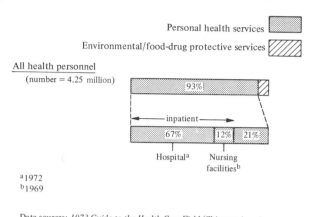

Personal health services

Environmental/food-drug protective services

All health personnel
(number = 4.25 million)

93%

←——— inpatient ———→

67%   12%   21%

Hospital[a]   Nursing
facilities[b]

[a]1972
[b]1969

Data sources: *1973 Guide to the Health Care Field* (Chicago: American
Hospital Association, 1973).
National Center for Health Statistics, *Health Resources
Statistics 1971* (Washington, D.C.: Department of Health,
Education, and Welfare, 1972).

INPATIENT AND AMBULATORY PERSONNEL

Hospital personnel of all types receive about 60 per cent of hospital budgetary expenditures, and thus are the largest single expense in hospital services, although they were not the major cause of hospital price inflation. In federal hospitals employees received two thirds of the budget; those in the general nongovernmental not-for-profit hospitals got 57 per cent; those in the for-profit hospitals got 49 per cent in 1972 (2).

Quite clearly, the hospital is the predominant workplace of the health occupations, both in terms of numbers of personnel and health expenditures. Thus the health occupations, paralleling the inpatient focus of the organization and financing of services, also emphasize the remedial, higher-cost aspects of health care; only about one fifth of personal health workers are not in hospital or nursing home settings. Further, the small number of environmental personnel also reflects the U.S. emphasis on the personal services approach to health rather than one of changing the choice-giving environment of people (Figure 6–1).

PERSONAL HEALTH OCCUPATIONS: TASK AREAS

The fact that the health occupations number about 125, with an additional 250 alternative job titles, speaks to the absence of planning and coordination in this aspect of health care organization. Nevertheless, it is possible to group them according to their main tasks, and thereby get some sense of what 4 million personnel attend to.

Diagnosis and Therapeutics Categorized roughly, just over one fifth of all personal health workers engage in the field of diagnosis and therapeutics. This includes physicians, dentists, optometrists, podiatrists, and related personnel. Physicians are 4 per cent of the 4 million (Table 6–1).

Care of the Dishabilitated About half of all personnel focus on the care of the dishabilitated, those patients or persons who cannot take care of themselves. This includes midwives, who attend to healthy women at childbirth, and various types of nursing personnel. About half of these are aides. Registered nurses are about 19 per cent of the 4 million.

Counseling and Education Those personnel whose task emphasis is the counseling and education of ill or healthy consumers comprise the smallest proportion, less than 5 per cent of the 4 million. These include social workers, health educators, and dietitians.

Machine-Related Technologies Those personnel engaged in machine-related technologies, including biomedical engineers, technicians, and surgical aides, make up less than 10 per cent of all workers.

Table 6–1 Health Occupations, United States

*Estimated Health Services Personnel Active
in Selected Occupational Fields*[a] *1971*

	No.	% of Personal Health Services Personnel
Total health personnel	4,250,000	
Environmental/food and drug protective services	268,000[b]	
Personal health services	3,992,000	100.0
Fields focusing on:		
Diagnosis and treatment		22.3
Physician M.D.	322,000	4.0
Physician D.O.	12,000	0.3
Physician assistant	450	0.01
Medical assistant	250,000	6.2
Ophthalmic assistant	17,500	0.4
Optometrist and optician	35,200	0.9
Podiatrist	7,100	0.1
Dentist	103,750	2.6
Dental hygienist	16,800	0.4
Dental assistant	114,000	2.8
Pharmacy	140,750	3.5
Occupational therapist	13,500	0.3
Physical therapist	24,000	0.6

Table 6–1—Continued

	No.	% of Personal Health Services Personnel
Care of the dishabilitated		51.9
Midwife	4,950	0.1
Registered nurse	748,000	18.7
Practical nurse	427,000	10.7
Nursing aide, orderly, attendant	875,000	21.9
Home health aide	22,500	0.5
Counseling and Education		3.2
Social worker	29,800	0.7
Psychologist	27,000	0.6
Health education/information and communication/library	41,500	1.0
Dietetic and nutritional services	37,000	0.9
Environmental health/food and drug protective services[b]	268,000	[c]
Machine-related technologies		6.9
Biomedical engineers and scientists	62,000	1.5
Clinical laboratory worker	150,500	3.8
EKG technician	9,500	0.2
Dental laboratory technician	31,150	0.8
Surgical and other aides	23,400	0.6
Organizational components and interrelations		10.1
Administration	48,400	1.2
Social science analysts	2,000	0.04
Medical records	54,500	1.4
Automatic data processing	2,500	0.04
Secretarial and office services	297,500	7.4
Total	3,848,800	94.4
All others	401,200	5.6
Grand total	4,250,000	100.0

[a] Categories are mutually exclusive.

[b] Does not include air and water pollution control personnel.

[c] Not included in personal health services.

Source: National Center for Health Statistics, *Health Resources Statistics 1971* (Washington, D.C.: Department of Health, Education, and Welfare, 1972).

Organizational Components and Interrelations   In the fifth task area, focusing on the organizational aspects of health care, are about 10 per cent of all personnel. Here, administrators and medical records personnel form the smaller proportion, secretarial and office workers the largest.

Many of the occupational groups are organized, and in a variety of ways. In governmental agency statistics the health professions are defined as dentistry, medicine, nursing, osteopathy, optometry, pharmacy, podiatry, and veterinary medicine. Allied health personnel were recently defined as those with training and responsibilities for supporting, complementing, or supplementing health professionals in the delivery of health care or assisting environmental health workers (3). These and other health personnel have formed their own associations or labor unions.

Who Enters the Professions?

Before looking at the interrelations of various occupational groups, an internal view of certain of them is in order, that is, who enters them, and who may go where within them.

Medicine

STUDENTS

Persons who enter the medical profession come most often from families that are affluent and live in large cities. In 1967, 63 per cent came from homes with annual incomes of over $10,000; this contrasts with the 34 per cent of the overall population with that level of income. About one fourth of medical students come from cities of over a half-million, compared with 16 per cent of the general population. The affluent family background of physicians has been historically a fact, and is increasingly so (4).

Very few medical students come from poor families, fewer in 1967 (9 per cent) than in previous years. Entry is at best economically difficult since average annual expenses amounted to $3,400 at that time; one fifth of this was met by loans or grants, over 70 per cent by families and spouses (5).

The proportion of black students entering medicine increased slowly, from less than 1 per cent in 1968–1969 to 3.6 per cent in 1971–1972, excluding the two black medical schools. Graduates increased by 0.5 per cent. Almost half of the blacks graduated from either the Howard or Meharry Medical Schools (90 per cent of black physicians graduated from black colleges). Enrollment of other minorities during the 1968–1971 period increased by less than 0.5 per cent (6).

Women have traditionally been admitted to medical schools as a small proportion of the students. This has not measurably changed and the proportion who are accepted out of the greater numbers applying has in fact dropped in the 1966–1970 period. The graduation rate remains at about 9 per cent (7).

At the graduate level, during the residency training period, the picture of physicians makes an interesting alteration. The proportion of women becomes somewhat higher and of blacks slightly lower than among medical graduates. This results mainly from the addition of those who trained in foreign medical schools, the foreign medical graduates (FMGs) (Table 6–2).

A small but increasing proportion of FMGs are U.S. citizens who were unsuccessful at entering U.S. medical schools (where applicants are

Table 6–2 Health Occupations, United States

Sex, Race, and Economic Characteristics of Medical Students and Practitioners, 1971–1972

	Total (%)	Women (%)	Black (%)
Medical students	100.0	n.a.	4.8[a]
First year	100.0	11.3[b]	7.2
Graduates	100.0	9.2	2.4
Residents in training	100.0	11.0	2.0
Foreign medical graduates[c] (FMG)	32.0	17.4	2.0
Type of Residency:			
General Practice/Family Medicine	2.4	8.4	1.8
General surgery	14.9	1.9	2.0
Pediatrics	7.4	31.7	2.0
Active M.D.s (*N* = 311,000)[d]	100.0	6.9	2.2
General practice	18.7	4.3	n.a.
Surgery and surgical specialties	27.7	2.5	n.a.
Pediatrics	6.0	20.8	n.a.

[a] All medical schools, including the traditionally black (88%) Howard and Meharry.

[b] 1970–1971.

[c] Does not include graduates of Canadian medical schools.

[d] 1970. Of physicians active in *patient care*, 21% are in general practice. [Chapter 4, Table 4–3 referred to active M.D.s in *office* (solo or group) practice.]

Sources: "Medical Education in the United States, 1971–72." *J. Amer. Med. Assoc.* 222 (Suppl.), Nov. 20, 1972.

M. Pennell and J. Renshaw, "Distribution of Women Physicians, 1970." *J. Amer. Med. Women's Assoc.* 27:197–203 (Apr. 1972).

Department of Health, Education, and Welfare, Division of Manpower Intelligence Rept. 74–86 (Washington, D.C., unpublished, 1973).

increasing more than twice as fast as enrollment spaces; about three fourths of those who are turned away are considered qualified) (8).

Most FMGs are foreign-born (4.4 per cent were U.S.-born in 1972). In contrast to the mid-1960s, most now come from the underdeveloped countries rather than the affluent countries for their residency training. By 1971 FMGs formed about one third of all such trainees (9).

More than half of the women in residency training and one third of the blacks are graduates of foreign rather than U.S. medical schools (10). Studies show that the trainee salaries of FMGs were on the average about four-fifths of what U.S. physician trainees were paid (11).

GRADUATE TRAINING

Type and Place   Among the most sought-after specialty traineeships are the surgical residencies indicated by the high proportion filled each year. The smallest proportion of women and ethnic minorities are in these traineeships (Table 6–2).

The least-sought traineeships are in general practice and family medicine. FMGs, blacks, and women fill disproportionately more of these positions (12). Further, among FMGs, those from affluent countries have been granted entry into the preferred specialties as well as placement in the most sought-after hospital settings, compared with FMGs from poor countries (13).

The most-sought locations for training are the university medical center hospitals; these have the highest proportion of their resident positions filled (91 per cent). Least filled (81 per cent) are those in the not-for-profit hospitals, which also have higher proportions of foreign, rather than U.S., medical graduates. The hospitals with the highest proportions of FMGs in residencies are the for-profit type (Figure 6–2).

Far less sought than the hospital-based specialties are those in public health or occupational health. Again, higher proportions of these are filled by women and FMGs.

Thus entry into the medical profession has been very limited for certain groups, particularly women, minorities, and the poor. Proportionately more women and blacks have gone to other countries for their medical education. In graduate training, women, blacks, and FMGs, particularly FMGs from the underdeveloped countries, have less access to the more preferred residencies generally.

The emphasis of this training is clearly on the hospital-based, surgical specialties, with concomitantly little focus on general or family or public health and environmental-related health care. Even the earlier, internship phase of training now has a specialty focus compared with its general

Figure 6–2 The Health Occupations, United States

Selected Physician Residency Traineeships and Settings: Total Positions Filled and Those Filled by Foreign Medical Graduates, 1971–1972

Residency positions filled by United States/Canadian graduates and foreign medical graduates

Positions filled by foreign medical graduates only

Residency training positions
(total offered: 50,200)

United States total — 32% / 85%

Hospital specialties

Total — 32% / 85%

Family practice — 11% / 57%

General practice — 70% / 46%

Neurosurgery — 22% / 93%

Pediatrics — 38% / 92%

Non-hospital specialties

Total — 10% / 44%

Public health — 14% / 46%

Occupational health (in-plant) — 50% / 14%

Type of hospital

Medical center — 23% / 91%

Federal government — 24% / 88%

Non-federal government — 32% / 82%

Non-government: not-for-profit — 43% / 81%

for-profit — 57% / 85%

Data source: "Medical Education in the United States, 1971-72." *J. Amer. Med. Assoc.*, 222:997, Nov. 20, 1972 (supplement).

nature in the mid-1960s (14). The point was reached by 1973 that internships were specialized to the extent that they were being credited toward certification in a specialty field. The internship is now officially known as the "first post-M.D. year," with the former first year of residency becoming the "second post-M.D. year" (15).

Following the patterns in education and training, the field of medical practice reflects a similar picture and gives, as well, incentive to the trends in education. Of the 311,000 physicians active in 1970, whether or not engaged in direct patient care, less than 7 per cent were women, and a lesser amount were black. One fifth were foreign medical graduates—about 2½ times more than were practicing in the United States 10 years earlier. FMGs are increasing 7 times faster than the supply of U.S. trained physicians, providing medical care here rather than in their own countries. About one third of physicians now licensed each year are FMGs (16).

Of all M.D.s, fewer than one fifth were in general practice, and that proportion is decreasing (16.3 per cent by 1972). About one fourth of the FMGs were in general practice (17).

PRACTICE AND INCOME

The largest proportion of M.D.s were in surgery and the surgical specialties (27.7 per cent); this field also had the highest average income and the smallest proportion of women (2.5 per cent). The specialty with the highest proportion of women, pediatrics, also had the lowest average income (Figure 6–3).

Highest incomes derive from partnership and group practice arrangements, more of which than other group arrangements are incorporated; about 5 per cent only of women physicians practice in group settings (18). Thus, by specialty and practice setting, women's income is considerably lower than men's. Black physicians also make less than white physicians.

In the 44 neighborhood health centers set up under the federal antipoverty program which had difficulty retaining its salaried physicians, there were higher proportions of blacks, women, and pediatricians willing to work in them (18a).

An additional aspect of practice, besides specialty and setting, which affects physicians' incomes and income potential is their hospital affiliation. It has been found that the type of hospital—whether prestigious,

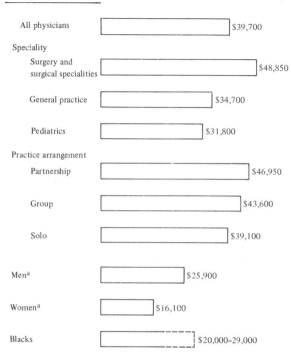

Figure 6–3 The Health Occupations, United States

Physicians' Income by Type of Practice, Sex, and Race, 1969

Average annual income

All physicians	$39,700
Speciality	
Surgery and surgical specialities	$48,850
General practice	$34,700
Pediatrics	$31,800
Practice arrangement	
Partnership	$46,950
Group	$43,600
Solo	$39,100
Men[a]	$25,900
Women[a]	$16,100
Blacks	$20,000-29,000

[a]Median income, 1964.

Data sources: American Medical Association, *1972 Profile of Medical Practice.*
G. Schway, "Selected Characteristics, NMA, Preliminary Findings,"
J. Nat. Med. Assoc., Jan. 1970, pp. 1-7.
C. Lopate, *Women in Medicine* (Baltimore: Johns Hopkins University Press, 1968).

church or nonchurch related—which accepts a physician on its staff bears some relation to the physician's ethnicity, as well as his or her medical school, residency placement, certification in a specialty, and sponsorship by other physicians. Those without this preferred background have had difficulty or outright failure at obtaining hospital ties (19).

Clearly, as these patterns in medicine show, one's race, sex, income, and choice of specialty are crucial in developing the preferred background, which in turn allows full access to the medical profession.

Nursing

Family background, sex, and race have also made a difference for those seeking to enter the nursing profession. Among the three types of programs which prepare students to become registered nurses, the four-year college program, in the later 1960s, was almost exclusively women (99.1 per cent). More of its students came from large cities; fewer came from low-income families, and half were from families who had more than a $10,000 annual income (20).

The three-year, hospital-based nursing program and two-year community college program each had proportionately more men, 2–5 per cent of all students, fewer large-city students, more coming from poorer families, and fewer from affluent families (about one third). However, more students in these schools received no loans or scholarship aid at all compared with students in the four-year college programs. In 1971 the community colleges graduated the most blacks (6 per cent), the hospital schools the least (2 per cent) (21).

PROGRAMS

Of the three types, the two-year program which grants an associate degree was growing fastest in the early 1970s; the hospital-based diploma schools were slowest, at about 1 per cent per year. Together, these two program types account for about 80 per cent of the schools and graduates in nursing (Table 6–3) (22).

An additional training program is the practical nurse school, usually one year. These schools are almost equal in number to all R.N. programs combined and graduate about 39,000 yearly compared with approximately 47,000 from the R.N. schools (23). More blacks (about 15 per cent) graduated from these programs than any of the others.

Other types of nursing personnel—aides, orderlies, attendants—usually have short-term on-the-job training, if any. Perhaps one fourth of these are men; one third or more are black (24).

REWARDS

It is clear (see Table 6–3) that the nursing personnel with longest training periods and in the more formal educational settings have the greatest potential for higher incomes when they go out into the world of health care work. Greatest potential earnings derive from a master's degree in nursing, for which the B.S. in nursing is prerequisite. Those with lesser potential for earnings are also those with lesser likelihood of entering the longer programs; these are more often persons with low-income backgrounds and blacks. They are, in effect, outcasts in the work settings of health services.

QUESTIONS

In the early 1970s hard questions were being asked about whether there was evidence that longer, and more costly, programs did, in fact, train persons more competent to render nursing care to the dishabilitated. That evidence was not available (25). Nor could real differences in training be found to justify the variety of the shorter-length programs (26). One study of East Coast two- and four-year college programs showed a blurring among them also in the purposes and content of their curricula; there was, as well, a wide discrepancy between what was taught the students and what nurses were required to do in the actual delivery of health services (27).

In effect, differences among all types of training programs centered on the types of persons who entered them, their income and race, and age (those over 35 were allowed in practical nurse training) and on the potential for socioeconomic advancement which the credential granted—whether degree, diploma, or certificate—allowed them (28). Moreover, there was evidence that those in the longer programs, of three or four years, had higher dropout rates, and that the graduates of the college schools were less likely to be engaged in nursing work, between the 25- to 50-year period of their lives (29). Another repeated observation was that nursing education, like medical training, focuses on the hospital care of patients, whether or not the school is hospital-based. And, like the physicians' focus, most employed nurses (70 per cent) are in hospital settings (30).

Allied Health Occupations

Indications are that the allied health occupations tend to follow similar patterns, although definitive information is not as readily available as in the older occupational groups, particularly concerning the ethnic character of the students and practitioners. However, it is fairly clear that jobs are sex-typed and that training is hospital-oriented. Training programs, perhaps expectedly, follow the patterns of the older professions, which

Table 6-3 Health Occupations, United States

Educational Programs and Student Background of Nursing Personnel

	Total Programs[a] (N)	Student Background[b]						Credential (Number Holding) 1972	Beginning[e] Salary or Range
		Women %	Residence: % Urban[c]	Family Income		% Black[d]			
				Under $5,000	$10,000 and over	Admitted	Graduated		
R.N. and LPN	2,654	97.8		17.1	37.9				
Training programs									
R.N.	1,363								
4 yr (college)	285	99.1	18.0	14.4	49.9	6.0	4.0	B.S. degree (80,000) M.S. degree (19,000)	$ 9,200 11,000
3 yr (hospital school)	587	98.2	10.1	17.6	33.4	4.0	2.0	Diploma (579,000)	5,400–12,500
2 yr (community college)	491	95.5	13.3	18.6	35.8	10.5	6.0	A.A. degree (22,000)	5,400–12,500
Licensed practical nurse 1 yr	1,291	97.0	n.a.	n.a.	n.a.	n.a.	15.5	Certificate	4,000–9,000
Nurse aide, orderly, attendant[f] On-job, wk./mos.	n.a.	78.0	n.a.	n.a.	n.a.	n.a.	26	None	3,500–7,500

[a] 1971.
[b] 1967.
[c] 250,000 population.
[d] 1968–1969.
[e] 1970.
[f] 1964.

Sources: National League for Nursing, *From Student to RN: A Report* (Washington, D.C.: Department of Health, Education, and Welfare, 1972).
American Nurses Association, Research Dept., *Facts About Nursing* (New York: ANA, 1970).
S. Altman, *Present and Future Supply of Registered Nurses* (Washington, D.C.: Department of Health, Education, and Welfare, 1972).
L. Lecht, *Manpower Needs for National Goals in the 1970's* (New York: Praeger, 1969).
"Salaries in Community Health Services—1973." *Nursing Outlook*, Dec. 1973.

in turn monitor the official accreditation of new training programs; the AMA does so for 22 types of allied health occupations (Table 6–4).

Interprofessional Patterns

Viewing the major health professions in relation to each other reveals a repetition of patterns which allow limited access to certain groups and disproportionate resources and rewards to others. It is clear (see Table 6–5) that the professions in which practitioners are predominantly (over 90 per cent) male and white are also those with highest incomes and those whose practitioners are in proportionately smaller supply; these also have fewest schools, longer and more costly training programs, and in medicine and dentistry expend disproportionately large amounts of training dollars. This picture is not likely to change very much in the immediate future because both the makeup of entering student groups and the allocation of federal health dollars is paralleling the established patterns (30a).

The health professions, in effect, form a pyramid, with predominantly white male medicine and dentistry at the peak, and nursing and the allied technical occupations, mainly women, farthest down. To this picture one should add the fact that more affluent persons are more likely to enter the more costly and more economically rewarding professions. The by-now-familiar cycle then becomes evident—how outcast groups remain outcast.

Health Training and Health Care

This situation in the health occupations, of uneven access to health care training, recalls the similar problem in education generally, reviewed in Chapter 2. Health care training also reflects the second major problem of education, that of making it socially useful and usable, properly relating it to the jobs in communities that need to be done, and using effective and efficient methods for developing those necessary skills.

Training Emphasis

The education of health personnel is hospital-based and specialized in focus when the day-to-day needs for personal health services involve, overwhelmingly, people who are ambulatory, in communities, and who require basic, primary, nonspecialized services.

Table 6-4 Health Occupations, United States

Selected Allied Health Occupations,
Educational Programs and Sex Composition, 1972

	Programs (No.)	Education Prerequisite (yr)	Minimum Length (yr)	Graduates (No.)	Accrediting Body	Women in Occupational Field[a] (%)
Occupational therapy	38	12	4	770	American Medical Association[b]	95
Physical therapy	60	12	4	1,460	American Medical Association[b]	92
Dietetics/nutrition	78	12	4	840	American Dietetic Association	n.a.
Medical technology	749	12	4	5,370	American Medical Association[b]	80–90
Medical assistants	44	12	1–2	415	American Medical Association[b]	Majority
Dental hygienics	102	12	2–4	2,270	American Dental Association	80
Dental assistants	179	12	1–2	2,700	American Dental Association	94
Certified laboratory assistant	194	12	1	1,970	American Medical Association[b]	80–90
Total	1,414			14,955		
Other dental and allied health	1,400			10,260		
Grand total	2,814			25,215		

[a] 1970.

[b] Council on Medical Education in collaboration with allied health group concerned.

Sources: Department of Health, Education, and Welfare, Report on Licensure and Related Health Personnel Credentialing 1971.

American Medical Association, "Allied Medical Education Research Review, Spring, 1973." (Chicago: AMA, 1973).

Hearings, U.S. Senate Health Subcommittee, May 19–20, 1970.

Women's Bureau, "Careers for Women in the 70s." (Washington, D.C.: Department of Labor, 1973).

The Profession of Dietetics: Report of the Commission on Dietetics (Chicago: American Dietetic Association, 1972).

Department of Health, Education, and Welfare, Division of Manpower Intelligence Rept. 74–86 (Washington, D.C., unpublished, 1973).

Table 6–5 Health Occupations, United States

Selected Health Professions and Allied Personnel, Sex and Race Composition and Shares of Resources

	Medicine	Dentistry	Optometry	Podiatry	Pharmacy	Nursing	Allied Technical
Students (%)[a]							
Women	12.8	2.8	5.1	1.4	26.5	98.0	80–90 (est.)
Blacks	5.5	3.9	1.0	2.1	3.5	7.7	n.a.
Other minorities	2.6	3.0	4.9	1.0	5.0		
Schools							
Number schools/programs	112	56	12	5	73	1,367	2,814
Training (minimum years post high school)	7–8	6	6	6	5	2–4	1–5[b]
Cost/undergraduate student /yr ($)	12,650	9,050	4,250	5,750	3,550	1,650–3,300[c]	3,680[d]
Share of all health professional educational expenditures (%)[e]	63	6	−1	−1	3–4	22	1–2 (est.)[f]
Share HEW allocation (%)[g]	76	7	1	−1	3	10	1.7[h]
Amount of net expenditures met by Federal capitation	29%	38%	26%	16%	26%	13–22%	n.a.
Practitioners[1]							
% all health personnel	4.0	2.6	0.9	0.1	3.5	18.7	24
Women (%)	9.2	3.4	4.0	7.6	11.9	97.3	33[j]
Blacks (%)	2.2	2.3	0.6	4.2	2.3	7.5	11[j]
Earnings (average annual, estimate)	$39,700	$29,500	$25,400	$21,400	$28,100 (self-employment) 11,600 (hospital staff)	$ 8,100–10,100	$ 6,000–10,000

[a] Various years, 1971–1973.

[b] 34% are in 2-year colleges.

[c] lowest in community colleges, highest in hospital schools.

[d] 1972.

[e] 2.6 billions of which $1.33 billion was from federal funds, 1972.

[f] $25 million was spent through federal funding 1969–1970.

[g] HEW was the largest federal agency supplying health training funds (77% of all such funds in 1972).

[h] 1969–1970.

[i] Various years, 1969–1972.

[j] For medical and dental technology only.

Sources: Department of Health, Education, and Welfare, Division of Manpower Intelligence Repts. 72-128; 74-60; 74-86 (1973) (Washington, D.C., unpublished).

Department of Health, Education, and Welfare, "Survey of Health Professions Student Financing, 1970–71." (Washington, D.C., unpublished).

Association of American Medical Colleges, Report of the Commission on the Financing of Medical Education (Washington, D.C.: AAMC, 1973).

Institute of Medicine, Costs of Education in the Health Professions Interim and Summary Reports (Washington, D.C.: National Academy of Science, 1973 and 1974).

American Association of Junior Colleges (Washington, D.C., unpublished, 1970).

Department of Health, Education, and Welfare, Inventory of Federal Programs That Support Health Manpower 1970 (Washington, D.C.: National Institute of Health, 1971).

American Medical Association, Education and Utilization of Allied Health Manpower (Chicago: AMA, 1972).

157

National studies record the commonsense observation that on any given day most people (perhaps 85 per cent) are unaware of illness, although during the course of a year about four fifths will experience some illness (31). Of the sicknesses that people have, possibly three fourths are self-treated (32). Of the ills for which people seek medical care, estimates are that 67–85 per cent are minor and self-limiting, resolvable without medical care (33); of the others which are medically treatable only a small proportion are major illness; the majority are common respiratory problems, gastrointestinal infections or disorders, obesity, or chronic ills such as arthritis, high blood pressure, and heart disease (34).

A recent national survey of acute conditions is the United States showed that less than 60 per cent are medically treated, and of those, less than two thirds were severe enough to restrict individuals' activities; over half were respiratory, another one fifth were digestive and infective, and another 15 per cent were injuries (35). In one assessment by medical specialists of the necessity for specialist care of ambulatory patients in a group practice, they found that just 9 per cent needed either physician or dental specialists; in a similar study of hospital emergency departments, 46 per cent, still less than half the patients, required specialists' services (36).

As a final example of the lack of fit between the emphases and focus of health personnel, particularly the physicians, who are in effect the gatekeepers for the system, with the personal health care needs of the general population is a report of patients in a university medical center teaching hospital. This study estimates that less than 0.1 per cent of ill persons reach such special facilities—which now, in fact, contain about half of all hospital beds. The important point is that it is from this tiny and unrepresentative fraction of persons who seek health care that virtually all medical students and most of the other health occupations learn how to provide services (37). This, in effect, gives health personnel a very narrow, skewed perspective of what the major needs are for personal health services—and for other environmental health services—and of what such services should consist (Figure 6–4).

In sum, the most common acute illnesses, such as upper respiratory infections, and the chronic illnesses, heart disease, arthritis, and asthma, when not managed at home require basic, primary medical care, that is, the diagnostic and therapeutic armamentarium available to the general or family practitioner in an ambulatory care setting (38). Such practitioners are, as noted earlier, an increasing minority. Even when internists and pediatricians are added, as they often are to the total of primary care

Figure 6-4 The Health Occupations, United States

Schema of Estimates of Illnesses Treated in One Year in Large Populations of Affluent Countries

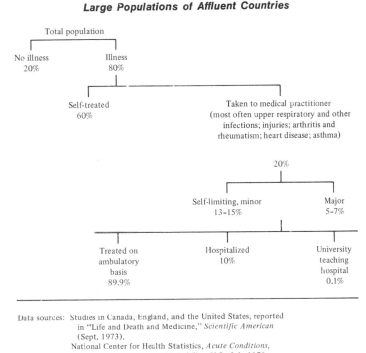

Data sources: Studies in Canada, England, and the United States, reported
in "Life and Death and Medicine," *Scientific American*
(Sept. 1973).
National Center for Health Statistics, *Acute Conditions,
Incidence and Associated Disability, U.S., July 1970-
June 1971* (Washington, D.C.: Department of Health,
Education, and Welfare, 1973).

physicians—those who provide first-contact assessment to adults and children—this proportion of primary care practitioners is diminishing (39).

Limits of Primary Care

As with the most prevalent types of facilities and services, the types and training of health personnel focus on inhospital and specialized care. Basic, primary health services, which are ambulatory by nature, are not only less costly both in the facilities and the types of personnel they require, but are also more closely related to the health care needs of most people most of the time.

Such services can undoubtedly prevent much discomfort and disability and some deaths, and could do so most effectively for certain outcast groups who lack any such services. It is important to recognize at the same time however that primary care is not likely to prevent disease of either acute or chronic types, except to a limited extent for total populations; that is, it is not likely to improve overall health. Disease prevention is by and large a problem beyond the capacity of health care practitioners and services as they have been and are organized and oriented. As reviewed in Chapter 2, disease prevention and also optimal health could best be effected by altering the disease-generating socioeconomic and ecological–technological conditions in the environments of people in their particular communities. Otherwise, the changes in life patterns and practices which even nonspecialist and non-inhospital-oriented health personnel advocate will not and cannot be accomplished by most patients, the consumers of personal health services.

Specialized Training and Its Effects

HEALTH CARE CONSEQUENCES

The fact of increasing specialization among physicians, the principal gatekeepers of personal health services, in contrast to the primary, nonspecialist needs of most people has created a gap in health services. This primary care gap in effect has produced a maldistribution in the types of health services available. It has also tended to produce disinterest in ways to best assist the chronically ill, disabled, elderly, and ethnic minorities where they live (40).

The gap, meaning lesser access to most needed services for many if not a majority of persons, then affects especially lower-income groups as specialists converge around specialist facilities and affluent populations. This further contributes to the uneven distribution of health personnel as well as the types of services and facilities available in certain locations. In turn, this process generates more specialty-oriented programs, almost always related to inhospital services. For example, in neurosurgery, the highest earning of the specialties, one review concluded that the 95 training programs (based in medical center operation theaters) exist at least in part to simply provide "clinical material" for the trainees but are not needed to supply the necessary neurosurgeons of the future (currently these practitioners perform only five or six major operations monthly) (40a). This inhospital focus and elaboration of services thus contributes to the emphasis on high-cost forms of care, further raising the costs of care, as previous chapters described.

Thus the health services problem, of providing geographic and financial access to an array of needed services, cannot be separated from the social question of access to the health occupations, access both within and between the more and the less prestigious professions. The process of increased specialization has the social consequences of limiting entry to those with preferred backgrounds and of ensuring socioeconomic advantages for the relatively few who have gotten in.

ECONOMICS

Historically, U.S. physicians, when they were predominantly general practitioners, officially repudiated the multiplication of specialists, viewing the new types as economic competitors. In the later nineteenth century when it became clear that enough people were willing and able to pay the higher fees of specialists, the official position of physicians was altered in favor of specialization as a form of higher-quality care (41). Recent findings also show how more physicians shifted into specialties during periods of general prosperity, and how increasingly, most physicians begin practice as specialists, favoring the more economically rewarding types (42).

International Comparisons

The issues of who can enter which of the health professions and what emphasis, whether primary or specialized, training and practice shall take are pertinent in virtually every country, the affluent and the poor. The extent of the problems of unequal access and of the lack of primary care differ widely, however.

Access

In the U.S.S.R., for example, as is well known, about three fourths of the physicians are women. However, at the highest decision-making levels, far fewer are women, while more than 90 per cent of the semiprofessional health personnel are women (43). Perhaps related to the femaleness of this field is the fact that salaries between the occupational groups do not differ as much as in most countries; nurses receive about 80 per cent of what physicians earn (44). Most of the eastern European countries have relatively large proportions of women physicians compared with western Europe and the Americas (45).

In the poor countries as in the affluent countries, women tend to be sex-typed for certain health services. For example, in Nigeria women physicians must have experience in maternal and child health; women physicians provide most family planning services in India; certain medical work is defined as unsuitable for women in Thailand (46). Sex typing in the affluent countries is apparent in England and Germany, for example, where relatively more women enter pediatrics; women dentists in Israel have relatively larger children's practices (47).

Further, a review of over 50 health-related occupations in Great Britain, The Netherlands, West Germany, Japan, and India showed a pyramid, with medical care at the top, followed by maternity and health information occupations, and then nursing and young child occupations. Those who worked at the top came from higher-income backgrounds, were predominantly male, and were from the majority racial or ethnic group. These groups also received the highest incomes and had the best chances for promotion on the job and for further education. Such prospects were less likely in the other types of occupations; these other workers, also, were more often women, those coming from poorer families, and relatively more from minority groups (48).

Access to the British medical, dental, and nursing occupations clearly illustrates the uneven prospects for ethnic minorities, non-British immigrants, and women (Table 6–6). Although women (13 per cent of all physicians) are equally represented in the hospital-based and nonhospital general practices, they compose more of the hospital house staffs (20 per cent) than the more prestigious and higher-paying consultantships (7 per cent). Similarly, foreign-born physicians (20 per cent of all physicians) form the largest part of the house staff (60 per cent); the vast majority come from South Asia (49).

Even among the predominantly female (82 per cent) nursing personnel, men occupy relatively more of the longer-trained and potentially more advantageous State Registered Nurse (SRN) positions (19 per cent) than the State Enrolled Nurse (SEN) posts (11 per cent) or auxiliary places (2 per cent). Foreign-born personnel are more often in the lesser trained and lower-paid categories.

Recent legislation has made certification of men as midwives legally possible. Although the foreign-born may be trained as health visitors, they cannot be so certified (50).

Within the British National Health Service, then, there is limited access by sex, ethnicity, and economic background as income groups are tracked differently through the required educational and training programs. The salary distinctions reflect this pyramid (Table 6–6). Nationally,

Table 6–6   Health Occupations

Selected Health Personnel,
Sex, Origin, and Earnings, England and Wales, 1972

	% of Total	Women (%)	Non-British Born (%)	Beginning Base Salary ($)[e]
Physicians	100	13.0	20	
Hospital-based	50	13.0	33	
Specialists[b]	(53)			
Consultants	(37)	7.0	13	15,250
Registrars (trainees)		15.0	33	7,000–8,600
House staff		20.0	60	5,000
Nonhospital	50	13.0	n.a.	
GPs[c]	(47)			14,000
Dentists[d]	100	7.6	n.a.	
Hospital-based	8	10.0		
Consultant	(2)	1.7		
Nonhospital: GP	92	7.6		11,000[e]
Nursing personnel[f]	100	82.0		
In hospital[g]	91	88.0		
State registrars (SRN)	(45)	81.0	19	2,750
State enrolled (SEN)	(22)	89.0	24	2,600
Auxiliaries	(26)	98.0		n.a.
Midwives (MW)	(7)	100.0	14	3,750
Total	(100)			
Nonhospital	9	est. 97–99		
Health visitors (HV)	(38)	n.a.	0[h]	3,400–4,000
District nursing (DN)	(26)	95.0		3,500–4,000
Other (SRN, SEN, ancillary)	(15)	n.a.		2,600–3,200
MW	(16)	100.0		3,750
Total	(100)			

[a] Does not include fringe benefits or other allowances; 1972 increases were 4–9%, with the largest at the lowest levels.

[b] Virtually all are hospital-based; types, as % of all M.D.s, are medical (internists), 13.4; surgery, 12; pediatrics, 4; obstetrics, 8.

[c] 80% are approved for obstetrics.

[d] 6.3% are specialists.

[e] 1971.

[f] Parentheses contain percentages of *sub*totals.

[g] SRN is 3-year training; SEN is 1 year.

[h] Foreign-born persons cannot be certified.

Source: Great Britain Department of Health and Social Security, unpublished data compiled through Oct. 1972.

women at staff levels in the health and social services received 56 per cent of the wages of their male counterparts in 1971 (51).

There is recent evidence that within the medical education system of Canada new students are being accepted without regard to family socio-economic background and in increasing proportions for women. However, despite similar admissions test scores, relatively fewer non-Canadian-born persons were accepted in 1968–1969 (52).

The pervasiveness of patterns of sex–ethnic–income limits for access to the various levels of the health occupations pyramid is quite apparent.

Emphasis

Almost as widespread is the problem of balancing primary care and specialist training and practice in relation to the needs for health services among populations. Concern has been voiced in The Netherlands about the increasing specialization of its physicians. Sweden recently began a pay policy which no longer rewards specialty credentials. A study of Israeli physicians showed how their increasing emphasis on specialty certification was a means to perpetuate their income level above that of other professionals (53).

In British Columbia, physicians voted a plan in 1971 to limit their net earnings; however, they did so on an average-for-specialty basis. So, while the plan may contain earnings now paid under Medicare (their national health insurance), it is not likely to slow the trend toward specialization. Under Medicare in another province, Quebec, specialists made $44,400 in 1971, about $10,000 more than the general practitioners (54).

These and other examples show clearly the relation of increasing specialization and economic rewards for physicians while other evidence indicates the fundamental need for emphasizing primary care services among populations (Figure 6–4).

An exception to this may now be occurring in England. Until 1969 the proportion of GPs was annually diminishing in England, a decline that began in 1929. The decline has apparently stopped at an almost 50:50 division between GPs and specialists. This probably resulted from measures taken to balance hospital and community practice settings, reallocating funds to ambulatory, primary care, a move that is to increase as the National Health Service is reorganized. The provision for government-supported practice settings for the GPs—the health centers—as well as special allowances for rural practice, larger payments for the care of elders, among other changes has brought the average GP income to almost 90 per cent of the specialists', where it was 75 per cent in 1965 (55). At the same time, specialists' earnings are limited by the salary method and their numbers indirectly limited by the number of specialist positions planned in the NHS hospitals where they practice. In addition, patients who make up the practice of specialists are referred from their own local GPs, who, as noted earlier, refer about 12–14 per cent of the patients for specialists' evaluation (56).

Summary

The interrelated issues of access and emphasis in the health occupations—the limited access for certain groups and the inpatient and specialized emphasis in training and practice—are related to the problem of assuring access to health services for all persons, especially outcast groups living in poor or isolated regions. Unequal access to the occupations tends to perpetuate the pyramids that exist both between and within the professions, tracking persons along sex, race, and income lines. The most prestigeful occupations are most easily entered by the most favored social groups. By specializing, these groups in effect widen the distance between themselves and those further down the pyramid, and retain the most favorable socioeconomic advantages. The provision of health services is then also affected as primary care services diminish for all, and as health services converge around urban and affluent areas where they are sought and can be supported—although such services may not be directly related to the real health care requirements of the people.

How the health care professions have dealt with these problems in the delivery of health services is the next question. Beyond that is the question of what effects their solutions have produced.

chapter 7

Solutions and Their Problems

Limited access to the health occupations and the specialist emphasis within them has contributed to major health services problems, namely, the uneven distribution of most-needed types and numbers of personnel and, less directly, to the rising costs of health care. At the same time, the health professions, in association with other types of government and non-government health care providers, have attempted to deal with these problems, specifically the lack of primary care, maldistribution, and high costs. These attempts have had certain consequences for health services and for certain social groups within the health occupations.

What follows is a review of these efforts and effects and an estimate of the future context for changes in the health occupations, an alternative interpretation of what is now happening, and a viewpoint for joining the pieces: efforts, problems, and context.

Medical Care Assistants: Traditional and Newer Varieties

As the dearth of primary medical care became increasingly and more publicly discussed in virtually all health-related circles in the 1960s, attempts were made to develop new types of primary care practitioners or to expand the task area of other health care practitioners into primary medical care. Many new job titles were thus created: the physician's assistant, Medex, family nurse practitioner, child health associate, pediatric nurse practitioner, ambulatory care associate, among others, and renewed interest in an older title, the nurse–midwife.

166

PROLIFERATION AND CLASSIFICATION

Developing new personnel types as a way of meeting problems in the delivery of health services was of course not a new approach. As early as the 1930s, when general medical practitioners began to decline among physicians, new workers were formally trained as assistants, such as the medical technologists and radiologic technicians. Similarly, as nurses were required to work in task areas other than the care of the dishabilitated, other personnel were trained in increasing numbers for that set of tasks, the practical nurses and aides.

This approach, of spinning off new types of personnel, was used rather than the alternative of training more primary care physicians and nurses and insuring their distribution where they were needed.

This process accelerated in the 1960s. Between 1963–1973, 15 new types of training programs were approved by the AMA Council on Medical Education alone (1). Each profession has its own array of assistants and technicians, in dentistry, optometry, pharmacy, and so on. And, those occupations which are assistive in primary and secondary (specialized) medical care now also have assistant types of personnel of their own, such as the assistants to physical therapists and dietetic aides (see Table 6–1).

As a way to sort out the types of personnel who directly work with physicians in rendering primary and specialized medical care, the Institute of Medicine in the National Academy of Science devised a three-group classification of physicians' assistants (2). Those who can provide primary care to children and/or adults without the immediate supervision of the physician are Type A, known as the physician's assistant or child health associate, among other titles. Type B are the physician assistants, who are trained in a specialized area of medical care and are able to work in that area without the immediate supervision of a medical specialist; these include the orthopedic and urologic physician assistants and, perhaps, clinical nurse specialists such as the cardiac nurse in intensive care. The third, Type C, are the traditional assistants who work in the presence of the M.D. and are under his or her immediate direction, as the medical assistants or ophthalmic assistants, that is, those who assist in either primary or specialized medical fields.

EFFECTS ON HEALTH CARE

Solo Practice   Traditional aides have allowed physicians in solo practice to increase the number of ambulatory patients they can see by about

8 per cent; and, should the practitioners increase their office hours, they can see up to almost one fifth more patients when assisted. Maximum productivity, measured by office visits per physician per week, has been estimated at 183 visits when the M.D. works 60 hours and employs two aides. However, what tends to happen in reality is that since aides do allow for a larger practice, physicians tend to work fewer office hours, thus without much of a net increase (and sometimes a net decrease) in patient visits (3). The exception to this is likely to be the very busy lone general practitioner in a health-scarcity area; such a practitioner is likely to work longer and, understandably, delegate more tasks to aides than solo physicians in nonpoor or urban areas or those in group practices (4).

In the specialist field of pediatrics (where over one fifth of physicians now also have a subspecialty), average weekly patient visits were 110 in 1967, half for illness episodes, during 35 office hours a week. Solo pediatricians had two aides, most often a clerical person and a medical assistant without formal training, and predominantly women. The third most common employee was a nurse; when this was so, pediatricians delegated more tasks, mostly telephone advising and routine history taking and patient instruction (5).

Group Practice   Physicians in group practices do see more patients per week and thus earn more. By employing assistants, however, they can increase patient visits by twice as many as when aides work in solo practice settings; longer physician hours also become more productive in a group setting (6). Relatively fewer tasks tend to be delegated to assistants in group than in solo settings, especially in regions where there are numerous physicians and nurses. These are, of course, the more urban and affluent regions, where, ironically, people are generally healthier and come more often for routine health supervision rather than for illness-related health services (7).

The Paradox   In other words, a paradox presents itself. In affluent areas more specialist health personnel work shorter hours providing services to healthier people who seek non-sickness-related health services. Health professionals thus perform tasks in these contexts which are commonly done by nonspecialist, less lengthily trained personnel in scarcity regions where more people are also more ill (8).

Numerous studies reiterate the paradox, reporting how 80 per cent of pediatricians' work could be done by less-specialized personnel (9); one third to two thirds of internists' medical work could be delegated (10); general practitioners spend more time in direct contact with patients than internists do (11); fewer U.S. physicians attend to the elderly at home than in any other country (12); physicians and residents perform tasks in ambulatory care which nurses could do, and nurses perform tasks that other personnel could do, in clinic settings (13), in office practices (14), in neighborhood health centers (15); or, conversely, others with less training do as well in certain activities as nurses (16) or as physicians in community settings (17).

Posing the Problem   In effect, health personnel overall are not trained in relation to the common needs of people, and health personnel are not practicing in ways and places related to the greatest needs. This enigma may be interpreted as a problem of overspecialization of the health professions, over- or inappropriate training of health personnel, under- or misplaced employment of practitioners. The alternative, and more common interpretation, is simply to view the effects: the gap of primary care and thus maldistribution of personnel and services as the problem, and as the solution, attempt to fill the gap with those who will go where the need is greatest.

The New Practitioners

The new primary care practitioners are then a major proposed solution to the problem so defined. Whatever their particular title, whether physician assistant, child health associate, Medex, Primex, or other, the training of these practitioners centers on the diagnosis, assessment, and management of common health problems in adults and/or children. Skills emphasize history taking, performing the physical examination, doing routine diagnostic tests and treatments, giving emergency care, record keeping, and counseling of patients. The longer programs include more basic, social, and clinical sciences in the initial classroom period. The focus in all programs seems, however, to be the *practice* of primary care under supervision (18).

TRAINING PROGRAMS

Of an estimated 80 physician assistant (P.A.) training programs in process in 1972, perhaps half were for specialized personnel in fields such as orthopedics, urology, or ophthalmology (19). These, almost by definition, could not help solve the problem of primary care; rather, they are more likely to aggravate the maldistribution problem, since their graduates are obliged to locate near specialist physicians and facilities.

The training programs for primary care practitioners vary widely in format; they include nine of the Medex type, those which recruit ex-military corpsmen. Although they range in length from a few months to 3½ years, most run one to two years. They report a capacity for 10 to 20 trainees most often, and usually award a certificate rather than a degree on graduation. There were about 400 such graduates in mid-1972 and about 800 a year later (20).

Another variation of primary care training, more often including those of the "expanded role of the nurse" than the above P.A.–Medex type, are frequently attached to the institutions in which they will and do work. In effect, they often approximate in-service training programs.[1] The majority of the pediatric nurse practitioner (PNP) programs were so reported in 1972. There were perhaps 200–250 PNPs trained in total (21).

In a similar way, some large city health departments were attempting to develop training for their public health nurses to staff neighborhood health centers as primary care practitioners. Medical schools have developed such programs to help provide ambulatory care to the chronically ill in university medical center clinics. Nurses have also been trained in clinic settings to do the routine pre- and postnatal assessments for normal women that is usually done by obstetricians (22). In addition, there were about 2½ times more nurse–midwives (1200) trained by 1972 as 10 years earlier, although fewer (37 per cent) were actually giving delivery service than in 1963 (52 per cent did so then) (23). And at least 24 programs were under way training nurses as "nonphysician family planning specialists." Most of the 450–500 graduates (1973) were taught to do gynecological examinations and testing and to administer oral and other forms of birth control (24). Finally, there were numerous workshop training sessions, lasting a few weeks, which sought to train nurses in the systematic physical assessment of patients. These programs have often been added to both undergraduate and graduate courses in colleges of nursing. These trainees also have been called "nurse practitioners."

A Pattern If there is a pattern to this proliferation of training programs in primary care, it is that of paralleling current medical practice, subdividing or segmenting basic health care into patient age, sex, or treatment types. Thus there were the child health associate and the family planning specialist in primary medical care and the urological physician assistant in secondary medical care. Such subdivisions in primary care services, following the typical segmented approach described in Chapter 4, is not likely to redistribute primary, first-contact care very easily. For example, to provide integrated and readily usable primary care to an isolated rural community or an urban ghetto, it seems more difficult to supply several primary care personnel for children, pregnant women, persons of child-bearing age seeking birth control, elders, and other adults than one or two general primary care practitioners capable of rendering services to all age–sex groups. At a minimum, the logistics of staffing, scheduling, and record keeping in the second, integrated approach

---

[1] Many of the specialist Physician Assistant programs have a similar purpose.

would be simpler for both providers and consumers. Moreover, training for primary care by institutions for work specific to their own settings may limit the capacity of their trainees to practice primary care in other settings in the future. Thus such programs, because of this limited flexibility, may make little impact on the overall availability of primary care.

Performance Whether their training has been of a general or segmented type, the new primary care practitioners in practice are providing services no less well and sometimes better than physicians according to increasingly numerous studies and other evidence. The general Medex practitioners, for example, were handling 80 per cent or more of health care, in remote practices especially, and were increasing physicians' patient-visit total by up to 1¼ times; other physician assistant–M.D. practices show 50–75 per cent increases in patient visits (25). In other words, P.A.s are improving physician productivity considerably more than did the addition of various types of traditional aides noted earlier.

The numerous types of nurse practitioners in ambulatory settings have clinically managed patients with chronic disease as well as physicians have, and often more effectively, in terms of results showing less patient disability, less discomfort and fewer complaints, and fewer broken appointments (26). They have also in some settings more effectively detected illness symptoms in apparently healthy patients (27). In obstetrics, nurse–midwives have delivered babies safely, and nurse–physician assistants have provided more consistently followed postnatal care and more effective birth control techniques. Similar results were found among the nonphysician family planning specialists (both nurses and nonnurses) compared with physicians (28).

Further, a somewhat less direct indication of satisfactory performance is the finding in a national report that the new primary care practitioners have not produced any significant problems of medical malpractice (29).

HEALTH CARE EFFECTS: IMPLICATIONS FOR PRIMARY CARE

The evidence thus far shows that primary medical care can be effectively taught in far fewer years than the current 12½-year average obtained by physicians; that relatively little of the weighty bioscience base of medical education is actually used in practice; and that persons with diverse backgrounds, including corpsmen, nurses from both hospital and college schools, and persons from other fields, can effectively learn to provide primary medical care (30).

This clearly has implications for making possible an increase of primary care practitioners, and at a lesser cost, through larger numbers, trained in shorter periods, at lesser costs per trainee. In addition, the primary care practitioners, virtually all of whom are salaried, had a starting salary between $6,000 and $15,000 in 1971 (31). Here, then, is the potential for increasing the supply and reducing the cost of primary care practitioners.

Distribution The important additional problem is to have such practitioners go where the need for primary care is greatest, thereby enhancing access to these services for outcast groups. Of the first 90 Medex practitioners, almost half (47 per cent) went to work in rural areas, particularly in the Northwest (32). Another survey of about 150 graduates of the non-Medex programs (18 in all) showed that they located themselves for their first place of practice near their training sites, just as physicians do (33). About one third went to nonmetropolitan areas, and into the South and North Central regions. The starting salaries were larger in rural areas generally. However, for their second jobs, these practitioners tended to move from rural to urban areas, where salaries also tend to equalize after two years of experience; they moved from hospital to private practice settings and took on more independent patient care and administrative activities, with less time spent in laboratory and clerical duties (34).

This suggests that the redistribution of primary care practitioners to scarcity areas may be only temporary and tenuous and that the private fee-for-service sector of health services may gain considerably. A survey of the first 100 graduates of a pediatric nurse practitioner program showed that about one third of them also went to work in private practice settings (35).

Economic Effects There has been a significant economic benefit to the private care practices, whether solo or group, through increased numbers of patients. In one rural medical partnership, the nurse practitioner's patient visits netted more than twice the income to the practice than those of the two physicians jointly, yet her salary remained at $5,300 (1972) (36).

This pattern, of attaching the new primary care practitioners to private practices, should it persist, is not likely to reduce the fees for health services paid by patients or insurers; it may, however, allow additional services, such as house calls, or more personal attention, especially in group practice settings (37). A more profound effect may be the bolstering of the fee-for-service system of medical practice, which, as reviewed in Chapter 5, tends to cost more and to distribute itself among more favored populations.

Thus, again, the new practitioners could deter basic changes in the organization and financing of health care that would improve access to services for all social groups. They may also have the effect of deterring, or making less apparent, the necessity to deal with the increasing specialization in medical education, its cost consequences, and its lack of relation to contemporary needs for health services.

Practice Restrictions   Another issue related to the new primary care practitioners, although not peculiar to them, is that they may not be employed to perform the tasks for which they were trained. Several reports show that a large proportion of nurses trained as primary care practitioners do not spend most of their time providing primary medical care; many, at best, combine their new skills with their traditional duties, particularly in health center settings (38). Those in private practice settings more often engaged in primary care (where consumer demand for services is greater), in all settings, involving more healthy than ill persons (39). Another limitation on practice occurs when, for example, the family planning specialists were forbidden by some county health officers to administer IUDs; only one in six nurses so trained worked full time in her new capacity (40). Other restrictions include credentialing requirements, which will be dealt with later.

These experiences illustrate how the arrangements under which practitioners work, the practice settings and other conditions, become more important for what they can actually do than the skills they were taught or the tasks they were intended to perform (41). This again speaks clearly to the necessity to consider the arrangement of delivery systems, including the kinds of services various settings make possible, and to relate the training of practitioners to delivery settings.

Dual Delivery   Another concern regarding the new practitioners is that they might accentuate the differences in health services between poor and affluent groups, a "two-class system." Medical professional groups have clearly stated that this is not their intent and that these distinctions, that the affluent shall have the M.D. while the poor are granted the new practitioner services, should not occur; however, no means have been suggested to prevent this from occurring (42). Although there is no ready evidence to suggest beginning trends, there is the hint of at least one pattern. It is possible that if the primary care practitioners who were trained in nurse practitioner programs tend, as they seem, to work predominantly in public health agencies and community health centers, while those trained in physician assistant and the post-corpsmen programs continue to move toward private practice settings, then a distinction under the present delivery arrangements is likely to occur (43). The poor, more likely to receive public services, will have female, nurse practitioners while the nonpoor will have male, physician assistant practitioners; and, the most affluent are likely to continue to have ready access to specialist physicians.

Prospects   At the same time, other conditions in health care delivery settings are pointing toward increasing support of new primary care practitioners regardless of their professional or other-than professional background. For example, under federal employment in the Veterans' Administration, Public Health, or Indian Health Services or the military, persons having one year of physician assistant training or work experience are given the same civil grade, whether their initial training was in nursing, physical therapy, medical technology, military corpsmen, or three years of medical school (43a). The 1972 Social Security Amendments allowed demonstration projects to devise means for paying nurse practitioners and physician assistants. Further, insurance companies are increasingly using nonphysicians—nurses, physician assistants, ex-corpsmen—to conduct basic physical assessments for their clients, estimated to reach 600,000 in 1973; this provides them with sufficient information on 90–95 per cent of their clients (43b).

Finally, as organized group health care settings develop, those who are rendering primary care are likely to be salaried at the same levels regardless of the avenue they used to acquire proficiency; more such practitioners are likely to be employed, too, because of the greater need for their services, their lesser costs relative to specialists, and the fact that they will have immediate access to supervision and consultation as well as the evaluation of their peers and of a fairly consistent group of consumer patients.

These and other changes that affect the ways in which health services are organized and financed may well influence the training and practice of primary care practitioners more than the decisions taken by the older occupational groups.

SOCIAL EFFECTS

Occupational Access An additional concern about the new practitioners is that so far they differ—beyond the possible patterned direction of service toward different socioeconomic groups—in their social origins.

The ex-corpsmen–Medex programs trained, among their first 90, about 12 per cent who were black, oriental, or Hispano; 2 per cent were women. In the civilian physician assistant programs, 7 per cent were blacks, and one fifth were women (half of whom were eye-specialist assistants in training to become ophthalmic physician assistants). The vast majority of these programs were directed by physicians and were under medical school auspices (44). Beginning salaries were lowest among the ophthalmic assistants, who also had the lowest rate of annual increase. Among all types of practitioners, the gap between men and women's earnings became wider with work experience following training (45).

In the practitioner programs that train for the various nurse practitioner titles, whether for segmented work, such as the pediatric nurse practitioner, or for integrated work, such as the family nurse practitioner, the trainees are, expectedly, women. Program direction was through the collaboration of colleges of medicine and nursing, or other physician and/or nurse leadership of varying degrees of influence. The salary of these practitioners was generally lower than for the physician assistants, often within the range paid to nurse personnel (46).

The effect of these patterns is clear. By attempting to fill the gap in primary care under current conditions in the educational and practice settings of the health professions, the new practitioners are being divided by sex, with physician assistants and nurse practitioners each respectively an offshoot of the medical and nursing professions. Perpetuating older patterns, salary and other potential rewards are greater for the predominantly male category, which may also have greater access to the more favored private practice rather than public service settings.

Further similarities to traditional patterns seem likely. As the physician assistant has a lesser status in the medical profession, relatively more blacks and women have been able to enter. Among nurses, the nurse practitioner title has taken on favorable higher status overtones, and so may well result in the unintended effect of having even fewer blacks than other nurse personnel types; blacks, as earlier described, have been most often in the less rewarded levels of nursing (see Table 6–3). And, if as often recommended (47), nurse practitioner training, conceived by some as an "expanded role," is tied to college undergraduate or graduate education, the effect is likely to further exclude lower-income groups and other nurses who were trained in shorter programs—again, those groups include relatively more minority persons.

Response by the Medical Profession Response to the new practitioners by the medical profession includes a caution that the need for them be documented by their potential employers (that is, by practicing physicians through the AMA) and a concern that licensed primary care workers may seek to become, or may in effect practice as, physicians; further, that the 250,000 medical assistants now employed by physicians be allowed to enter such training—this, in fact, is what is happening when the ophthalmic assistants are so trained (48). Since most assistants currently work for specialists, their use of physician assistant training programs is of course not likely to add to the supply of primary care practitioners. Internists, pediatricians, and obstetricians are most interested in hiring the new assistants, while family practice physicians and GPs are least interested, contrary to the intended aid which new practitioners were to be in primary care (49). Physicians were also interested in the economic impact these new personnel would have for their practices in terms of income and expenditures (50).

Such responses suggest that physicians in private practice might be more likely to support the development of specialized assistants, rather than primary care practitioners who could conceivably, under certain conditions, become a lower-cost substitute for providing basic health care (51). However, the development by the AMA of accreditation and certification procedures for the new training programs, as it had done for the older allied health professions, is likely to limit this possibility for competition (52). The AMA has also recommended that physician assistants not be allowed to practice as they were trained when they are employed and paid by other-than-private physicians (that is, hospitals or salaried physicians); and second that physician assistant services, when reimbursed by government or private insurers, be paid directly to the employing M.D. (53).

INTERPROFESSIONAL EFFECTS

While the AMA and American Nurses Association (ANA), each representing 50 and 33 per cent of those respective types of health care personnel, were dealing with questions about the new practitioners under their respective umbrellas, AMA–ANA interprofessional relations were also affected (54).

To the ANA, the physician's assistant (P.A.) was not the same as the nurse practitioner (NP); the P.A. extended physicians' services, while the NP was regarded as extending nursing services and therefore was a member of the nursing profession. In turn, the ANA claimed jurisdiction over defining the scope of NP practice, training requirements, and interpreting their legal relations with physicians (55). Further, several state nursing associations held that nurses would not follow medical orders written by physician assistants and that nurses could practice "independently," making diagnoses and prescribing treatment for nursing care problems, that is, those problems and practices regarding the care of the dishabilitated (56).

Another variant of the interprofessional disagreements generated by the new primary care practitioners was the opposition to licensing trained nurse–midwives. This occurred, for example, in one eastern state where specialists and nurses are heavily concentrated. Both the official obstetricians and nursing groups opposed such a law because of their concern that midwives might compete with them (57).

Historical Bases The turmoil within and between the nursing and medical professions precipitated by the development of new primary care practitioners is but a recent example of a long history of tenuous intergroup relations. The bases for these difficulties are fairly clear, considering the social origins and working conditions of doctors and nurses as groups. Male physicians with affluent backgrounds and very large prospective social and economic rewards have traditionally worked in the rigidly organized setting of the hospital with nurses who were female, of middle or lower-middle class backgrounds, and with relatively delineated futures. Economically, nurses were salaried; physicians, entrepreneurial. Administratively, hospitals accepted physician-led direction, while nurses were medically and organizationally in subordinate positions. Thus, while all health care providers espoused the ideals of responding humanistically to patients' needs, the underlying conditions for delivering health or medical services made joint efforts, teamwork—which requires something other than pyramid-like relations—very difficult and usually nonexistent (58).

In response to these conditions, nurses organized themselves, as many occupational groups have, into a professional group, following the pattern set by the medical profession's AMA. Stating their intent to improve the quality of patient care, they developed strategies aimed at influencing the decisions about how nurses should be trained and under what conditions their work should be regulated (59).

Interestingly, most professions in their historical development, including medicine and nursing, moved their training programs to universities and pressed for state licensure laws for themselves before they formulated codes of ethics (60).

Professions as Dual-Interest Groups

This chronology of development perhaps speaks to the dual and sometimes contradictory purposes and actions of professional organizations—their intent to improve the quality of services to people and also to defend and improve the socioeconomic interests of their members (61). These dual aims often conflict, resulting in patterns that do not improve the delivery of health services and are socially discriminatory as well (62). These effects were clearly evident in the process of specialization described earlier (Chapter 6), and in the development of the new primary care practitioners.

Professional Education

Other paradoxes present themselves, stemming from the actions of the professional groups. For example, they subscribe to a lengthy, university-based education intended to instill a people-oriented focus in students, based on sound knowledge. Studies of health education students, however, show that the ideal of human service tends during the education process to recede; students attempt rather to gain the approval of and model themselves after their faculty—in medicine these are most often male, research-oriented specialists (63). In nursing they are women who are sometimes personally unskilled at dealing with current problems in providing care to the dishabilitated or at analyzing the issues involved. This may be because their experience was in former years, or because they are very young and have done little or no work as nurses prior to their employment as teachers (64).

Perhaps most important is the common trait of teachers in the health professions—that they have tended to see the problems of providing health services and of training health personnel from the viewpoint of the interests of their own professions, and have had little if any experience in intergroup sharing of ideas and efforts. This narrow vision, then, the part rather than the whole, is passed on to students, to the new health personnel, to the new teachers (65).

Further, the fact that training is longer and begins at an earlier age than is true for the health personnel who are not regarded as professionals, tends to ensure that the socialization process, the students' adoption of the professions' patterns of thought and behavior, will be more firmly rooted and less likely to be questioned (66).

Having a professional self-image, graduates of the longest and most costly programs tend to pursue those activities which their professional group regards as prestigious. Among these are further academic studies, research, and specialization, which in turn allow greatest economic rewards and career potential (67). Further, involvement in the professional organizations, gaining visibility and contacts through its activities, gaining and maintaining the approval of older and more influential members, can open up options to advance professional careers (68). Conversely, of course, those who do not have the approval of their colleagues cannot expect these kinds of options.

Professionalization

In sum, the process of professionalization, socializing persons into a profession, has usually begun at the point of allowing entry of certain social groups into certain training programs, continues through the period of education and beyond, into the postgraduate settings of work and profession-related activities. In effect, professionalization is a process, like specialization and the proliferation of new personnel which are related to it, that limits the access of certain groups to the health occupations.

Another effect, however unintended and unplanned, which this orientation-to-the-profession has in practice is that the "most professional" and most professional-aspiring persons and groups of health personnel tend to avoid contact with outcast consumers, thus diminishing further their chances for meeting the greater needs of outcasts for health services. This effect has been reported among specialist physicians particularly, and nurses and mental health personnel, among others (69). So the paradox: the very process for entering a professional field intended for human service in effect deters such service for many, and also denies to others the chance to serve.

Credentialing

The professionalization process has its underpinnings in the ability of the professional organizations to control credentialing, that is, the formal accreditation of training programs and conditions for legal licensure and certification to practice. Since 1970 particularly, credentialing procedures have been given increasing scrutiny nationally, and, as a result, harsh criticism.

THE PAST

In decades past, professional education occurred in relatively small, autonomous schools and hospitals, supported by private funds. States, regions, and populations tended to be more isolated from each other. It was perhaps natural for private groups to set up standards for accrediting training programs, to certify practitioners who met their standards, and to press for licensure laws, passed on a state-by-state basis, which would assure a perhaps unsophisticated general public of adequately trained professionals.

Those conditions no longer exist. Public funding and public viewing is the direction for educational and services organizations. These organizations are growing increasingly large. Institutions and regions are irrevocably intertwined and interrelated with surrounding population groups. They have a nationwide viewing population through the media as well. This public is not only mobile and knowledgeable, it is also less willing to accept the old mystiques, paternalistic professionalism, or the high costs which they as taxpayers and consumers must pay.

INTERLOCKING PROCESSES

It is this social reality which most likely led the Congress to mandate a study of health personnel credentialing by the Department of Health,

Education, and Welfare in 1970. The major finding in that report was that credentialing is, in fact, an interlocking, closed, and socially discriminatory set of processes. The accreditation of training programs, the certification or registration of practitioners (by definition done through nongovernment agencies), and individual licensure (done by definition through government agencies) are tied together: (1) by sitting the same individuals on accreditation and licensing boards, (2) by having certification and/or licensure depend upon graduation from accredited programs, and (3) by allowing little outside, other-than-professional intervention in these processes (70).

There are well-known patterns to these interconnections. For example, the professional organizations, having their own bodies to approve training programs, also, at the state level, either nominate or submit members' names for appointment on the State Boards. Each such board examines and licenses nurses, or physicians, or other personnel. The boards are also responsible for accrediting educational programs but may, and do, accept accreditation decisions by other state or private agencies, principally those tied to the professional organizations (71). The state associations of professionals collaborate with the licensing boards and with state legislative committees to initiate or amend credentialing laws (72). There may, in addition, be an exchange of resources, whereby fees collected for licensure go to the state association, or the state association may help fund the regulatory functions of the licensure board. This has been especially questioned because most boards have no public members to provide alternative views to what this mutually supportive link decides.

In half the states, in fact, membership on the Boards of Medical Examiners is exclusively of physicians, and similarly so for osteopaths, podiatrists, and physical therapists. Some boards limit themselves to members of certain few professions only, such as those for dentists, optometrists, and pharmacists. Usually boards that license dental hygienists, practical nurses, or midwives have no representation from those occupations on their boards at all (73).

The composition of these legally prescribed boards of examination and licensure thus has the effect of controlling the entry, education, and ability to practice for various professions (all states require licensure for at least 11,[2] and up to 25 health professions and occupations) (74). They thereby help perpetuate the pyramid-like relationship between professions. Their decisions are cushioned against the diverse views of less prestigious personnel groups or of consumer–taxpayers.

[2] Including dental hygienists, dentists, practical and professional nurses, optometrists, pharmacists, physicians, podiatrists, and physical therapists (M. Pennell and P. Stewart, *State Licensing of Health Occupations.* Washington, D.C.: Government Printing Office, 1968, updated).

Accreditation procedures have become increasingly complex, numerous, multitiered, overlapping, and thus costly; a means for furthering competition and economic control of one professional group over another; and they have not been successful in their mission, which was to control the unneeded expansion of new training programs. These were the findings of a joint AMA–Allied Health study with the National Commission on Accrediting (NCA) (75).

The NCA has since 1949 been the nongovernment agency which recognizes the authority of other agencies to accredit education programs in many fields. Most importantly, its views have been accepted by the U.S. Office of Education, which requires accreditation before programs can qualify for federal funds (76).

The AMA now is recognized as the accrediting body for 22 allied health occupations. However, its report, cited above, declares that intergroup collaboration is limited or nonexistent (77).

The American Dental Association does the accrediting for a number of dentistry-related occupational training programs.

In nursing, the state licensing boards each set standards and accredit their state's programs. Nursing programs may also voluntarily seek accreditation by the National League for Nursing, which also approves practical nurse programs, collaborating with the National Association for Practical Nurse Education and Service (78).

LICENSURE AND CERTIFICATION

In many of the health occupations, including those which are licensed,[3] certification or registration[4] from one's professional group may or must be obtained in order to reasonably expect to be employed in that field. Requirements for certification often include graduation from an accredited school, additional qualifying examinations, and supervised periods of practice. Certification in the medical specialties is done by the specialty boards; it is done in the allied health fields by each occupational association (79). The American Nurses Association began in 1973 a certification program

---

[3] State licensure laws are *compulsory* for some occupations (that is, persons cannot work without a license), such as for physicians, dentists, dental hygienists, optometrists, pharmacists, osteopaths, and podiatrists; licensure is *voluntary* for others (that is, persons cannot use a title without holding a license) as for R.N.s, licensed practical nurses, physical therapists, social workers, and psychologists.

[4] Registration means that persons who meet certain qualifications are listed on an official roster maintained by a government or nongovernment agency.

in specialized areas of nursing care, such as geriatrics, pediatrics, and psychiatry (80).

Several of the allied health associations have in recent years developed new types of technician–assistive personnel, as well as accreditation and certification programs for them within each association. Assistants in dietetics, occupational therapy, and physical therapy are examples (81).

SOCIAL AND HEALTH CARE EFFECTS

Thus the newer groups are tending to follow patterns established by the older professions: specialization on the one hand, and proliferation of new assistive personnel on the other, all tied into the credentialing systems set up by the original group. The effects of this pattern, regarding access to and emphasis within the health occupations, are similar to those of the older groups.

In other words, credentialing mechanisms, because they are tied to time spans of formal education in specific types of institutions as well as to written examinations, have had the effect of limiting entry to and passage within and between the health occupations. These procedures have often sifted out those whose skills were learned in nonformal training settings or who do not readily express their capacities in written language. These persons, as described in Chapter 2, are more likely to be the poor, of other races than white, women, and older adults (82). Moreover, professional licensure has not been found to have a strong reliable correlation with the delivery of quality health care (83); physician examination scores have not shown a relationship to the quality of actual practice (84); accredited educational programs have often not turned out the types of practitioners that were intended (85). In these cases, the conditions under which people work were always more important than were their formal credentials for affecting the standard of health care they rendered.

Further, the nature of licensure, as a legal rule, tends to be rigid and slow to change. Its usually narrow definition of duties has incurred violations. It has impeded geographic movement as well as interoccupational transfer at a time when health care is undergoing pervasive and rapid changes (86). It is not a guarantee for continuing competence, and it has not been effectively enforced (87). In short, it has not been found to work.

The design of credentialing mechanisms, then, lodged within the professional organizations, is another enigma resulting from the dual-purpose nature of these organizations. Credentialing is aimed both at assuring standards of good health care and at preserving and improving the social and economic potential of the possessors. The second purpose has been better met.

THE NEW PRIMARY CARE PRACTITIONER: A CASE STUDY IN
CREDENTIALING AND DUAL INTERESTS

An apt illustration is again recent experience with attempts to increase primary care practitioners. Ensuring competence in the new practitioners while preserving a place for the older types has led to some anomalous results.

Types of State Licensure   In 1973, 33 states had laws which allowed physician assistants to practice (88). At least 18 of these laws were of the regulatory type. Such laws create a regulatory body that sets up rules— which may be broad or very specific—for the training and employment of physician assistants. The advantages of this type of law include some, although limited, flexibility for rule changing, and assuring consumers of a given range of competence of the practitioner. On the other hand, the regulatory body must somehow acquire the expertise, if indeed it is available, to supply the necessary examination and approval procedures to include the competent and exclude the incompetent applicants. And varying requirements between states may make geographic mobility difficult and unlikely (89).

In contrast is the general delegatory type of law which simply amends the medical practice acts to permit physician assistants to work under physician supervision (90). The AMA advocates this type as the means for allowing nonphysicians to participate in the practice of medicine (91). The advantages here are the latitude for experimentation while ensuring patient safety by the presence of the physician. The limitations are, however, that physician assistants would very likely not be used in regions where there are few or no physicians; and physicians may be reluctant to hire such personnel if they fear the risk of malpractice suits (92). Early experience has not brought greater legal risk, however (93).

In the 18 states where physician assistants are not regulated solely by their physician–employers, the regulatory agency most often responsible for them has been the state board of medical examiners (in 14 states). Most of them require that applicants be graduates of accredited programs and be supervised in practice by a physician. Many of them specifically prohibit physician assistants from performing tasks in the fields of optometry, dentistry, and pharmacy, among others. These limitations came as a result of objections to P.A. licensure by the professional organizations in those fields (94).

National Certification As the states developed legal regulations for physician assistants, the federal government through HEW funded the National Board of Medical Examiners, which now devises and monitors virtually all types of physician testing, to develop a national proficiency examination for primary care physician assistants. The intent was that knowledge and skills were to be tested—that is, proficiency—regardless of the particular type of learning and work experience of the applicants (95). In other words, the aim was to avoid some of the usual rigidities inherent in formal accredited program and written examination requirements.

When the first national testing was done at the end of 1973, it was a seven-hour written certifying examination and was open only to the graduates of certain programs, those accredited by the AMA or funded by HEW (96)—on the face of it, a contradiction of its intent, and a repetition of some of the credentialing weaknesses cited by both AMA and HEW studies.

Other less direct effects of this national examination are that it can test to some extent the variety of training programs, and it allows graduates from the family nurse and pediatric nurse practitioner programs, Primex, Medex, and others to take the test. In effect, it equates the practitioners and training programs based on the tasks they perform, not on the auspices of their professional organization or school.

Licensure for Primary Care While the development of credentialing for new primary care personnel was under way at state and national levels, several state nursing associations moved to expand their own legal capacity to render health care. They did this by pressing for revisions of state nurse practice acts, but in quite divergent directions.

In certain western states, nurses became legally able as a group or as individuals, and under rules set by the state board of nursing in collaboration with other licensure boards, to both diagnose and treat illness, including prescribing certain types of drugs (97). In other words, the laws made explicit that nurses as health practitioners, and with certain additional training, could render primary medical care.

In contrast, in an eastern state where physicians are abundant, the nurse practice act was amended so as to explicitly separate nurses from physicians and thus the nursing care tasks and their control from those of medical care. In this state, diagnosis and treatment by nurses was applied to the problems of nursing care, or in effect was defined as the problem-solving process necessary to provide care to the dishabilitated (rather than the problem-solving process as applied to determining the existence or extent of illness, which is medical care). In addition to the nursing regimen, the act includes the carrying out of any prescribed medical regimen and says that the former is not to be inconsistent with the latter.

Nurses are expressly denied the authority to practice medicine (98). The state nurses association specifically sought such independent status (99).

At about the same time and in this same state, new legislation providing for registration of physician assistants also made nurses, depending on their experience, qualified for that task area and title. In so doing it did not, of course, disallow nurses from being able to work under the Nursing Practice Act (100).

Thus although they belong to the same professional group, certain segments of nurses regard the task or practice area of health care known as primary care in at least three distinct ways. There are those, as in some of the western states, who regard it as it has been customarily understood to be, medical care, which nurses with some additional learning are capable of performing. Others regard it as an expansion of the task area of nursing care. In either case, they view it as a step upward for nurses, whether or not a specialized area of nursing practice. The third perspective, like that in some eastern regions, is that primary care is not nursing care and should not seek recruits for its practice among nurses. There is, however, among nurses, general, but not unanimous, agreement that new sets of tasks, whether extended to primary care, or in certain age- or disease-related areas of nursing care (such as geriatrics or psychiatry), ought to be learned on an advanced, formal education level and/or officially recognized with certification (101).

It is important to observe that among the states legislating changes in nursing practice, official physician support for what physicians saw as nurses' extension into primary medical care existed only where physicians were in very short supply. In the other states, where medical societies opposed such changes, concerted efforts were under way to train physician assistants under the more direct tutelage of physicians; in such states, although rural physician-shortage areas existed, the overall physician-to-population ratios were higher. In other words, physicians sought legal support for nurses to give some medical care only in the most doctor-poor regions (102).

The differences in views among nurse groups are not unlike the past and current disagreements within the medical profession concerning specialization and subspecialization, primary general physicians and non-physician primary care practitioners—a step down from the vantage point of physicians—and the credentialing related to these changes.

These developments, somewhat confused on the surface, become fairly understandable when they are viewed as the responses, if somewhat belated, of professional groups to a problem in health services, the dearth of primary care. Their responses attempt a dual purpose, to both improve primary care and to retain or improve the socioeconomic potential of their own group members in relation to older or newer groups.

The newer types of primary care practitioners in turn have now begun forming their own organizations, again following older patterns. The physician assistants have formed an expectedly male national group. The various types of nurse practitioners have formed local groups so far, and a special section in the national ANA (103).

Use of Noncredentialed Personnel

The familiar pattern, followed by both older and newer professional groups —of developing new types of health personnel to fill health care gaps, demarcating them through new forms of licensure or certification and so protecting them economically from others—has had other consequences. That is the increasing use of noncredentialed personnel, who in effect must fill the gaps left by increasingly segmented and specialized credentialed groups.

Traditionally these have been the hospital aides, as noted in the previous chapter. Many, many new types, however, were trained beginning in the 1960s, primarily in ambulatory care settings. Their work was found to be at least satisfactory compared with credentialed personnel in areas of mental health, maternal child health, family planning, health education, and community organization (104). Thus their tasks were similar to credentialed professionals in similar settings; their training was far shorter and without formal recognition; they worked most often where professionals worked least, in ghetto and isolated regions, and in publically funded settings; and their salaries, in an analysis of 26 such programs, ranged from $3,700 to $6,700 (105). Most were from low-income backgrounds, of other than white races or non-English speaking, and women (106).

Professionals often resisted or resented delegating tasks to these personnel, some because they feared potential replacement or because they competed for "patient-teaching material" for their health professional students (107). Even in settings where noncredentialed personnel were offered planned training and advancement, including a certificate representing a level of skills, their jobs became "dead-end" because no recognition was given them in the credentialed occupations' education programs, nor was the certificate usable outside the immediate health delivery system (108).

In the view of low-income workers, economic advancement was of course found to be as important an aim as among credentialed professionals; this was expressed in part through unionizing, now found among a wide spectrum of personnel, older and newer types, credentialed and noncredentialed.

Other Solutions to Services and Personnel Problems

The search, then, for ways to provide more and better primary care has brought to light again the inequitable effects of current credentialing processes, effects that spread both between and within professions and between professions and noncredentialed personnel. As a result, many proposals have been made to change the credentialing processes.

Credentialing Reforms

Since there is general agreement that changes are needed, proponents usually focus on one of two approaches, either improving the credentialing of individuals or establishing some form of institutional credentialing for health services organizations.

INDIVIDUAL APPROACHES

Those who support an individual credentialing system have advocated one or more of these steps: (1) concerning the accreditation of training programs, approval standards should be set for clusters of occupations, thereby eliminating duplication in administrative and other educational resources expended in small programs as well as the time and costs involved in accreditation itself; (2) control over accreditation should be vested in the community rather than the current nonpublic organizations, which perform quasi-governmental tasks (judging program eligibility for federal funds); (3) standards should be tested in relation to the public interest; and (4) education equivalency tests should be developed to allow persons who have learned through work, life, and other nonformal learning experiences to enter formal educational programs at an advanced level (109).

Regarding the certification of skills, written examinations should not be required following graduation from an accredited training program; proficiency examinations should be developed to allow recognition of the skills of persons regardless of their educational background (110). On the issue of state licensure, the HEW report and others called for a temporary moratorium on licensing any new types of personnel in order to develop more organized credentialing processes. Some suggested that (1) national examinations be accepted by state licensing boards with a uniform pass–fail level; (2) licensure boards within each state be integrated or form a single board, following a model law, and include the professions to be licensed and consumers as well; (3) boards be sufficiently funded to carry out all their tasks; (4) current health practice laws be broadened to allow greater delegating authority; (5) accreditation of one's training program not be a criterion for licensure; and (6) relicensure or recertification be based on specific continuing education requirements or evidence of continued competence (111).

INSTITUTIONAL APPROACHES

The HEW report also recommended demonstrations to test institutional licensure. Those who advocate this approach to assuring the competence of health care personnel propose the licensing of health services organizations, including hospitals and other delivery arrangements, by a state board, and the repeal of individual licensure laws. The board, with non-health members in the majority, would also register all health service organizations and practitioners, would certify noninstitutional personnel, would set up regulations for delegatory authority, and assess state needs for personnel and evaluating personnel competence; health organizations would assume legal liability for all services rendered by their staffs and come under regulations to prevent worker exploitation. They would be required, prior to licensure, to give proof of the competency of their personnel and adequacy of their facilities, and would report all employment and terminations, including the reasons (112).

The individual licensure approach stresses professional responsibility for maintaining standards of health care, freedom of movement, and career advancement. It is likely to help preserve current distinctions within and between the professions and other types of health personnel, in terms of training, practice, and rewards (113).

The institutional licensure approach emphasizes flexible work patterns based on proved abilities, gives freedom of movement to those now restricted by individual licensure, and emphasizes organizational rather than physician liability for malpractice risks. It is likely to enhance the influence of organized delivery settings, principally hospitals, but in time, of HMO-type arrangements. Under current patterns it could cause difficulties for physicians who work in more than one hospital, and for health worker unions which are organized by specific job titles (114). The hospital association, among others, supports this approach. The medical and nursing associations oppose it for physicians and nurses, although not for other personnel (115).

A third approach advocates an integrated system for assuring practitioner competence and institutional high standards (116). Among the more recent variations of this approach is a proposal for a federal commission to assist organized health care settings to set up mechanisms to evaluate practitioner and institutional quality. Quality would be based on certain criteria, including the actual effects of services on health, and personnel and consumer views of services. This proposal would preempt state licensure laws except for physicians and dentists, and would exempt health care settings from other federal quality regulatory standards (117). In effect, the assurance of competence would become primarily a public responsibility. This would mitigate the sometimes conflicting dual purposes of professional organizations; these groups could then focus on their socioeconomic interests (118).

It seems likely that the credentialing of health training and health services will become more integrated nationally, more publically accountable, and tied to governmental agencies. This is because of general dissatisfaction with current ineffective practices, in turn related to changing patterns of organization and financing. Courts have increasingly and clearly held hospitals responsible for the services rendered to patients (in addition to the attending physicians), in effect saying that a service institution is accountable for the validity of practitioners' educational credentials (119). Such institutional responsibility is likely to spread as more tax dollars are used to allow the development of and payment for services in organized ambulatory care settings. This impetus will be even greater as federal funds pay for increasing proportions of health services, whether by the gradual extension of Medicare/Medicaid or through a national health insurance program.

As already discussed, the development of new primary care practitioners as a solution to the primary care gap is still a question. Under current patterns of education, credentialing, practice, and financing, their impact on adding to the amount of primary services available, rendering such services in health-scarcity areas, or effectively reducing costs can be only minimal. Minimal, too, can be their effect on improving the access of outcast groups to the health occupations.

Redistribution of Personnel

Many other means, of course, have been tried to increase access to primary health care. Among these are efforts to redistribute health personnel to scarcity areas by financial inducements. However, these have been generally ineffective except among those personnel who are in a low-income class to begin with (120). Another is the development of government-sponsored service facilities or decentralizing of training centers into those regions. This has been done because of evidence that physicians and dentists tend to set up practice in their home and/or school region or similar socioeconomic area, and, among physicians especially, near specialized and inpatient facilities. This information, however, is based on middle- and upper-middle-income practitioners; low-income persons who live in poor or isolated areas may not follow the same patterns when they become practitioners (121).

Loan forgiveness of student aid for those who work in scarcity areas after graduation is another method. Since this has been ineffective (students repay the loans in cash), a new federal training bill *requires* payback of the loan by a period of national service with several options, including work in a shortage area (122).

Other newer proposals also are being formulated in more stringent terms than previous voluntary inducements. For example, the AMA resolved that half of the new enrollments should be in primary care specialties since the design of family practice as a specialty has as yet had little appeal for medical students (123); the surgeons' organization has proposed ways to limit the number of surgeons and surgical specialties, including allowing only board-certified physicians to practice (124); one state with a large physician population, but many doctor-poor areas, has required its state-supported medical schools to reserve almost one third of their enrollment spaces for those who will work in shortage areas (125). Another method, to develop ambulatory care settings in order to broaden physician skills, has been slow and has as yet been virtually absent from medical school curricula (126).

Increasing the Supply

Other efforts aim at increasing the numbers of practitioners. This may be done by enlarging the enrollments of health schools through federal funds tied also to requirements for telescoping training time. The estimate is that on the average training time for physicians could be reduced by at least two years, and student–faculty ratios could be increased from 1½ to at least 2½ students per teacher (127). Another approach was to develop a national corps that could be sent to shortage areas. The results of this program, however, have so far been limited because local medical and dental societies, whose approval is necessary, have often not agreed with the local population about the existence of a shortage of dentists or physicians; further, health professionals have not readily offered to join the Corps (128).

Retraining older or retired practitioners has been tried, as well as recruiting students from scarcity areas, which would, in effect, mean low-income and minority persons. Here, however, effects on rates of new graduates have been minimal, as noted in Chapter 6. Moreover, only about one fourth of the 68 national health professional associations had initiated minority recruitment programs by 1973 (129).

The effort to increase the supply of primary care practitioners has been offered as an additional reason, beyond equity, for encouraging women to enter male-dominated professions. Compliance with anti-sex-discrimination guidelines were required by June 1973 for private as well as public schools receiving federal aid in both student and faculty policies; plans for policy-program transition were to be in effect at that time (130). However, none of the HEW Health Opportunity Training Grants programs were directed at women (131).

Further, some educators were using sex-related reasons for predicting that the very need for primary care physicians would mean that the acceptance of women in medical school, having risen slightly, would again slow. The explanation given was that women have had a higher attrition rate in school (although excel in clinical practice), and have worked fewer hours, owing to marriage and family demands; they would therefore be greater financial risks to medical schools (132). Along this line, others said that support for women in medical schools was likely only when school capacity greatly increased and the demands for medical services became less urgent (133). That these predictions were realistic was supported by the fact that financial aid through scholarships, family support, or part-time jobs has been less available to women students than men (134).

As an additional source of medical services, the AMA favored continued support of foreign medical graduates (FMGs) and the development of new medical schools by local initiative and with ample commitment of financial support to avoid reliance on federal funds (135).

A New Physician

As a final proposal for filling the gap in primary care, a new type of physician training has been put forward, a five-year ambulatory care, community-based, group-practice-oriented program. The graduate would be a "medical practitioner" or "doctor of primary medicine." Training, however, would occur in centers affiliated with, but not part of, medical schools. Medical schools would then be free to fully attend to the training of medical clinician/specialists and medical scientist/teachers (136). Emphasis has been on these for some years; medicine is, in fact, the only health profession with more than half its students at graduate-specialist levels; other professions have about 10–12 per cent at those levels (137).

Ad Hoc Solutions in Sum and Deficit

In sum, the solutions proposed for granting access to primary health care range wide and are numerous. They include the development of new non-physician primary care practitioners and a new type of physician primary care practitioner. They suggest allowing movement of able practitioners within and between certain occupations through alternative credentialing processes such as equivalency and proficiency testing. They aim at redistributing personnel geographically by financial incentives or obligations or by relocating or developing new health services and health education centers in shortage areas. They would seek to change the emphasis on types of services available by limiting the numbers who may enter certain specialties, by requiring certain numbers to enter so-called primary specialties, or by developing family practice as a specialty. Others focus on the reorganization and development of primary care practice settings.

Another approach seeks to increase the supply of practitioners by decreasing training time, adding to enrollments, granting better access to training for minorities and women, supporting more FMGs, retraining or upgrading retired practitioners, or finally, building a mobile national health corps.

Measures undertaken to increase the supply of personnel have limited potential for several reasons. They are usually based on projected "shortages" of particular types of personnel. These projections, in turn, are computed on past or present ratios to population, and so assume that those ratios are satisfactory; there is, in fact, no evidence that health personnel-to-population ratios are related to better health for people. Shortages are also often defined as deficiencies in "qualified" personnel as determined by professional credentials (138). Projections about needed personnel often then in effect serve to support the claims of promoters of certain training programs (139). Further, the focus on increasing the supply of personnel usually fails to take into account changes in the makeup of population in future years, changes and improved efficiency in health care delivery arrangements, in alternative personnel patterns, in the composition of those entering certain occupations, and of other ways that may improve health unrelated to the delivery of personal health services. They in effect seek solutions within current limiting conditions

(140). In addition, they avoid the question of redistributing personnel geographically and changing the emphases in the very structure of the health occupations, in its inpatient–specialist and noncommunity–nonenvironmental focus.

Similarly, the numerous other attempts to make primary care readily available have had and can have only limited effect, if only because of their very *ad hoc* nature. They are neither interrelated nor tied to the conditions and changes in the health care delivery network—which is itself little more coordinated or planned. Even a combined set of solutions that may seem successful in a given situation is almost assured against having wider effects because of the sporadic nature of health training and health services programs.

Changing Conditions

Nevertheless, as earlier chapters described, major changes are in the offing in the financing and organization of health services. Increasing support from public funds will require a public accounting, at least to some extent, of how that money is spent and how efficiently. The cost study of educating health professionals is being followed by a proposed national cost study on all other allied health personnel training (141). Health personnel training acts of 1971 not only supported new training facilities and more students, they also encouraged, but did not require, new efforts by the professional schools to devise ways for shifting emphasis: from inpatient to community-related training, from urban to rural (decentralized) settings, from rigid to flexible entry and exit requirements, from narrowly professional to health-system-oriented curricula, from autonomous to cooperative teaching and training programs within and between professional groups (142).

The wide-ranging and far-reaching intent of the legislation was clear and portends further Congressional approaches to health care training. The 1973–1974 revision of the Public Health Service Act, which encompasses most health services and education legislation, is another step toward developing a framework for national health policy. Impelled by the necessity to account for the use of public funds, measures are likely to be aimed at ensuring the relevance of health training to an enlarging health care system, one based on the real needs for health services in communities and accessible to all communities; at the same time, all social groups must have access to the health care occupations, whose services and training are increasingly paid by public funds.

In line with this potential national imperative, with its economic and social ramifications, and in contrast to uncoordinated *ad hoc* solutions, other less-seldom-heard proposals have been made. These suggest a more coherent approach to health personnel planning, development, and distribution, an approach tied to the system of health services delivery (143). While various such approaches differ in scope, virtually all advocate a planned system of joint, shared, or core studies, with multiple routes for entry and exit from training, and cross-professional mobility and flexible movement within occupational groups, implying less rigid forms of credentialing (144).

Some attempts have been made to implement more systematic and flexible training. But these have usually been limited to particular groups of occupations, each tending to reflect an economic group, such as aides or community workers, allied health personnel, or certain health professionals (145). Their effects have been minor, again in part because of the uncoordinated ties between programming for training and for the delivery of services. Evaluation, too, has been limited.

However, beginning research efforts in the early 1970s have suggested a sound basis for core approaches to health care training (146). This view is that certain definable sets of tasks exist, requiring sets of skills that become the focus of types of jobs or occupations, and that these task sets or task areas are also interrelated. This then forms the basis for ways to assist persons to enter and move within and between health, and possibly other, personal services occupations.

Under a federal feasibility study grant, one school has developed a prototype School for Health Professions plan, which may or may not be implemented. It proposes an initial nonstructured training period in which students from diverse backgrounds may assess their own skills and foci of interest and then be guided by faculty in a curriculum plan that would emphasize ambulatory health services in such areas as primary medical care, dental care, social–mental health work, or coordination (reception–clerical–assistive tasks). In addition to the skills and knowledge essential to these tasks, interpersonal communication and self-learning processes form the curriculum. The content would integrate various disciplines by focusing on patient or community health problems; and groups of learners, although they would focus on different tasks in their work experience, would learn jointly and have a common instructional and advisory faculty (147).

Such approaches to training would seem to offer the best possibility for dealing with the central and interrelated problems of the health occupations: access—entry and advancement for all social groups; emphasis

—focus on most needed primary care services; and efficacy—the type and place of training that will produce competent and usable practitioners.

Integrated Health Training

For example, an integrated training program for the health occupations would allow entry by both credentialed and noncredentialed health personnel, persons working in nonhealth fields, as well as young students who are beginning their vocational preparation (Figure 7–1). Ways of assessing the applicants' knowledge and skills would include a combination of written and oral testing, observed trials, and interviewing. Conclusions reached mutually by entrants and faculty would then result in a curriculum plan within an estimated time span and might include remedial and/or financial aid. Entry would be limited to the numbers of personnel needed in the various fields of practice, particularly in the region in which the training center is located. Priority might be given to those social groups least represented in certain practice fields. Federal funding could give priority to centers that so selected their trainees, and a national clearinghouse could inform interested applicants of vacancies.

By focusing on the entrants' actual skills and knowledge rather than the means by which they acquired them, the process of entry into health training would avoid the sex–race–age–income group discrimination now associated with formal educational prerequisites.

All students would take certain core studies, although some students, depending on their backgrounds, could omit some aspects. These studies might be taught in a combination of academic and less-formal, experiential teaching styles to mesh with the variety of learning styles which socially diverse groups of students are likely to represent. The difficulties of such joint teaching and learning, and the individual and group search for ways to deal with them, are of course very like the interpersonal and intergroup problems faced by diverse types of health personnel who must render coordinated health services. Thus the experience of working to learn together and to teach together is a necessary, but not sufficient, component to providing health services together (when and if the health care delivery system is so devised as to emphasize group over independent services), and to dealing with the broader problems of health services delivery and other means of assuring the health of populations.

The settings for the core studies, as for all phases of training, would include, to varying degrees, the necessary quietude of academic settings, and the equally needed involvement in community, through individual, tutorial, and group experience.

Among the essentials of the core studies would be the basic, social,

Figure 7–1 The Health Occupations, United States

Schema for Integrated Health Training

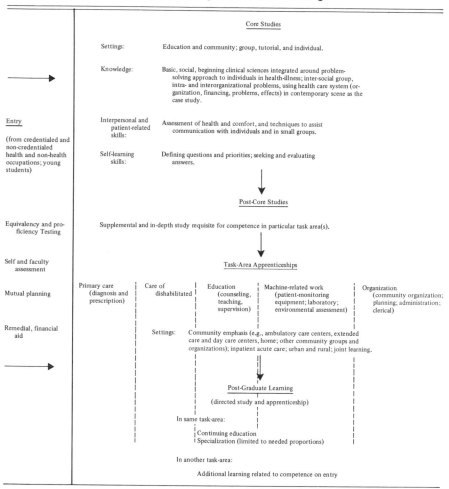

Data sources: After concepts in E. Gilpatrick, *Suggestions for Job and Curriculum Ladders in Health Center Ambulatory Care*, Research Rept. No. 4, 5 (New York: Research Foundation, City University of New York, 1972); Nancy Milio, University Assembly Lecture, University of Missouri Medical Center–Columbia (Oct. 30, 1972); "Highlights of an Educational Plan for a School of Health Professions" (San Francisco: University of the Pacific Medical Center, Aug. 1973), working document.

and beginning clinical sciences learned, not as separate disciplines, but drawn on to solve or deal with personal health or community health problems. This would include the typical or most common spectrum of health and illness in individuals and also those patterns characteristic of various kinds of communities. Using as the fundamental case the problems involved in health care delivery to persons, communities, and nation, various interpersonal and intra- and interorganizational concepts could be taught and various alternative patterns of health care pursued. The practical field work would in effect monitor, moderate, and refine the conceptual ideal.

Other learning would include the interpersonal skills necessary to relate on a person-to-person level to colleagues and clients, individuals and groups. Further, the beginning skills of evaluating health, care, and comfort requirements of individuals and the basic techniques to assist them might well be introduced to all personnel who will work in any phase of health care.

Throughout the curriculum, as is, of course, the ideal aim of any education program, would be an emphasis on self-evaluation—defining the question, setting priorities, seeking and testing answers—to foster the critical consciousness, the practice of continuous learning. The diversity among students and among faculty should foster an attitude of questioning and answer seeking.

A core of studies, in effect, acknowledges the fact that all health personnel must deal with problems concerning the organization and delivery of health services at, primarily, a single level at a given period in their working life. This may be at the one-to-one, interindividual level, or the internal organizational level, or the interorganizational, intercommunity level. At whatever level of such problem solving (or more modestly, answer seeking), they must, to be competent, have skills in applying basic, social, and clinical science knowledge; they must have interpersonal sensitivity to their coworkers and to patients and other persons in the community; and they must be able by self-evaluation and supervision to continue to learn from day-by-day experiences.

Following the core studies, postcore learning would be a necessary supplement to the core and may be done jointly by some student groups entering the more closely related task areas.

The task areas, then, are simply those areas of health care which focus on certain sets of activities essential to the delivery of health services. They rely on fairly definable skills, and use, more often than other areas, certain kinds of knowledge. None is exclusive, however.

For example, primary health care focuses on diagnosis and prescription of treatment; this set of tasks has been applied to general physical care (medical), dental (dentistry), eye (optometry), or foot care (podiatry), and to different age and sex groups (pediatrics, geriatrics, maternity). Care of the dishabilitated focuses on ways to ensure the comfort and support the fullest recovery or the humane dying of those who cannot care for themselves. Although the foci of these two task areas differ, as do the skills most often needed, they clearly share the need for certain kinds of knowledge and might more competently discharge their tasks if they shared some basic skills—thus the inclusion of that base in the core studies.

A third task area, labeled education, includes the skills necessary to counsel, teach, and supervise individuals and groups. Clearly, again, these are skills which other task areas need to use and therefore need to have some competence in, but in which such skills are not the focus. These educational personnel could develop [in ways that personal health services practitioners cannot, since their major efforts must be directed toward rendering one-to-one services] community-wide, small and large group, or communications-media formats for teaching self-health measures. Such measures may well include necessary environmental changes. The arrangements for staff education would also be their responsibility. Other such personnel might provide continuing counseling services, to patients, as individuals or in groups, whose health problems are not primarily physical in nature.

Machine-related work centers on tasks related to diagnostic testing, or other equipment-tied procedures for evaluation or treatment of health-related problems, including those of the physical environment.

A fifth task area, organization, concerns the problems dealt with by the other task areas, but focuses on the organizational and social group level. It includes such activities as community organization, planning, or administration.

Thus each task area may encompass a number of occupations (now defined by a variety of titles) which persons who have been trained in that task area might be prepared to undertake. Their apprenticeship—the focus of their supervised practical experience—would be in one task area, although of course they would also be using skills which were the predominant mode of those in other task apprenticeships. To the extent that numerous job titles for similar tasks now have a discriminatory effect on certain sex–income–ethnic groups, integrated training could help eliminate such non-competency-based distinctions.

Postgraduate learning, following at least a minimum of work experience, could be pursued in the same task area as continuing education. Some persons could specialize in some facet of their task area, but their numbers would be limited to the proportion of such specialists needed in a given region or of a given type.

Others seeking postgraduate learning might, on the basis of their changing interests and perspective, pursue training in another task area, having already gained familiarity with it through core studies and perhaps other less formal modes of learning, such as experiences in their work situations. Such postgraduate study would be an individualized combination of directed study and apprenticeship.

By thus limiting specialization and allowing interoccupational movement, integrated health educational programs would help shift the emphasis in the health occupations to primary and community-based care givers. It would also improve access by all types of health personnel to all task areas. By emphasizing apprenticeships and skill-based competency in community settings, it would also become more effective in preparing persons for the work that most needs to be done.

Further, since all the task areas are essential to the delivery of necessary health services, the range of social and economic rewards granted those practicing in the various task areas, or those within a given task area, need not be as disparate as they have been traditionally.

If such integrated training programs were accredited or otherwise certified, and graduates worked in approved or certified health care settings, this would reasonably assure competency to the public in the provision of health care, especially if such program certification involved public as well as health care provider representation.

Building from an integrated health training base, certified health care delivery organizations, whether of the ambulatory HMO type or inpatient, could develop more flexible opportunities for their personnel to render services according to the needs of the populations served. This conceivably could be safely done through competent on-the-job supervision and other continuing education programs.

Further, integrated training in combination with certified health delivery settings (which might indeed be required to have built-in mechanisms for on-going education as well as for personnel and consumer input into programming prior to certification) would make possible, and in fact necessary, the team concept, a notion not very usable under present training and services patterns. This would be a realistic expectation, especially if rewards among the task areas were equitably distributed.

NECESSARY ADJUNCTS

The potential that integrated health training may have for dealing with the interrelated problems of access, emphasis, and efficacy in the health occupations could not of course be realized, even following a trial of substantial size and effort, without mechanisms to develop and implement health personnel policy. These steps, in turn, would have to be tied to the needs for health personnel in a coordinated system of health care delivery. Otherwise the distribution of the most useful mix of health personnel could not be assured. Ideally, such policies, further, would be tied to policies related to general education, which might well include far more teaching of self-health measures and of the complex of socioeco-nomic–political–environmental aspects of health. In addition, environmental and social policies, once developed, would find a needed synergy with health.

A final aspect to the framework in which integrated health training could realize its potential social and health services contributions is a planned transition phase. This would have to encompass national to local levels, and include all groups to be affected—health personnel, educators, students, and, in time, new entrants, who may well then enter the health care field with new and realizable expectations.

REALITY

The realistic prospects for planned and integrated training for health personnel is to date slight, given the historical and current thrust toward autonomy by groups of health providers. At the same time, as described earlier, various facets in financing, organization, and education for health care are moving toward consolidation. Beyond the effects of necessary economy efforts and public accountability for public financing, other changes, depending on their speed and size, could make integrated health training more feasible and more necessary.

In the delivery of health services, for example, prototype HMOs, by placing all personnel on salaried earnings, broadening employee decision making, and in effect, requiring more teamwork in a relatively small, face-to-face setting, could help level the pyramid between occupational groups, that is, those working in the equally essential health care task areas. Consumer involvement in more publically subsidized programs would also add to interoccupational cohesion, for the call for access to services and to education for occupations is not likely to be stilled until means are found to grant access to more than token numbers.

Further, in the health occupations themselves, changes described earlier may be interpreted as pointing toward new possibilities. For example, the training of increasing numbers of varieties of assistive personnel in short time spans to do essentially the same work as longer-trained professionals is tacit admission of overeducation and overspecialization. So also are reports of little discernible differences between educational programs claimed to be geared to different levels of ability (148).

Another portent of necessary changes is that health personnel do, in fact, cross over from one task area to another. Historically, for example, nurses, especially in doctor-scarce rural and ghetto areas, have rendered primary medical care, the tasks now legitimized in some states under

Nursing Practice Acts or through formal training programs, as in the physician assistant, nurse practitioner, or similar programs (149).

Further, recommendations and planning within the medical profession suggest the eventual separation of training for primary care from the medical schools, as envisioned in the doctor of primary medicine, and now more possible with the training of new primary care practitioners. Under a recent proposal, medical schools would focus on the training of specialists, and graduates would qualify for a license to practice independently *only* after specialist residency training is completed (150). Thus medical school graduation would no longer produce physicians as that label has been ordinarily understood. As wholly specialist institutions, medical schools would presumably receive public education funds only for the training of needed specialists and providing they would grant access to primary care practitioners trained in other settings.

Shape and direction may indeed emerge as these changes occur, sporadic and *ad hoc,* planned and unplanned as they are. However, the effects on the delivery of health services and on various occupational groups may mean small gains for a few, but most often inequities for those who have long had limited access to services and jobs, the outcast groups. In other words, unplanned, uncoordinated, and unmonitored changes may lead to a new system which nevertheless perpetuates less favored treatment of certain income, ethnic, sex, and age groups.

International Comparisons

Like the United States, most nations are taking steps to assure the efficacy of their health personnel systems—both in terms of the relevance of the occupations to changing societal needs for health services, and of the educational methods used to produce basic, and ensure continuing, competence of the practitioners. Compared to the United States, these problems are perhaps less complex in many countries because they began to deal with them earlier.

Many nations have developed national mechanisms, to varying degrees, for defining and resolving health care issues and monitoring the effects of those decisions. Such mechanisms are part of the variety of national health service organization and financing programs which exist in most industrialized and poor countries, and are also related to their more developed social, educational, and economic policies.

These national conditions are then responsible in part for the relatively fewer types of health personnel in most other countries. That is, the nations' development of more planned and integrated ways of dealing with changes in health services has precluded to some extent the sporadic proliferation of many job types for similar types of work. The U.S.S.R., for example, has less than one third as many paramedical personnel per physician (and more physicians in relation to population) as the United States (151). Further, varieties of new personnel are not as necessary because of the relatively greater numbers of general physicians to provide primary medical care.

In addition, other traditional primary care practitioners have continued to render services. Midwives in The Netherlands, for example, deliver more than one third of all babies, more than two thirds of whom are born at home; as earlier noted, The Netherlands vies with Sweden for the world's lowest infant death rate (152).

Other policies, such as free postsecondary education, and traditions of widespread adult education, as in Scandanavia, along with previously noted fiscal and planning policies affecting the distribution of health personnel and the limitation of credentialed specialties, have also served to deter the formation of substitution personnel (153).

Use of Alterprofessionals

However, in virtually no country has the problem of distributing professionals to rural or isolated areas been solved, as discussed in Chapter 2 (154). One of the most frequent ways for dealing with this, then, has been the training and/or use of *alter*professionals, persons skilled in certain task areas by means other than the ways professionals attained their skills, and at lower cost. A review of six European and Asian countries showed a patterned contrast in 64 health-related occupational groupings. There was an average of two alterprofessional types to one professional grouping. In contrast with the professional categories, the alterprofessionals on the average entered at an older age, were required to have work experience but less prior formal education; they received fewer years of training, were taught by professional rather than their own occupational peers, and their credentialing (formal or informal) and later on-the-job supervision were also most often done by professionals. Alterprofessionals were less likely to live in and be trained in urban areas, and less often worked in urban areas than professionals. They were thus more likely to render services to rural, ethnic-minority, low-income, or otherwise outcast populations. Finally, compared with professionals, their incomes were lower, and their opportunities for advancement through further education or on-the-job promotion were far less than for the professionals. Greater proportions of women, ethnic minorities, and low-income groups filled the alterprofessional job categories (155).

Training Patterns

In an attempt to relate the training of health personnel to the planned delivery of health services, several countries have developed to some extent integrated and more flexible educational patterns.

The U.S.S.R. has perhaps the most experience with these. The greatest proportion of its trained personnel, the "middle medical workers"—feldshers (or nonphysician primary care practitioners); nurses; midwives; pharmacists; dental, x-ray, and laboratory technicians; and sanitarians—are trained in middle medical schools following their secondary education. Auxiliaries, who are trained on the job, may also qualify to enter such schools (156).

The length of study is about two to four years, depending on previous education and field of study. The faculty are physicians, and in the clinical settings all types of personnel are equally responsible to the physician in charge. In fact, however, in rural areas, teams of two to four middle medical workers attend to most health services with but monthly supervisory visits from a physician (157).

Medical schools, which are institutes offering customarily a six-year training for physicians, give priority for entry to middle medical workers (who make up 20–30 per cent of students); they also may begin medical studies through evening classes (158).

In the late 1960s, Sweden developed integrated and modular alternative-path training for auxiliary and nursing personnel. Under this system, core studies and later additional training prepare persons to work in general or geriatric inpatient facilities, in general acute or long-term care, primary ambulatory or home care, or in occupational therapy or radiology services. A proposal has also been made for all health practitioners to be trained together under a comprehensive national educational strategy (159).

Japan has a more limited but graded system for a variety of nursing personnel, which is currently undergoing revision.

Credentialing

Beyond education policies and programming, most countries have continued to use traditional methods of credentialing individual practitioners. However, licensure is often based on national, rather than regional or local examinations, particularly in countries that have a national health service. Sometimes, as for English physicians, licensure is granted following graduation, without further examination (160). In England, too, public members sit on the national professional councils which determine basic education requirements for the health professions (161).

With the increasing attention to planned health services in many countries have come also proposals for altering traditional means of credentialing personnel. In Canada's 1972 proposal for major reorganization of its health services were recommendations for policies to integrate the training and supply, educational funding and curriculum planning for health personnel, and to include public representatives on province-level professional licensing boards (162).

Changes in Great Britain required in the 1965–1972 period a thorough national exploration of health personnel policies, including the effectiveness and aptness of educational and credentialing patterns. Studies showed that there was need to have personnel who could be more flexibly deployed in hospital and in community settings (163). Personnel were not being appropriately trained for the kinds of health services problems that changing communities presented (164). New health services patterns were allowing more patients to remain in community facilities, including their own homes, and the numerous new health centers were allowing physicians and nurses to work together in new ways (165). Finally, having joined the European Common Market, with its reciprocity policies, which include intercountry occupational mobility, Great Britain was required to plan to mesh its training requirements with those of the Continental countries (166).

As a result, and following testimony and recommendations of the various groups of practitioners and other health care providers involved, an educational plan was proposed, to be fully implemented by 1977. It includes common basic training and modular sets of skills allowing entry–exit flexibility for nursing and midwifery personnel, who compose three fourths of all health care personnel (167). In noninstitutional settings, the traditional health visitor would emphasize primary health care tasks, while the district nurse will continue to emphasize the care of the dishabilitated, including therapeutic applications in homes and in the health centers. Both types will assume new titles in the future. Nursing and midwifery credentialing bodies will also be joined.

Other recommendations not included in the final plan called for common training for all health personnel and a joint credentialing board that would encompass all health services practitioners (168).

Professional Organizations

It is perhaps a fair generalization that as national health programs have emerged, the task of the professional groups, of forthrightly attending to the economic interests of their members, has assumed greater importance. In many affluent countries they, in effect, openly bargain with governments, through coalitions or joint organizations, in setting pay policies (169).

Their other major task, that of the competence of their practitioner members as developed through educational programs and licensure, has become a process joined with the public. Thus their professional perspective and expertise tends to serve an advisory, rather than an independent regulatory purpose for health policy. Their position remains one of great influence but not of control (170). Even in their economic goals, the professional groups have shown responsiveness to wider social concerns and movement toward equity. For example, in line with growing national support for an alternative to fee-for-service payments, the Canadian Nurses Association called for nurses working in an expanded role to be paid on a salary rather than fee-for-service basis (171).

This illustrates also the point of view taken by nurses, physicians, dentists, and others who have been in positions to see the effects of traditional decisions in the health professions. Through the World Health Organization and International Council of Nursing, they have called for flexibility rather than autonomy by the professions; for integrated and continuing education; and, in a recent and pointed report, for a separation of personnel interests in health care planning so as not to thwart the public demand for equity (172).

The Poor Nations

While many affluent nations are having to reshape their traditional ways of providing for health services, the poor countries are in many respects attempting to build systems of health care for the first time. The question facing them, concerning primary personal health services, like so many others, is whether or not they should follow the traditions of the richer nations.

They may, as many have, focus on training professionals with the formal educational requirements and expense which that entails. Such a focus, however, in Thailand, for example, excludes about 95 per cent of the population from entering medicine, nursing, or midwifery (173).

Further is the chronic and worldwide problem of getting such personnel into rural and health-scarcity areas. The overpopulation in urban areas of all health personnel, including dentists, pharmacists, and technicians, is creating their unemployment, underemployment, and often emigration to affluent countries. These personnel, clearly from the more affluent social groups, have also become vocal in calling for further university education credentials in their own professional fields (174).

Alternatively, the poor nations may limit the professionals' options and focus resources on alterprofessionals. Proposals to limit professional use of social resources include ending the building of medical schools and regionalizing current medical schools on an intercountry basis. In the 1960–1970 decade 75 per cent of all medical schools built were in the poor nations, which then had about the same population-to-school ratio as the affluent countries (175). Other proposals are to require general practice prior to specialist training and rural practice in lieu of military service, and to make urban practice more costly through a monthly licensing fee (176).

Focus on the training and practice of alterprofessionals has been strongly recommended by WHO, particularly because no study has yet showed that physicians are better able to render effective service in the rural areas (177). By shifting resources to alterprofessionals, some social inequities could also be ameliorated, of course, both in employment and earnings, and in greater access by the rural poor to needed health services.

The training of such personnel, drawing them from current auxiliaries and from rural or other outcast populations, is planned as being community, rather than classroom-based, and flexible. Plans and proposals include giving all ambulatory care workers six months of training in primary diagnosis and therapeutics, or giving nursing personnel primary care training and leadership in rural health centers. Others suggest core studies with task area modules, and most include decentralized training facilities and health services centers (178).

The changes in primary care training and practice have been more fundamental in China. In addition to having many alterprofessional primary care practitioners—the nonphysician "barefoot doctors"—physician training also has been altered. In addition to focusing curriculum on the most prevalent needs for services, the recruitment—and thus composition of the practitioners—has changed. Local regions, rural and urban, send their hardest working and most socially committed young people to the schools, which, in turn, interview and select their students using other-than written-examination criteria. Further, since administrative responsibility for health care delivery is inclusive of rural and urban districts, all graduate physicians regularly rotate their service in urban and rural health centers; they thus work with the alterprofessionals, who, in turn, serve the communes where they live (179).

Summary

The nature of the health occupations—increasing specialization and the proliferation of similar job types—has had the effect of limiting the access of certain social groups, predominantly women, minorities, the poor, to the more favored positions within and among the various occupational categories. These patterns have also contributed to limiting access to health services by less favored population groups through the concentration of specialist personnel in urban-affluent areas, the related encouragement of high-cost forms of health care, and relative disinterest in most-needed primary care.

In their attempts to deal with these health services problems, the health occupations groups have chosen—rather than examining the basic nature of the occupations—to focus directly on *ad hoc* measures for increasing the amount of primary care personnel available. Such attempts seem to be perpetuating traditional discriminatory patterns within the occupations, and to have only minimal potential for improving access to primary health services.

Greater impact on the problems of unequal access to both the health occupations and to health services is more likely to occur through more fundamental reorganization of health personnel patterns, recruitment, training, and deployment, tied to similar planned reorganization of health services delivery.

Whether the thrust of future efforts will continue to be of an *ad hoc* and uncoordinated type, or whether more substantive and far reaching, will depend on the decisions taken by the major interest groups and organizations, the subject of the next section.

Images of Access

The vignettes that follow, concerning a northern Indian village and a Kyoto ghetto, as much mirror the problems of creating full access to health-serving occupations as they show a modest improvement in access for some groups. Beyond access, they clearly reflect efforts to refocus training in health-related occupations, literally going outside university walls, tying environmental to personal services, relating trainee learning to the everyday problems that support or stifle health, for communities and for their individual members.

iv For Rural Women, Northern India

Beyond the Qutb Minar, one of the magnificent architectural remnants of Muslim rule, is the little agricultural village of Mahsudpur in Haryana, the small state contiguous with Delhi's south border. Although the villagers' monthly income is less than $15, they are better off than their urban counterparts. Mahsudpur is considered well off because many of its families own a small plot of land and one or two cows.

Most of North India's wheat farmers, over 80 per cent, own small plots of less than 8 acres, enough to sustain their families, but often not enough to get out of debt. According to some analysts, should the central government continue its farm policy of high price supports and large-scale mechanization, many tiny farmers, such as those of Mahsudpur, will be bought out and left homeless by the large agriculturalists—the top 5 per cent who own 20 or more acres—mainly upper-caste Brahmins and Rajputs.

Mahsudpur's eighty households dwell in mud-dung or brick huts set along a few narrow, often muddied paths. These quarters are loosely surrounded by a low brick wall giving way to the well and pond and a grazing area for the cows. The poorest families live in one or two rooms and a small court where the mud stove, the *chula,* burns throughout the day, boiling water or making butter-like ghee from milk. Joint families share a larger courtyard, each having its own living–sleeping area and cooking stove. Most people in India live in joint or supplemented nuclear families (including parents, unmarried children, and single, or widowed, relatives).

The well-to-do villagers like to exhibit their signs of wealth, perhaps wearing a large number of silver ankle bracelets or even keeping visible a sewing machine, all parts of dowries. The poor make do.

Viewing the rural poor, a Westerner is tempted to describe them as "passive" and attribute their resignation to a religious hope for a better life in the next incarnation. But after awhile, sharing in some of what they encounter—through the supreme luxury of choice which they do not have—I began to see them differently. They are not "passive," not indifferent about changing their circumstances. They are accepting of the unchangeable, of an otherwise overwhelmingly intense environment, the onslaught of sheer numbers of people, animals, insects, infestations, their sounds and smells, the extremes of nature, downpours and tidal waves, and searing, blinding heat. They are tired from the daily struggle to survive another day and weakened by limited food and ever-present disease. In such a world, there is little energy remaining for anger against what cannot be controlled; the inevitable frustration would soon be self-defeating, suicidal. So acceptance becomes a realistic attitude for those who have no choice but to face that life. Better to save one's anger, one's fighting spirit for the moment, should it arise, when there is some hope that struggle will produce change. That moment may have come for some minorities in the Western world, but not yet for much of India.

One of the village's poor whom I was taken to see was a young mother, looking older than her 18 years. As is the custom, she was kept separated on her hemp bedstead during the six weeks following childbirth. Her only food was *pinee,* balls of ground wheat, nuts, and ginger, and jaggery—hardened sugar cane juice—nutritious and tasty, although not delectable when taken as the sole source of food eaten in dark isolation amid a constant buzz of flies. Her premature infant fed at her breast. Her older children, toddlers, kept their distance.

Well-off or poor, the villagers share the uncertainty of the future, the hazards of the environment—from the lack of drainage for sewage to eye-burning conjunctivitis caused by their ever-smoking stoves—and, especially the women, their isolation from health and other personal services to enhance their day-to-day living.

To deal with this part of the troubles of India's rural outcasts, the central government incorporated a child welfare component into its vast Community Development Program in 1963. The purpose was to set up *balwadis,* literally "gardens of children," or day care programs in every Community Development Block (each comprising about 100 villages with about 75,000 people). There are about 5,000 such Blocks in India.

Mahsudpur's *balwadi* meets at the village *chopal,* a kind of central porch approached by steep steps and having roofed, columned areas on each side. All the village's fifty preschoolers, three- to six-year-olds, come for four hours each morning. The official maximum is thirty, more than enough for the energies of their caretakers, a village *ayah,* "helper," and a *balsevika,* "servant of children," or child care worker.

Mahsudpur's *balsevika* lives in an adjacent village and brings her baby with her to work each day. Like most *balsevikas* she came from a low-income family and was eighteen when she began the child care worker training course following her basic education.

Over 90 per cent of the 3,000 *balsevikas* who have had this 11-month course—all women—continue to work even after they marry, which virtually all of them do shortly following training. They can earn up to $35 per month—probably more than their fathers earned—working in Community Development. Although this still leaves them at the "low-income" level, they are earning more than most in nongovernment day care programs.

Training centers in eleven of India's fourteen states are under the guidance of state officials from Community Development, Social Welfare, Health, and Education, and are staffed by a social worker, teacher, and public health nurse. The prescribed program is evenly divided among classroom theory, classroom practice, and village fieldwork.

Mahsudpur's village *chopal* becomes ordered, after some initial running, climbing, and song—some of it invented by the preschoolers—when the lesson drill in counting begins, the children seated on mats, sandels off, in four long rows. Then follow some questions from the *balsevika,* to which the children quickly respond: "Where do you live? Who is your leader? Whose daughter is she? Who is your village leader? What animals can you domesticate?"

At lunchtime on the porch, the children bring their metal dishes and tumblers for their boiled egg, milk, and groundnuts (peanuts). This is another way in which the Ministry of Community Development is trying to increase the protein content in the diet of rural youngsters, recognizing that as being more basic to their general health and growth than health services. These children are lucky. For this most expensive of all nutrition programs reaches only 6 of every 100 preschoolers.

The *balsevika's* supervisor, who is from the State's Balsevika Training Center and can earn up to $120 per month, circulates through the villages where the graduates work, over a three-year period. This is a kind of inservice education to enrich their broadly based training in child development, group work, teaching techniques, recreation, and nutrition and health—including learning how to make a smokeless cooking stove. But the limitations of terrain, transportation, and time make these visits infrequent.

Before the village day care program was begun, the Block Level Community Development officials first met with the *panchayat,* the elected village council (which must include one woman to "represent" all the women). After its approval, the officials went to the *mahila mandal,* the woman's organization, to enlist their cooperation, meaning their willingness to use the program.

In addition to the child care program, Mahsudpur's village organizations also accepted a Rural Community Extension Program from the national University of Delhi. This is a two-year Master's Degree course to train middle-class, city-bred young women for Community Development work. While the expense of a graduate program for this work might be questioned, especially since few of the graduates actually go into extension work, the learning process itself seems to approach an ideal, for it requires learning by both faculty and students.

About half of the students' first year training is in the village, twice weekly and for two ten-day periods, conducting a survey and getting to know the people. The second year, extension work is done in child care, health, and home management with village families and groups. For this to be possible, the university faculty had to first come to terms with the village council and women's group, as did the students, once they were allowed to enter.

Thus the heart of community work, negotiating the approval and developing the means for participation by the consumers, is learned for what it is in reality, an open-ended process, not a set of textbook principles. Moreover, every two or three years the faculty "adopt" a new village, and so keep the process a living one. Program, teachers, and students then are aware of the continuous rhythm of initiation, negotiation, and acceptance (or rejection), a process which keeps the rendering of service relevant.

At one o'clock, as Mahsudpur's *balwadi* ends, an extension student picks up a drum, and with a song begun by a woman wearing a bright orange headpiece, calls the village women to the *chopal*. Within minutes, about twenty women and twenty of their children are seated on the rug. One of their songs is about the village boy who has gone to Delhi and now he wears a shirt and pants, no longer the traditional loose-fitting tunic and *dhoti*.

Today's demonstration–talk, requested by the women, was on stain removal. The rug was crowded, except for the area where I was sitting. Seeing this, the woman in the orange headpiece—the president of the *mahila mandal*—moved to sit next to me, and immediately the others followed her example, to everyone's comfort.

The demonstration was conducted with an easy dialogue between students and women. By way of evaluation, one woman said in Hindi, "Yes, my son comes home with ink stains. It is good that you teach me these things."

The young women faculty members who head the university extension training accompany their students to Mahsudpur by Jeep. They are welcome in the village households and are unobtrusive observers of the extension work. They want their students to dissolve the "elitism" that has been characteristic of child development programs in India, and in the teachers and preschools set up for the educated class. They want to break down arbitrary sex-role and caste distinctions, and erase as well the "great-personism," the affectations of writing and speech that are often evident in the formally educated. They think that village training, direct contact with the grass roots, helps reveal to students, and teachers, the uselessness of social barriers and jargon. Their approach is not common in India, nor probably anywhere, although it may exist in corners everywhere (1).

v For an Ancient Minority, Kyoto

Along the railroad tracks, a few minutes' walk from Kyoto Central Station, where the New Tokkaido Line's "Bullet" Train quietly and punctually and comfortably brings its Tokyo passengers, is a small neighborhood, once called a *buraku*. It seems uncharacteristically smudged. Its dried-out wood housing is tightly packed and cramped and uneven, not compact and pleasing as one becomes accustomed to seeing in Japan. Refuse sometimes clogs the narrow canals fed by the River Kamo, which flows among 1,500 households, producing stench.

These families have been here for centuries, since the days when they were relegated the lowly tasks of animal butchery and leathercraft, and so ostracized by Buddhist rulers. In time these outcasts became a ready supply of underworld workers, willing to do the unlawful bidding of the people in power. They are still called *eta* and *hinin,* less-than-human. Thus branded by history, they remain outcasts. Now some 2 million in Japan, they are heirs to some of the least desirable living conditions in Kyoto and to jobs that keep them at no higher than a lower-middle income.

This *Do-wa* district is one of nineteen which the City of Kyoto is trying to upgrade, attempting to counteract discrimination by special funds and programs. The core of this effort in the neighborhood is at the Soijin Community Center, a municipal subcenter begun fifteen years ago. It also houses a day nursery.

"Day nursery" in Japan means all-day care for children up to six years, who then enter the public school system (which is compulsory through grade nine). "Kindergarten" is preschool education for three-, four-, and five-year-olds, usually lasting four hours.

Soijin Day Nursery now takes care of about half of the *Do-wa* community's 700 preschoolers, infants to school-age, during their parents' working day, about eight to ten hours. Parents pay $2.50 per month, in contrast to the $6–10 charged in other districts.

The nursery is housed on two floors, crib and crawling rooms upstairs. Downstairs, many rooms open onto a playground for small groups of three- to five-year-olds. About three-fourths of the children are over three years old. Unlike other city-run nurseries in middle-income areas—which each care for only about 100 children—this one has somewhat of a gray cast (and is perhaps grayer during *tsuyu,* the rainy season, when I saw it). The walls are child-marked, the floors worn, the playground is barren earth, not as is usual a yard of flowers and grass; there are no polished wood-block floors or mosaics on the walls, no public address and music system or other electronic equipment, no tile bathing pools, no full-time public health nurse.

Yet, the essentials for comfort and health are present, as is the grace of Japanese form, removing one's shoes at the door, low bows of greeting, the sipping of light green tea. Most importantly, the mothering of children receives greatest emphasis, in terms of time and money and personnel.

Greatly exceeding national standards for adult to child ratios (1:10 for children under two years, 1:30 for those over two years) the Soijin nursery has one child care worker for every 15 three- to five-year-olds, one for each group of 5 one- to three-year-olds, and one for each group of 4 children under one. These workers are the *hobo-san.*

Hobo-san are the primary caretakers of young children in Japan's almost 13,500 day nurseries. They receive two years of junior college training. The health and welfare of preschoolers is stressed in the classroom as well as during weekly one-day fieldwork in a day care program and an extended period during the summer. Local governments are responsible for licensing them according to standards set by the national Ministry of Health and Welfare.

In Kyoto, during their first year of work all *hobo-san* receive a special orientation to the *Do-wa* districts by the city's Child Welfare Department and must see to their own continuing education through the local Hobo-San Study Group, a worker-oriented group of alterprofessionals. This group, among other things, has put together balanced meal patterns which are used in the city's nurseries.

Following some work experience, the *hobo-san* may take a civil service examination which then qualifies them for promotion to supervisor, with a salary that eventually can almost triple their initial $100 per month wage. Thus young women, or older women who have raised their families, may in two years train for a job based on a secondary education (more than 75 per cent of Japanese students now enter high school). They are then in a position, rather unique among vocations and professions, for qualifying themselves by whatever style of learning suits their sensibilities, emphasizing informal study or direct experience, for a sizable promotion in terms of responsibility, variety of work, and income.

The *hobo-san* are at something of a disadvantage, however. Their counterparts in kindergarten programs are *kyoyu,* preschool teachers. The training of *kyoyu* is very similar to that of the *hobo-san.* The two types of workers are often taught in the same institutions by the same educators—mostly *kyoyu* who have had four years of college—for the same period of time, two years. The teaching of the student teachers emphasizes methods of education and that of the child care workers emphasizes health care, although the amount and types of practical experience for the students is similar. *Kyoyu* and *hobo-san* may work in either the all-day nurseries or half-day kindergartens. Even in terms of salary, the child care worker can be earning the same as the preschool teacher within two years.

The *kyoyu* may qualify themselves for promotion to supervisors or teachers of *kyoyu* by taking two more years of college; but the *hobo-san* cannot crossover into the realm of preschool teaching except by starting at the beginning of *kyoyu* training.

Probably one of the main reasons for this rigidity, as well as the somewhat anachronistic pattern of having two separate types of workers, similarly trained for similar work, is the territoriality problem. That is, the child care workers are trained and licensed under the jurisdiction of the Ministry of Health and Welfare. The preschool teachers are under the Ministry of Education. Should both types of workers be joined under one department, the other ministry would lose authority and power, including a portion of its budgetary allocation. The distinction between the *hobo-san* and *kyoyu* also makes for a separation of social classes, routing less privileged women into the less prestigious *hobo-san* training.

The need for *hobo-san* and *kyoyu* will increase, in line with a 1968 national government report which recommended group day care for children over three months of age for urban families in which parents work or are unable to care for their children. Kyoto is seeking to increase its day nurseries by ten each year, not only for working parents, but especially for all families in *Do-wa* areas.

The Soijin Day Nursery, encapsulated in the Community Center, does more than oversee the health and safety of preschoolers, more than allow parents to work, more than deal with individual problems when the *hobo-san* visit parents at home or talk with them at the monthly parents' meetings. The wider programs of the Center make the day nursery a more effective means of freeing people from social constraints in the long term. The Center's program for improving the environment, housing, and drainage will make individual health care and medical treatment longer lasting. Special employment for women—even if it is janitorial work, a not uncommon sight on Kyoto streets—will alter their traditional homebound place and economic dependence, as will the educational programs for young people and older women offered there. The Center also has been building a grass-roots organization of *Do-wa* dwellers, aimed at influencing city policy, demanding more changes, faster, in the district—including the assignment of a full time physician and nurse in the Center instead of the present twice-yearly visits to examine the children (2).

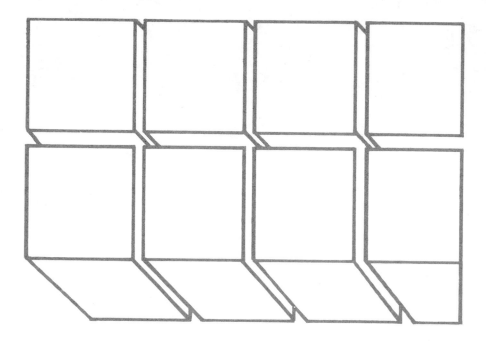

part four

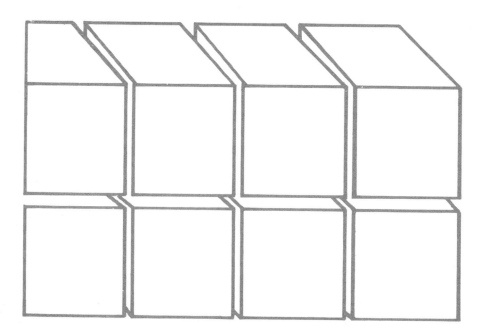

Access to
Decision Making

chapter 8

Making and Implementing Decisions

The problems of delivering health services and of organizing the health occupations are intertwined. Further, both networks share the interrelated problems of unequal access and specialist emphasis, as well as the associated question of efficacy: whether current patterns are related to contemporary needs for health services of various social groups, and whether present methods and techniques in the provision of and training for health services, at the organizational or the individual levels, are, in fact, filling their intended purposes (Figure 8–1).

The choices of approaches to deal with these problems, clearly, as the previous chapter illustrates, may limit how thoroughly issues can be dealt with. The decision making involved in one sphere of health care usually has ramifying effects in other areas. Most important, the policy decisions made for health-care-related issues are tied to conditions in the societal environment, viewed in the broadest sense. This includes sociopolitical economics and the ecological and technological considerations of the sort discussed in Chapters 1 and 2.

Decision Making as Bargaining

In the final analysis, decisions concerning health-related issues, as for any other social question, mean generating resources of certain types (funds, facilities, personnel, expertise) and amounts and allocating those resources. Since no social groups, whether they are formal organizations (such as hospitals, insurance companies, or professions) or demographic groupings

219

Figure 8–1 Health Care Decision-making Schema, United States

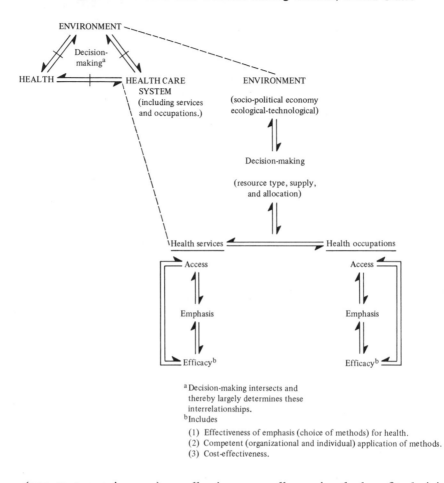

a Decision-making intersects and
thereby largely determines these
interrelationships.
b Includes

(1) Effectiveness of emphasis (choice of methods) for health.
(2) Competent (organizational and individual) application of methods.
(3) Cost-effectiveness.

(sex–race–age–income) equally give or equally receive the benefits deriving from these decisions, the process of decision making is one of bargaining. The aim is simply to acquire resources or assure the potential for acquiring resources in the future, in effect to ensure the growth or at least survival of the organization or group. This might mean, for example, for a health care organization, acquiring more personnel, equipment, facilities, or the funds to purchase these; or it may mean none of these in return for concurring in a decision, but rather the assurance of certain *strategic* resources, such as access to policy-making channels and timely information, which would allow for an effective gain in resources in the future (1).

Power

Such bargaining is the nature of power relations, power being the capacity to bargain effectively. The most powerful, of course, are those who for various reasons have most of the bargainable resources, and thus have the largest array of effective choices. They may choose among alternatives in confronting an issue in a bargaining situation, and their choice will enhance their resources or resource-getting capacity.

Prerequisites

Effective bargaining between groups has of course many prerequisites, especially concerning interorganizational decisions, which in health-related as well as other social matters are increasingly taken at the national and governmental level. This means that the major organizations and groups involved include certain segments in the legislative and administrative branches of government, and their constituencies as well. These include those who receive tax health funds, state and local health agencies and hospitals; fiscal intermediaries, the insurance companies; drug and equipment firms; universities and training centers; and groups of individual practitioners, such as physicians, dentists, pharmacists, and nurses, among others. Any may be public or private nonprofit or for-profit.

ORGANIZATION AND FUNDS

Necessary to their bargaining capacity is first organization, which also implies the funds to form organizations. Groups representing the interests of certain health care providers, such as physicians, dentists, hospitals, and insurers, have been among the most influential and largest spenders among the registered national lobbies, particularly since the late 1940s, when consideration of extensive national health legislation began (2).

Effective bargaining also requires access to policy-making channels—the points at which the posing of the problems are made, the alternatives for solution considered, and the criteria for making choices determined. Such channels, in the formulation of health policy at national or local levels, are, as earlier described, scattered and not integrated regarding programming or in time, from one administration to another (3). This often allows a *de facto* form of policy making, that is, policy shaped by those who have best access to the various stages of decision making at any given point in time.

Various means have been used in the hope of gaining easier access to such channels. For example, until the early 1970s at least, more than 80 per cent of political campaign contributions came from the largest corporations, and health-related industries were among the largest givers (4). Professional groups have also formed overtly political arms (5). Further, informal, but organized, contacts have also been used, such as between physician and patient–Congressman (6).

INFORMATION EXCHANGE

In addition or alternative to direct access is access to the information to be supplied to decision makers, and/or the information on which decisions are to be based, and/or the probable and early decisions made before public announcement. Analysis has shown that policy and legislation are often not based on systematic research but on information limited to what is made available to decision makers (7). Further, other than public interest considerations have been emphasized, such as the benefits of using technological solutions to health care problems for those who manufacture and are trained to use technological equipment and processes (8).

The larger lobbying groups often become, in effect, the information-gathering arms for those who write legislation. For example, the report of the Commission on Hospital Care, set up by the American Hospital Association, led to the Hill–Burton legislation allowing hospital construction with public funds (9).

Further, the additional funds for information gathering done by groups of health care providers are sometimes granted by private foundations. The subsequent reports of findings have then been influential in both public and nonpublic health care policy. For example, funds from the Rockefeller, Kellogg, and Russell Sage Foundations have had great impact on the type and direction of physician and nursing education. In the early 1970s, foundation health-related funds were primarily directed toward hospital-related interests (10). Such foundations, as private institutions, have of course no means to account to the public for the direction of their allocations and the eventual influence which their study projects may have on the public.

Congress, in 1973, in recognition of the limited types and sources of information on which to base its legislative decisions, was considering other means for establishing a data base, at least concerning complex technical and scientific matters (11).

SOME EFFECTS OF ACCESS

Access to the formal and informal decision-revision processes can also be very important in affecting approaches to and the effects of health care decision making. Such access can assure a bargaining outcome which increases the resources or future bargaining capacity of the bargainer group. Organizations of health care providers have, for example, been able to shape the federal regulations prior to the implementation of certain national health legislation such that they were allowed generous loopholes; or such that the time period for response to regulations[1] was extended and they were allowed unusual legislative hearings on the administrative rules with eventual rules revision; or such that they were able to have new laws amended so that they were more to their liking (12).

Once the regulations have been determined, the implementation of policy embodied in law and executive order has not necessarily resulted in the intent of prior decisions. For example, although mandated by the Congress, the Department of Health, Education, and Welfare had in the early 1970s failed to report studies that could have shifted hospital construction allocations; had not placed a physician in counties where no physician was available; had not allocated most of the community mental health center funds designated for poverty areas; and had not evenly distributed funds for area health education centers (AHEC) because of vying for such funds within HEW (13).

As a case in point, the AHEC program was intended to provide in rural areas training for a variety of health personnel, and continuing education for health personnel working and living in the localities. Initially funding was to be in line with a regional plan for health services worked out under the Regional Medical Programs (RMP) and tied to Veterans Administration (VA) medical support facilities. Both programs, RMP and VA, envisioned uncertain futures if they pursued their traditional acute care, hospital-based emphasis. By seeking to sponsor AHEC programming, they would thus have a place in the presumed primary care, non-hospital-focused health system of the future. The AHEC allocations, when finally made, however, granted $10 million dollars to 10 university medical schools under a third HEW agency, separate from RMP or VA. Thus the medical centers had the use of more AHEC funds than RMP and VA—which continued to sponsor small similar programs, called area health education activities (AHEA) (14).

At other than the national levels of implementation of course, the intent of decisions to provide health services may also be deterred, altered, or subverted. Numerous examples exist, including one where it was necessary to locate maternity and infant care programs—intended for poor families —at medical centers because of the difficulties in getting specialists to go to ghetto- or rural-based facilities; this was done to assure the continued participation of medical schools, which wanted patient "teaching material" (15).

[1] Usually 30 days after publication in the *Federal Register*.

Such untoward effects are not, of course, limited to publically financed programs. The efforts of any health organization to retain or acquire resources may lead it to establish, implement, or refuse to give up programs, with the effect of limiting its intended and stated health care purposes. Examples might include how many facilities set up costly and underused cardiac or dialysis units rather than regionalizing such equipment, or similarly, refuse to share other special services such as underused pediatrics wards (16). In practice, retaining such equipment and services helps them, in turn, retain specialist practitioners and a specialist or prestigious public image, which further attracts private donations, research grants, and other means for acquiring new resources (17).

A Set of Processes

As it exists then, decision making is a set of interorganizational/intergroup and political processes. Quite clearly, other constituencies of government, the voters, taxpayers, the consumers of services, do not ordinarily have comparable means to enter these decision-making processes.

Access to decision making means the opportunity for those affected by the decisions to be made to influence the *posing* of the problems to be decided, the *alternatives* from which the choice for solutions are to be made, and the *criteria* on which selection is to be based. Then, following the *selection* of "a solution" or set of proposed actions—the decision—comes (if decision revision does not intervene) the implementation or *control* phase—in other words, assuring the effectiveness of the decision through setting administrative policy and regulation.

To participate in the full decision-making cycle means also to have input into the feedback mechanisms, which in effect are the responses to the decision—whether the decision accomplished its purpose as well as how it was received. This is, in a word, *evaluation*.

Finally, with evaluation, comes the decisions as to how to deal with those effects or outcomes of decisions, in other words, whether and what new decisions or *changes* must be made. These latter aspects of decision making, evaluation and changing the system, will be taken up in Chapters 9 and 10.

The processes of decision making—from the posing of the problem, of alternative solutions, of criteria for choice, through making a choice, effectively implementing it, evaluating feedback, and considering changes—clearly involves many decisions, any of which may affect the outcome and effectiveness of a single decision. Such processes, in the realm of health care as well as any other set of human activities, are repeated at national (and international) and local levels; they occur between organizations, between groups within organizations, and between individuals,[2] as well as between individual and group. In the field of human services, of which the personal health care system is part, the organizations involved are most often health care providers, whether fiscal, institutional, or as practitioners; the individual is most often the consumer of services, unrepresented by an organized group.

These pages will now focus on the decision-making processes related to issues of control, particularly among health care providers at the inter-organizational level, second, between providers and the consumers of health services, and then briefly, between groups within health care facilities.

Making Decisions Effective: Controls and Providers

Control deals at the broadest level with the question of how to make a system of health services effective in contributing to the health of populations. In somewhat different terms it means asking whether the outcomes in better health so attained are worth the resources invested in the system. If not, there follows the question of whether those resources might be better invested elsewhere or in other ways in order to bring about better levels of health, or the same levels of health to more of the population.

In any case, the point at issue is the balance between social costs and the quality and amount of benefits—in particular, financial costs—in relation to gains in health. Finances, as the universal liquid resource, relate, of course, to all major health system problems. In recent years, particularly since the increase in public financing of health services, the search for control mechanisms to implement effective health care has focused on the most immediate and apparent problem, that of limiting rising costs. Other kinds of controls, focusing on the competence of individuals and other institutional standards of quality of health care, such as licensure, certification, and accreditation, were discussed in the previous section, as were some of the decision-making processes between and within organizations which led to these forms of control.

Provider-Determined Methods

Thus under the traditional and current views of priority problems in health care, forms of control—that is, means of implementing standards of ef-

---

[2] Only here, between individuals, is there really the human possibility for having decision-making processes based on something other than a bargaining or political relationship.

fectiveness and efficiency—have focused on competence or quality (the predominant method in the past) and more recently on cost. In other words, *these* are the emphases which resulted from decisions concerning the posing of problems, priorities, and methods, and not alternative foci for controls, such as assuring full access, need-based emphasis, and population-based efficacy of health services.

Cost Controls

FISCAL MEANS

Cost control measures discussed earlier (Chapter 5) were of the fiscal or monetary type. These included the ones directed at consumers, such as cost sharing through deductibles and copayments, and the ones aimed at providers, as salaried earnings or the risk sharing involved in capitation payments, or the limitation of payable "reasonable"[3] charges (18).

NONFISCAL MEANS

Nonfiscal consumer-directed cost controls included limitations on services which could be covered by insurance and/or limiting the eligibility of certain groups to certain services. That is, at an extreme, insuring the healthiest groups for the least-costly services would mean lowest expenditures by the insuring organization.

Control over rising costs by nonfiscal means aimed at providers of health services, rather than consumers, has received increasing attention recently because of their hoped-for greater potential impact on costs and quality of services. The health maintenance organization (HMO) described earlier is one attempt at combining cost and quality controls with a system of delivery. A discussion of other combined cost and quality methods, and some of the decision making that produced them, follows.

Cost–Quality Control Mechanisms

The time is past when the question of *whether* to have controls on health care providers was at issue. That debate ended in the late 1960s as a result

[3] Newly defined in 1972 as not to exceed the 75th percentile of actual charges for similar services in the area during the previous year, and charges for medical supplies and equipment that do not exceed the lowest levels at which such are widely available in the area [Social Security Amendments of 1972 (P.L. 92–603)].

of the compromises that were needed to pass the Medicare–Medicaid amendments to the Social Security Acts. Medicare, Part A, granted to the hospitals full cost reimbursement and to the private insurance companies the prerogative of acting as fiscal intermediaries with cost-plus reimbursement for their services to the government, and relieved them of the unprofitable burden of health insurance for the aged and poor. Part B guaranteed to physicians fee-for-service payments based on their own determination of charges, and made the insurance industry the carriers for the supplemental nonhospital benefits of Part B. Further was the stipulation that government was in no way authorized to interfere in the patterns of providing medical services (19).

Thus it was apparently necessary—in order to enact a national policy of assuring health services to the aged and poor—to guarantee to private providers, open-ended payments and noninterference. The result of these guarantees, however, contributed heavily to accelerating costs that have required increasingly stringent efforts to bring under control.

This situation meant, then, that policy questions, the posing of the problems, no longer involved whether, but rather what kinds of cost controls should be used, directed at which group(s) of providers, and administered by whom.

By the early 1970s, mechanisms for control over the development of health services—initially of a voluntary type and focusing on planning and coordination—had been revised. The new emphases were on compulsory participation of health care providers receiving social security financing—Medicare, Medicaid, and maternal–child health funds—and on methods to withhold funds for services and facilities that were adjudged unnecessary. Most of these more stringent measures were enacted through amendments to the Public Health Service and the Social Security Acts (Figure 8–2).

PLANNING

Comprehensive Health Planning Agencies In 1973 comprehensive health planning (CHP) agencies, after about five years of development, existed on a statewide level [(a) agencies] in the 50 states and at more than 200 related areawide levels [(b) agencies]. Their purpose was to assess, on a geographic–population basis, needs for facilities, services, and personnel, in cooperation with all types of public and private health care provider and consumer groups (who were to be represented on their policy-making boards). Half the funds for this program came from the federal government, a fourth from state and local government, and much of the remainder from hospitals, hospital associations, and insurance companies (20). In practice, the areawide (b) agencies consisted of about

Figure 8–2 Health Services Controls, United States

Major Organizational, Statutory Mechanisms

Organizational Entity	Total Number	Method	Legal Authorization
Hill-Burton State Hospital Planning Agencies	50	Planning and coordination; hospital services; state-wide; voluntary.	Federal Public Health Service Act, Amendments for Hospital Survey and Construction, 1946 (1949, 1954, 1961, 1964, 1967, 1970).
Regional Medical Programs (RMP)	56	Planning and coordination; primary and specialized services; regional, in-stitutional and non-institutional providers; voluntary.	Public Health Service Act, Heart Disease, Cancer and Stoke Amendments of 1965 (1968, 1970).
Area Health Education Activities (AHEA)	57	Planning and coordination; areawide training; voluntary.	Public Health Service Act amendments as above.
Area Health Education Centers (AHEC)	10	As above.	Public Health Service Act, Comprehensive Health Manpower Training Act of 1971.
Experimental Health Services Delivery Systems (EHSDS)	19	Planning and coordination; areawide services deliv-ery; all provider types; voluntary.	Public Health Service Act, Partnership for Health Amendments of 1967 (establishing National Center for Health Services Research and Development.)
Experimental Medical Care Review Organi-zation (EMCRO)	10	Evaluation of quality of services; areawide; all provider types;	As above.
Comprehensive Health Planning Agencies: State ("a") agencies / Areawide ("b") agencies	50 / 208	Planning and coordination; state and areawide; pri-marily institutional services, authorized to plan for services, fac-ilities, personnel; voluntary.	Public Health Service Act, Comprehensive Health Planning Amendments of 1966, (1967, 1970).
with certification of need authority[a]	20	Capital expenditures control over institu-tional facilities for changes above a given dollar amount; mandatory.	State certification of need laws in 20 states.
as Designated Plan Agencies (DPA)[b]	47	Capital expenditures control over providers receiving federal financing for Medicare, Medicaid, or maternal and child health services over program revisions of $100,000 or more for facilities/equipment; mandatory.	Federal Social Security Act, Amendments of 1972, Sec. 1122.
Utilization Review (UR)[c]		Peer review; institu-tional services of pro-viders receiving federal financing for Medicare and Medicaid services; mandatory.	Social Security Amend-ments of 1965 (Medicare); 1967.
State agency sample-resurvey of JCAH-approved hospitals[d]		Certification review of Medicare-approved hosptials; mandatory.	Social Security Amend-ments of 1972.
Professional Standards Review Organizations (PSRO)	41	Claims review; insti-tutional and non-institu-tional services of providers under Medicare, Medicaid, maternal and child health services financing; mandatory.	Social Security Amend-ments of 1972.

[a] In a few states this authority is given to the Hill-Burton or other planning agency.

[b] The Hill-Burton agency was so designated in six states; the statewide Comprehensive Health Planning agency in four states by 1973.

[c] Required, but not fully operative in Medicare-certified hospitals (numbering 6,700).

[d] Joint Commission on Hospital Accreditation is the private agency that certifies hospitals as meeting minimum standards in order to receive Medicare financing.

Data sources: *Compilation of Selected Public Health Laws*, Vol. 1 (Washington, D.C.: Government Printing Office, 1971).
Comptroller General of the United States, *Study of Health Facilities Construction Costs* (Washington, D.C.: Government Printing Office, 1972).
W. Curran, *National Survey and Analysis of Certificate-of-Need Laws 1972* (Chicago: American Hospital Association, 1973).
National Center for Health Law.
Health Planning Memorandum, Department of Health, Education, and Welfare, Feb. 1973.

six persons with a $110,000 budget, who were required to spend an appreciable part of their time seeking assurances of annual funding from their donors. Perhaps as a consequence, fewer than one in five were able to develop the beginnings of a master plan, which was their mandate (21) (Figure 8–2).

Certificate-of-Need Laws In addition to problems of finding adequate and disinterested financing were the lack of hard criteria to determine the health care needs of populations and the power to prevent the development of what was not needed. In an effort to remedy some of this, a number of states, 20 by 1973, passed certificate-of-need laws. These usually gave the (b) agencies review-and-approval authority over applications by hospitals and nursing care facilities for any expansion costing anywhere from $50,000 to $350,000 as a minimum; a few states extended this control over ambulatory facilities as well, while, however, exempting physicians' offices or services (22).

With this authority, CHP agencies prevented unnecessary expanded or new facilities construction in about two thirds of 115 applications by 1973. This kind of a restriction was seen as an improvement not possible under the earlier voluntary methods of state hospital planning councils (set up to administer Hill–Burton funds) (23).

State certificate-of-need legislation has been supported by the hospital associations, the not-for-profit insurers, Blue Cross, the health planning agencies, and state health department and insurance rate control commissions. In opposition have been the for-profit hospitals; medical societies, who feared a legal base for hospital power; and nursing homes, most of which are for-profit. These groups sought voluntary, cooperative approaches (24).

The American Hospital Association, basically composed of the not-for-profit hospitals, further advocated, under a certification-of-need method, a public utilities approach to control over inpatient facilities. This would amount to franchising not-for-profit hospital corporations in given localities, producing a "monopoly" similar to that of public utilities (25).

The likelihood of this step in the near future seems limited. One reason is that in states where proposed certificate-of-need legislation included authority over long-term, and usually for-profit hospital facilities, the laws often failed to pass, an indication of the decision-making influence of for-profit hospitals (26). Second, a recent state supreme court ruling declared such a law unconstitutional because it tended to create a nonprofit monopoly, and further, that public utilities monopolies are controlled not directly but indirectly by state rate setting[4] (27). Such developments on a state level, limiting the power of certificate-of-need methods, could lead to vesting cost control instead in rate-setting commissions similar to those regulating insurance companies,[5] or, alternatively, to revising CHP agency authority as a fully legal agency with elected, and thus publically accountable, members (28). Such an agency could then be empowered to act in ways similar to local school boards (29).

Federal Government Action In spite of CHP agency control activity, however, fully 40 per cent of U.S. hospitals were planning new construction in 1972, even though bed-occupancy rates had continued to decline each year since 1966 (30). This fact among others brought a significant change in CHP control potential through federal government action. Under the 1972 Social Security Amendments, states could name a "designated plan agency" to carry out capital expenditures control over all health care providers (except individual practitioners) receiving social security financing, when such expenditures exceeded $100,000. This amounted to a national certificate-of-need law, for without the approval of the designated plan agency (whose mandate included development of a state health resources plan), federal development funds would be withheld. Most states were naming their CHP agencies for this responsibility; a few named the state hospital planning (Hill–Burton) council (31). The funds for such "cost containment" activities were to come from the Social Security Trust Fund, thereby assuring additional, consistent, and out-of-state support for such regulatory tasks (32) (Figure 8–2).

Thus comprehensive health planning agencies were moving from an initial voluntary, planning, and coordination approach to areawide health services development toward an increasingly mandatory, cost-control focus, first through state and then federal government empowerment. Among the issues that persisted were those of reconciling their status as nonlegal agencies with public accountability for their decisions affecting the allocation of public funds; whether control of capital expenditures could indeed control the costs of health services, much less bring about the array of locally needed services; and whether this regulatory agency approach could, in fact, regulate, and avoid becoming dominated by the health industry (33). In the few years of CHP operation, there has been a direct relationship between the time spent on hospital bed control and the amount of funds contributed by hospital interests to the CHP agencies (34).

---

[4] This does not, however, accurately reflect the *direct* methods of control over television-radio broadcasting or air travel [see W. Curran, "A Severe Blow to Hospital Planning: 'Certification of Need' Declared Unconstitutional." *N. Eng. J. Med.* 288:723–4 (Apr. 5, 1973)].

[5] Pennsylvania, Maryland, Washington, Connecticut, and California were among states moving in this direction in 1973.

Regulatory Agency Methods This question of the relationship between the regulators and regulated has some of its answer in the history of regulatory agencies. Most, if not all, such agencies were sought by the industry to be regulated. For the processes involved in regulation tend to bring competitors under control. The regulator–regulated relationship, opponents claim, amounts to a bargaining process that has resulted in accommodation with industries' interests rather than decisions in the public interest; and public, decisive, planning is not compatible in such circumstances (35).

The influence of the regulated on the decisions of the regulators has been found to come not primarily from such questionable practices as enticement with high-paying industry jobs following tenure in the regulatory agency, or through extensive hospitality, or by inducing governmental executive or legislative branch intervention. Rather, it comes from the continuous exposure of the regulators to the industry's point of view, a result, in part, of the regulatory process. In effect, this means frequent and ready access to the regulatory decision makers by the regulated industry in contrast to infrequent and difficult access by the public, the consumers of services and products (36).

Thus, whether a certificate-of-need agency, limiting capital expenditures, or a state rate commission limiting insurance premiums, the potential for effective regulation in the interests of economical and needed services for use by the public could be limited because of the health industry's representation in, funds for, and frequent access to decision-making agencies and the information and alternatives used in their regulatory decisions.

These fears of what can become a kind of self-regulation have been borne out to some extent in the self-regulatory processes of the health professions, earlier described, while malpractice suits increase; in the certification, by a joint physician–hospital association commission (JCAH), of hospitals whose patient services nevertheless have been of less than acceptable quality; or in other attempts, mandated by federal legislation to encourage the regulation of cost and quality of health services (37).

PEER REVIEW

Utilization Review One of the earliest such federal government efforts was the establishment of hospital utilization review under the Medicare insurance program in 1965. It was to be a continuing review by each hospital of its own patterns of services, particularly the necessity of certain services to a sample of patients, and a means by which to recommend improvements. Such a review procedure was required before a hospital could receive JCAH approval, which in turn the Social Security Administration accepted as certifying its adequacy to receive Medicare funds. The fiscal intermediaries such as Blue Cross or other insurance companies, which were to process Medicare claims, were, with state health departments, required to assure that the hospital would, in fact, carry out continuous utilization review (38).

Studies of the results of this method of control by the Social Security Administration and the Congress in 1969, 1970, and 1972 showed numerous breaks in the implementation of Congressional intent. Program regulations were framed in the interests of hospital management; JCAH approval was granted without hospitals meeting certification requirements; fiscal intermediaries ignored their responsibility to assure utilization review; hospitals reviewed only 60–90 per cent of the required items (39).

Beyond problems of assuring implementation in the 6,700 hospitals involved, the outcome of this review technique for controlling overutilization of hospital services, and therefore costs, showed a limited effect. Overuse was controlled primarily where hospital beds were in short supply to begin with (40). Second, few studies examined whether the quality of services was improved by this approach (41). Further, there was no coordination between reviews of Medicare and Medicaid services, or integrated reviews of inpatient and outpatient services (42).

Based on these findings, the 1972 Social Security Amendments required the States to do a sample resurvey of JCAH-approved hospitals, and, further, that hospitals found not to have an effective utilization review of Medicaid services would lose a portion of their federal funding (43). Reimbursement for services thus became tied to institutional review of utilization practices.

CLAIMS REVIEW

PSROs: Gatekeepers to Provider Resources   A potentially more rigorous and extensive control mechanism in the 1972 Amendments was the Professional Standards Review Organizations (PSRO). The PSRO approach differed from utilization review in a number of ways. It was not only to review the process of medical services to patients, but to do so on an area-wide basis, and could include all health care providers—health maintenance organizations, group practices, public and private clinics, independent practitioners, as well as hospitals and nursing facilities—receiving Medicare–Medicaid funds. Further, it was to review all claims and could stop payment for medically unnecessary services or for inpatient treatment that was possible on an outpatient basis. Finally, if it were operating effectively, the PSRO was to supersede all other forms of review and control. That is, the Department of Health, Education, and Welfare could waive all other prerequisites for Medicare–Medicaid payments to health care providers in a given PSRO area, including hospital utilization review (44).

PSROs as a concept were derived from the foundations for medical care (FMC), which confined themselves to reviewing the claims of private physicians for health insurance carriers' payments, including government insurers as Medicare (which pay most of the claims now) (45). In addition to cost control, a hoped-for emphasis was to be the assurance of quality of services, in terms of necessary, appropriate, and effective treatment related to diagnostic and age–sex–regional criteria.

The necessary research for establishing such criteria, the "patient profiles" and "provider profiles" against which to judge patterns of services, had just begun in the early 1970s in 10 experimental medical care review organizations (EMCRO) under the HEW National Center for Health Services Research and Development (46). These EMCROs were new or in fact ongoing claims review foundations for medical care. Their profile-development research was not part of the policy decision to implement PSROs nationwide, although their findings would presumably be fed to PSROs in time (47).

The claims-review type of FMCs were sponsored by medical societies, and EMCROs were state or county medical society affiliates. Thus the new PSROs were to follow this model. The explicit intent of the Congressional authors was in fact to view the PSRO, a cost and quality-control mechanism, as the perhaps last best chance for physicians to retain control over medical practice (48).

Initially, the AMA sought a less rigorous and statewide form of PSRO insurance claims review. Other physician groups supported certain changes, which were ultimately enacted. These included county or areawide PSROs rather than a single statewide agency with subunits; notification to all area physicians by HEW of a pending HEW–PSRO proposal, with an option to poll all physicians as to the PSRO's representativeness of area physicians; the stipulation that organizations other than hospitals and nursing facilities need not be under PSRO control unless specifically agreed to by HEW; and that a two-year trial period exist prior to final and full designation of the official control agency (after which an alternative, not necessarily physician-run group could be set up) (49).

Following the 1972 enactment, the AMA pressed for several amendments, including one that did not limit the number of physicians who could be included in PSRO membership, and thus, in effect, permit statewide PSROs (50). Six months prior to the scheduled implementation of the PSRO program, 27 state medical societies had sought designation as statewide PSROs (51).

Physicians and HMOs The activities surrounding the development of PSRO legislation, having a four- to five-year history, clearly suggest the potential which this type of control mechanism has for affecting the future resource-getting options for health care providers. It is perhaps evident why physicians in HMOs, or those in university medical center facilities—all of whose practices and federal reimbursements would be reviewable by PSROs—would seek to ensure that other than solely medical society physicians, representative of private, fee-for-service practitioners, be a significant part of PSRO control. These nonprivate practitioners would thus be likely to support such safeguards as local rather than statewide organizations, a poll for judging representativeness, and not making mandatory the review of ambulatory nonhospital services, such as those in HMOs.

Conceivably, a PSRO, by judging the pattern of services given by an HMO, for example, to be below a necessary amount, could then prevent its receipt of Medicare–Medicaid funds, jeopardizing its economic viability. Conversely, if the HMO were required to render more services to meet a level determined by the PSRO, that would raise the HMO's costs, and thus its premiums, thus placing it perhaps at a competitive disadvantage under current typical conditions with other forms of health care delivery. Such circumstances might then even prevent others' attempts to develop new HMOs or other new forms of health care delivery (52).

PSROs and Hospitals Beyond the interests of various groups of physicians, other kinds of health care providers sought to affect the design of PSROs. The American Hospital Association called for physicians who belonged to PSROs and were also affiliated with hospitals to be responsible first to the hospital board. Under the legislation, a PSRO could accept the findings of hospital utilization review committees, if it found these to be effective. PSROs were, however, given the authority to inspect premises and all records in the carrying out of their mandate (53). Thus the primary allegiance of physicians and the ultimate control over review were at issue as an unsettled negotiable matter in PSRO policy at the end of 1973, prior to the January 1974 scheduled implementation.

The PSROs also must determine and publish their findings as to the types of health care delivery that are most effective and efficient in their region. This would have the effect of good publicity for certain types of delivery and/or methods of financing health services. Thus PSROs could have an effect on the resource-getting capacity, the growth potential, of conventional insurance companies.

PSROs and the Insurance Industry The health insurance companies, as earlier described, were unwilling to become either dependent on earlier claims review FMCs or to be replaced by HMOs (as combined delivery–financing systems) (54). So they developed formal sponsorship and development of both types of organizations. Following the establishment of

PSROs—the equivalent of claims review FMCs for publically insured health care—they offered a proposal to the medical profession. Their proposition included the formalizing of agreements between insurance carriers and medical societies as to the design of PSROs, prior to contracting with the federal government. Insurance companies would, then, with other types of health care providers in the area, sit on the governing board, be a part of peer review committees as nonvoting consultants, and have access to the results of the peer review process. They would also take part in developing the guidelines for necessary services and publishing these for consumer use. They proposed that the PSROs merge with the AHA plan for retaining hospital utilization review with the PSRO as overseer. They sought consumer involvement in PSRO policy in the form of board representation from business management and organized labor. Finally, the baseline "profiles" of services, against which PSRO panels would judge necessary and reimbursable charges, would take into account the "experience-rating" method and data used by insurance carriers, as well as by government programs (55). Such an approach could lessen the amount of necessary, and therefore reimbursable, services.

The advantages of this type of PSRO physician–insurance carrier collaboration to the insurance companies include access to decision making over the control process, and to review findings to enhance their own planning; influence in the publicity activities; and—because all types of delivery as well as both public and private patient services would come under review—the expected results of lower utilization, and lower payable charges, would accrue to the private insurance carriers as well as Medicare–Medicaid. For if the costs for public patients were lowered, health institutions' unit costs could remain high for a long time, costs which then would ultimately be borne by private patients and their private insurance companies (56).

The insurance industry, then, in order to retain or improve its options for acquiring health care funds, framed this proposal in support of the PSRO as a regulatory mechanism. Similarly, it had supported the development of comprehensive health planning agencies with certificate-of-need authority and hospital rate review commissions (57).

PSROs and Comprehensive Health Planning Agencies   The PSRO's counterparts in cost control, the comprehensive health planning agencies, whose mandate includes the regulation of capital expenditures by health care facilities, early determined their posture in relation to PSROs. They, as a national association, sought to obtain from HEW review-and-comment responsibility over PSRO applications and area designations within the various CHP areas (58). This has similarity to the late 1960s, when newly forming CHP agencies experienced jurisdictional confusion, if not territorial disputes, with the previously formed Regional Medical Programs

(RMPs), which, since then, have been given changing and wide-ranging planning and coordination, health services, and educational authority.

One federal effort to form an amalgam of this variety of control-by-planning agencies began in the early 1970s. The National Center for Health Services Research and Development funded 19 Experimental Health Service Delivery Systems (EHSDS). These new umbrellas were to join in a mutual planning and deployment network all types of health care providers, insurers, and delivery units, institutional and ambulatory care settings, public and private, independent and organized. This was to be a purely voluntary cooperative effort (59).

Because this voluntary approach to unity was not capable of much impact, a new legislative proposal was made by 1974 to combine into one regional or statewide health authority all federal mechanisms used for local health planning: the EHSDS, RMPs, CHPs, AHEAs, and the Hill–Burton state hospital planning councils. The new authorities would be private, nonprofit organizations charged with planning and implementing a health care system and financed by federal funds on a capitation basis; their boundaries could be coterminous with PSRO regions (60).

DIRECTION

Thus, whatever the merits and potential effects of the form, or of those groups which have access to designing and implementing it, the signs of direction are clear. Within the Congress and HEW, movement has accelerated toward more and longer range, as well as more integrated approaches to control over health services, through planning and coordination, cost-containment procedures, and other means.

This direction was in line with other federal efforts to curb inflation in the early 1970s. Attached to the Cost of Living Council was a Health Industry Advisory Committee. Its purpose was to recommend ways to control health care costs, slowing the rise of inhospital care costs, selectively limiting capital expenditures, providing incentives for developing more ambulatory care, promoting state administration of health care controls, and for cost-saving health care delivery alternatives such as HMOs. Members of that 18-person committee included two executives from aircraft and auto corporations; 3 labor leaders; 4 representing hospital interests, 3 insurance companies, 4 physicians; one of the 18 was a woman (61). Thus as health care services use more tax dollars, the decisions affecting the provision of services are likely to be more closely tied formally and informally to other national concerns, not necessarily related to personal health.

A Cost–Quality–Delivery Control

HMOS

The HMO, discussed in detail earlier, is an organizational cost-containment device which results from combining health care delivery and financing. For properly working HMOs have a built-in set of cost and quality controls through financial risk sharing by providers as well as both formal and informal peer review processes which become possible when people work together in a common setting.

Controlling Its Development Most of the groups of health care providers who would stand to gain or lose from further development of HMOs had by the early 1970s more or less accepted HMO existence as social fact. The policy issues were then not whether, but to what extent, how rapidly, and by whom were they to be developed (public or private dollars) and operated (for-profit or not-for-profit)? Most important was whether they were to be pervasive and fully accessible, if not the predominant, forms of health care delivery, or whether they were to be alternatives that would exist only if they could compete economically with traditional delivery patterns.

Some groups opposed any public subsidy whatever for HMO development. These included certain private physicians, private hospitals, and proprietary pharmacists (62). Others supported public funding for HMOs under certain conditions, such as allowing other than salaried earnings for certain practitioners, or requiring provision of certain services, often those of their own group, while making other groups' services optional, in a minimum benefits package (63). Still others—training institutions—supported HMOs with the suggested addition of federal payments for training staff who would supervise student health care practitioners in HMOs (64). The state insurance commissioners' association supported state-level rather than federal regulatory control over HMOs, following current state-by-state insurance rate commission practices (65).

The position taken by the organized voice of a given group of health care providers on the central HMO policy issue—whether HMOs should become a sustained and readily accessible alternative to traditional health care delivery patterns—set, in turn, its stance on the type, amount, and distribution of federal resources that should be made available. This meant principally: How much money and under what conditions should it be allocated? The answers would determine the shape and definition of HMOs, their distribution and the access of social groups to them, and how likely such entities would be to persist.

Some of those funding conditions at issue included whether or not federal entitlement should override state laws prohibiting HMOs, whether funds should be limited to "demonstration" projects, whether profit-making HMOs should be eligible for funds, whether health-care-scarcity areas should have more extensive funding and lower-income consumers receive a subsidy for their premium payments (without which premiums would be higher for HMO users in poor regions, making less likely "competitive" prices in relation to traditional providers); whether HMOs should be required to have a minimum or a flexible benefits package, to have "moderate" rather than "minimum" copayments, or to have "open" or "closed" enrollment, limited to certain groups of eligible users; and whether or not they should have advisory councils, with or without consumer representation (66). These questions centered on making the HMO competitive within the current system of health services organization and financing. They required answers that would attract some support from physicians, hospitals, insurers, and consumers. Thus the resulting shape of HMOs became an acceptable compromise among those who were sufficiently organized to gain access to decision-making channels.

Posing the HMO policy issue alternatively, the central question might be, for example, under what conditions could HMOs effectively render needed services to populations regardless of their income, ethnic, age, sex characteristics, or where they live—in effect, regardless of their health problems? Then, answers to the questions regarding amounts and types of resources, and the conditions for their allocation and distribution, would flow from the policy perspective.

Policy would not, of course, necessarily result in effective implementation unless all phases of decision making were accountable to policy.

Controls as Critical Resources

These policy and program decisions, concerning comprehensive health planning agencies, professional standards review organizations, and health maintenance organizations, among others, are of course important for their immediate effects on the provision of health services and on health care providers. But clearly, to the groups of providers whose resource-getting capacity—that is, bargaining power—they affect, those decisions have further significance. It is a matter not simply of what decisions are made, but a matter of what decisions about who is to make decisions, that is critically related to future resource getting for all types of current providers. In other words, who, which groups—public, private; not-for-profit, for-profit; national, local; institutions, individual; insurers, deliverers; academics, practitioners; providers, consumers—will manage the controls?

This question becomes increasingly important as the myriad facets of health care become interconnected nationally, and greater efforts at control over implementation of health care policy are made, however such policy is determined. As earlier chapters show, these efforts extend to the organization of health care delivery, consolidation of financing, coordination of planning, and cost containment in both training and services.

These efforts are pointing to the perhaps most significant health services decision, of the decade at least: national policy as to the financing if not reorganization, of personal health services. Its significance lies in what it will do or fail to do—by establishing national patterns of services—for which of the groups of providers and which groups of consumers.

Shaping the Future Controls

NATIONAL HEALTH INSURANCE*

Although decisions being taken between 1965 and 1975 may result simply in an incremental, *de facto* national health program which a future decision will simply ratify, the realistic possibility of a definitive national health policy remains nevertheless.

Awareness of the impact of such policy and program gave impetus to national activity by the largest health care providers in the early 1970s. This included, by each of them, the formulation and Congressional sponsorship of national health bills, and developing organizational alliances with other groups of similar interests.

Their legislative proposals represented a means, through various approaches to a national health insurance program, for allowing each group to retain or improve its resource-getting capacity in the future (67). That is to give it the widest options possible and allow it to retain access to decision-making channels which determine the supply and distribution of resources, funds, and personnel.

The Private Practitioners' Plan　The AMA bill, for example, emphasized current delivery patterns, solo or group private practice without formal attachments between primary or secondary, inhospital or outpatient services, or between the delivery and financing of services. It continued the fee-for-service reimbursement method. It did not include mechanisms to redistribute health care geographically and disallowed federal inter-

* See Chapter 10 for detailed analysis.

ference in the patterns of medical care. It provided for physician dominance in statewide regulatory agencies and on a national advisory committee (68).

Approaches by Hospitals and Private Insurers   The bills of the American Hospital Association and of the Health Insurance Association of America both emphasized organized ambulatory care delivery patterns on the general HMO model. The AHA has these attached to and controlled by areawide, hospital-based, not-for-profit, and franchised corporations (69). The insurance companies used a sufficiently broad definition of HMO to include for-profit and not-for-profit delivery as well as financial institutions. Both bills encouraged capitation methods of prepayment and allowed other than a salaried basis for reimbursing physicians.

They offered some *ad hoc* measures for redistributing health personnel and training lower-cost and ambulatory care personnel. Under the AHA bill, planning, monitoring, and evaluation were centered in the areawide hospital corporation with review on a state level. In the insurers' bill, regulation and rate control was at state-level CHP agencies and insurance commissions, with a White House health policy advisory council, including insurers, at the national level (70).

The proposals of each of these private health care providers included the continuation of private health insurance methods of financing health services, except for the higher-cost care of lower-income populations and elders, to be paid out of public funds. They also included consumer-directed utilization controls through deductibles and copayments.

A Contrasting Measure   By contrast, groups with somewhat other interests at stake sponsored an alternative approach to financing. Large labor organizations, certain university- and community-based physicians, other health personnel and agencies, as well as certain consumer groups supported a single financing program, combining social insurance and public revenues for all social groups. It emphasized not-for-profit, direct-delivery HMOs or comprehensive types of medical care foundations, prepaid capitation methods of insurance, with alternative nonsalaried bases for physician reimbursement. It included mechanisms to redistribute health care resources, funds, facilities, personnel, and to relate, to some extent, health personnel training to the needs for personnel in health care delivery. Funding was directed toward not-for-profit health agencies, other community groups, and university medical programs. There were no deductibles or copayments. There were co-consumer planning, monitoring, and control methods to help assure necessary care and contain costs (71).

Organizational Alliances   Having submitted legislative proposals, certain of the largest organizations among the private health care interests have also sought to press for Congressional and other support for their positions. To this end, the National Health Council reorganized itself in the early 1970s to include for the first time profit-making corporations, thus attempting to represent the voice of the private sector of the health industry. In addition to its traditional members, such as the AHA and AMA, contributors included the association of insurance companies and the petrochemical industries (72).

Another organizational alliance, the Committee for Economic Development, represents the largest corporations in the country and so the largest institutional purchasers of employee health insurance plans (73). It issued in 1973 a report and plan for a national health policy and program, as it periodically has done on selected foreign and domestic policy issues. Its health plan is very like the Congressional bill sponsored by the insurance companies, the largest of which are part of the Committee for Economic Development (74). Labor, community, and other consumer groups had also begun to organize, although in a much looser, and less well financed manner (75).

Quite clearly, the attention by affected groups given to the national policy approach to health insurance is warranted. For passage of national health insurance legislation will mean a redistribution in new or traditional directions, of health care resources—between types of providers, facilities, services, personnel, and regions. It could increase the premium income of private health insurers by 30–50 per cent, and of drug sales by 20–25 per cent, for example (76). It also will mean a restructuring, or a reinforcement, of patterns and methods of decision making, influence and control over policy making, implementation, monitoring and evaluation, and future changes.

Consumer Decisions and Health Care Controls

In terms of numbers and dollars, the group most affected by decisions about health services is the consumer, both as citizen and less often in the role of patient. Decisions made through bargaining processes among organizations at national or local levels in effect set the options, the range of the possible, for consumers. As earlier chapters showed, those decisions allow or disallow financial and/or geographic access to health services and to the health occupations, and make possible or impossible effective access to decision-making processes which determine the shape, cost, and quality of health care.

If access to decision-making processes requires such resources as organization, funds, and timely information, it then becomes clear why consumers—citizens and patients—have had little impact on the shaping of health care, on the collective and individual decisions which affect them. Consumers of health services are not organized and do not have the comparable potential for financing effective organization—even if they had a common health care cause around which to unite—as have provider groups. Consumers, before they are consumers-of-health-services, are members of income, ethnic, occupational, sex, and regional groupings, with other problems taking priority over health services. The point at which they have most in common—illness—is the point at which they can least organize. The most influential and affluent among consumers most often enjoy ready access to all the health care options they desire. Those with fewest options, those outcast by income, race, sex, age, or living place—the outcast groups—have also fewest resources to join into effective organization.

Health Care Consumers-as-Citizens

ORGANIZATIONAL DECISIONS

Increasingly, decisions taken at the national level are becoming as or more important than local decisions as to what services are available in communities. This contrasts with earlier times when local, affluent consumer–citizens determined through philantropic funds and volunteer board membership the kinds of health care available to patients. That approach made for very wide differences in the fortunes of patients, depending upon who they were and where they lived.

Mandated Access to Decision Making In recent years, national decisions have not only affected local community delivery and financing of health services, but also the access of consumers to local decision making, access intended to include all social groups. Mandated in federal legislation as including consumers representing the population served, such community decision making is part of federally funded neighborhood health centers, some health maintenance organizations, Indian health programs, and comprehensive health planning agencies (77).

Provider Gains Certain health care provider groups have accepted this requisite for reasons that can be explained as their need to improve their resource-getting capacity and enhance their future bargaining positions. For example, some medical schools accepted the requisite consumer participation in order to add to their dollar inflow as federal research funds decreased. Second, consumer participation attracted more patient "teaching material" for their students through providing community-based ambulatory care services, for they were losing medically indigent patients who could now, under Medicaid, go to other than university hospital outpatient clinics (78). This organizational logic may or may not have been part of the thinking of the physicians who actually carried out the programs (79). Similarly, health insurers and hospitals accepted the stipulation of consumer input in their federally supported projects in exchange for gaining experience in HMO delivery and CHP agencies; for this meant little financial risk to their own organizations but had the potential for developing HMO expertise which they could use in future bargaining (80).

In another example, consumer participation was the requirement set by city health authorities in order for private hospitals to receive public operating funds; such funds were essential to their survival after federal funds were cut back. To enforce the agreement, the city health department became observer, inspector, and reporter of hospital decision-making processes and problems. In other words, the fact of consumer input became a countervailing force which helped public officials bring about changes in hospital conditions; they had previously had no such leverage (81).

Consumer Gains In some of the individual health care facilities in which consumers have had formal access to organizational policy and program decisions, the effects have benefited local populations. These include the addition of primary care services (82), less restrictive staffing policies (83), more comprehensive and better-used services (84), less physician-employment turnover (85), and more innovative problem solving (86). The recent addition in a few places of consumers to state health personnel licensure boards may bring changes in ways to approach credentialing problems (87).

CONSUMER–PROVIDER POWER BALANCE

The problems faced by providers and consumers in joint decision-making situations center on their varying perspectives, priorities, and bargaining resources. All of these affect how they will pose the issues and the alternatives for solution. Providers have been found to emphasize research and professional expertise in their approach to problems, and to favor changes which call for better coordination of community providers. In contrast, consumers favor application of present knowledge based on community needs, and call for basic changes rather than coordination (88).

Since bargaining is not possible without exchangeable valued resources, consumer views have often been overlooked in provider–consumer decision making; that is, consumer participation has been token. This is primarily because of the design for consumer input and the resources thus made available to them. This has resulted in their not attending health facility board meetings because of time or work-loss conflicts, because of transportation problems, or because of other priorities of family, and especially low-income family, life. Further, at meetings, their position has been compromised because of the greater experience, articulateness, access to information available to providers, or the consumers' hope of and need for future employment in the facility (89). Finally, the strongest restraint on consumer input is that often the providers control all budgetary funds, including those to be used to cover the costs of consumer participation (90).

CONSUMER BARGAINING RESOURCES

Without bargainable resources to influence the outcome of health care organizations' decisions, regularized, formal consumer participation is, for consumers, an impotent device for access to decision making. It is, under such conditions, an ineffective control mechanism.

Taken to the extreme, when certain local consumer groups have become aware and resentful of their powerlessness, the consumer–provider situation has become politicized. That is, the focus of decision making has shifted. No longer concerned with the provision of health services, it emphasized the question of the decision making itself—how and by whom decisions were to be made. At that point, consumers heightened their own bargaining position because, at some risk to their own interests and to the health professionals, they could jeopardize the survival of the health facility. As a result, some health professionals have simply quit. Other outcomes have been that, through administrative means, consumers were granted independent funds to sustain their own community board for negotiating the operational decisions for the health facility (91).

In other similar situations, consumer community groups have used the one resource which a federally mandated requirement, like consumer participation, assures them, the courts. In recent cases, charging that (1) local health centers could not alter either the process of community participation without consulting them, the consumers, and (2) that the centers had to provide the conditions to make consumer involvement meaningful, community boards won. The courts ruled, among other things that the health centers had to provide training and assistance to build local leadership, and that the community boards were to participate effectively throughout the entire decision-making processes in the centers (92).

REPRESENTATION IN CONTROL PROGRAMS

Under Mandate In the areawide comprehensive health planning agencies, as nonpublic entities receiving half their funds from federal revenues, their policy-making boards must have a consumer majority. Studies have showed that only about 5 per cent of CHP funding came from consumer groups. As to their representation on the boards, consumers were a 55 per cent majority, with physicians and health administrators making up most of the provider members. Five per cent were consumers representing labor unions, clerical, skilled, or unskilled occupations. The vast majority of consumers were white and had family incomes of more than $10,000 (93).

The nature and impact of this kind of consumer representation is suggested by these findings: (1) The community groups with which CHP agencies most often had formal ties and shared resources were medical societies and hospitals or hospital associations; the groups with which they most often had no ties whatever were consumer groups. (2) The more often the CHP agencies had shared board members with medical societies, the less likely they were to disseminate information to consumers. (3) Half the agencies had engaged in consumer information activities in a minor way only; a quarter of them had no such activities at all. (4) Half the agencies held no public hearings or did so occasionally only. (5) Sixty per cent of their time was directed toward environmental, nonpersonal health services activities, and this was closely related to frequent contacts and feedback from local neighborhood health centers (94).

The courts again have been used by consumer groups seeking effective voice in the CHP agencies, which as suggested earlier could have a far greater impact on the delivery of health services than any individual health care facility. Recently, a Federal District Court has ruled that it had jurisdiction to hear consumers' complaints on the decision-making arrangements in CHP agencies (95).

Without Mandate Other statutory mechanisms intended to control some aspect of health services, described above, have not required consumer participation. Thus the Regional Medical Programs—with widespread impact on patterns of services and training—have on their regional advisory boards less than one fifth of their members drawn from the public; these, in turn, were not necessarily or even likely to be representative of the groups most likely to use RMP services (96).

Likewise, state boards of health, most of which are empowered with policy making and administrative authority, have on 70 per cent of the boards, physicians as one third or more of their members. This is in spite of the fact that public funds, state and federal, were paying for one fourth of all physicians' services in 1970, compared with 7 per cent in 1966, suggesting possible conflicts of interest. Just over half the boards had consumer representation; on the average this amounted to 12.5 per cent of their members (97). The virtual absence of consumers from those other important control entities in the credentialing system, the boards of accreditation, certification, and licensure, was noted earlier.

The most recent and potentially enveloping control mechanism, the professional standards review organizations, has little provision for other-than-physician input. The federal law calls for statewide PSRO councils empowered to coordinate, administer the expenses of, evaluate and publish their findings on PSRO activities, as well as help replace ineffectual PSROs. Of a minimum of 11 on each Council, 4 may be "persons knowledgeable in health care," of whom 2 must be recommended to the Secretary of HEW by the governors, and would represent the public (98). A national PSRO Council was required, composed of 11 physicians, one of whom was to be recommended by consumer groups and other nonphysician groups. Other groups, who would be affected by PSRO decisions, such as insurers, health planning agencies, other health professionals, called for consumer involvement as well as their own in local PSROs (99).

NEW OPTIONS FOR ACCESS

Although consumer access to PSRO decision making remained unlikely, other recent federal legislation opened new possibilities for consumer–citizen impact on other health care provider controls. The 1972 Social Security Amendments granted access to the public to information on the performance of the state agencies, insurance carriers, and fiscal intermediaries who administer Medicare–Medicaid programs. Further, the findings from the sample resurvey of Medicare–Medicaid facilities, principally hospitals and nursing facilities, must also be available to the public. Such findings would also include an evaluation of hospitals' utilization review practices (100). Access to such information would be essential to any nonprovider, that is, consumer voice, regarding what does or should happen within health care institutions.

Another new set of options was opened with the recent passage of the Occupational Safety and Health Act. This allowed workers in over 4 million workplaces to actively obtain an assessment of the safety and healthfulness of their work environment, which could include personal health services. It also granted them administrative and legal tools to press for changes necessary to maintain their health. Such authority was quickly put to use by some organized work groups, both white and blue collar (101).

Consumers-as-Patients

INDIVIDUAL CHOICES

Clearly national health policy, embodied in legislation or executive order, sets the options, the limits and the possibilities, for access to health care decision making by consumers-as-citizens. Likewise, national and local law, and administrative policy of government and nongovernment provider organizations, affect the choices available to consumers-as-patients. That is even after they have reached the point of receiving health services, granting that distant organizational decisions regarding the financing, location, type, and control of services may have made this point difficult to reach, especially for certain social groups. This, in other words, is the point where consumers are least able to formulate a collective voice on their own behalf. They stand as individuals in encounter with health organizations, whether as inpatients or outpatients (102).

Administrative Constraints The question of birth control services is a recent example of how administrative policy and institutional practices limit the otherwise-intended range of choices of consumers-as-patients. Certain concerned physicians have pointed out how a proposed HEW plan to administer family planning services through welfare organizations could create at least the inference of coercion by low-income women seeking family welfare payments, but who may or may not want birth control services (103). Further, studies have shown that significantly more women of other than white races and the poor received sterilization along with abortion procedures than white and nonpoor women; and women who were sterilized were more likely to receive the costlier hysterectomy than the tubal ligation method if they were poor (104). Such patterns may well reflect institutional and professional choices concerning funds and medical learning experience than patients' preferences.

Consumer Preferences Health care providers have often had little regard for the preferences and choices of consumers-as-patients, judging patient-choices by their own preferences and priorities (105). A number of studies point out some of the differences. Physicians judge good family physicians by their knowledge and ties with specialized backup facilities and colleagues. Patients want the family doctor to be effective and readily available (106). Consumers-as-patients have been accepting of new patterns of health care by health personnel, and have readily accepted non-physician practitioners or have voiced no preference when they were satisfied with the services rendered (107).

Further, the poor placed high importance on health, as did other social groups; they spent less on health services because their scarce dollars had to be spent on the prerequisites to health, the essentials of food and housing and earnings; their use of health services differed from other income groups because the services available to them differed; and they wanted to know more about their illnesses than their doctors told them, including the presence of incurable or terminal illness (108). A national poll showed that 62 per cent of the public think that a terminally ill patient should have the option to tell the physician to allow death to come; only 37 per cent, however, thought that a physician should be allowed to practice euthanasia (109).

These questions, the choices of consumers-as-patients once they enter the health care delivery setting—concerning choice of practitioner, of treatment, of knowing or not knowing, of dying, or further, of the use of their person or of information about their person—have recently received increasing attention. This is, in part, because of the need to control the potential of interlocking computers and medical technology for invading privacy and taking prerogatives in individual lives.

Efforts have been made to make explicit the rights of patients, including the right to know the alternatives available and their likely consequences; to give or refuse consent; to access to information about themselves and their treatment, and control over the disclosure of that information to outsiders (110). Advocates of patients' rights have said that it is not for health care providers to grant rights that already belong to patients (111). They have sought various remedies to make those rights real, including the courts and new legislative measures. Experience with litigation concerning failure to obtain informed consent has been difficult, however, and therefore will be an unlikely route for the redress of patient grievances (112).

National legislation was being considered in 1974 for requiring informed consent for the use of experimental drugs. This would include requiring an explanation to the patients of nonexperimental alternatives, of the possible risks and benefits of the new drug, assurance that their immediate refusal or later refusal would not prejudice their future care; it would disallow any agreement that would waive their rights or release others from liability for negligence (113).

Other proposed legislation would control the transfer of medical information. Health insurance applicants who were denied insurance coverage would have access to all information relevant to that denial and would have to authorize the transfer of that data to any third party (114).

The Department of Health, Education, and Welfare further proposed a plan to protect those who have limited capacity to give fully informed consent to drug and clinical research—children, prisoners, and institutionalized mentally infirm patients (115).

Other proposals intended to allow informed choices to the consumer-as-patient include allowing patients to retain a copy of all their medical records—physician credentials as well as charges for services (116); this could then reduce the proportion of the one third or more of patients who do not understand or follow physicians' directions (117); it might also avoid the problems resulting from patients taking drugs prescribed by two or more physicians (prevalent among perhaps 40 per cent of the patients in some regions); others suggest that written drug information should be provided with all prescribed medications (118).

Broader efforts have been aimed at consumers-as-citizens, informing them of their rights as patients, of some of their alternatives in choosing health care providers, and to some extent of the decision-making processes that have shaped current health care patterns. For these purposes, television has been rarely used. More rare, even when focusing on approaches to the prevention of most prevalent diseases is "equal time" or even consideration given to environmental programs—taken in the broadest socioecological sense—which could improve the health of populations. Prevention is often limited to traditional efforts at changing the personal habits of individuals and obtaining regular primary care. This approach, again, avoids the economic and political decisions that set the conditions for individual habits and practices.

The print media, and more recently paperback books, have made informed offerings to help individuals in the self-evaluation of their health, ways to deal with problems before seeking medical help, as well as criteria on which to judge help that is given (119).

Decision making between and within organizations at various levels, as continuous bargaining for resources, results in the distribution of those resources—whether money or facilities, personnel, improved access to decisional processes—usually in patterned ways. This, in turn, affects the options available to consumers, as citizens and as patients, for having a voice in the conditions and decisions which affect them.

Health Services Organizations: Internal Effects of External Decisions

Similarly, bargaining between provider organizations also sets the options for the interrelations of groups inside those organizations, for the internal decision making, the formal and informal bargaining for resources, and the control of resources, that go on continuously. This has been shown to exist between the professions in a health facility (120), between the administrative personnel and the professionals (121); and between management and the noncredentialed personnel (122).

Group Bargaining Potential

One example of a national decision affecting the bargaining capacity of an inhospital group was the Medicare provision to pay for resident physician and intern services to elders. Less than 5 per cent of hospital budgets is allocated to support these physicians, yet most of the funds now come through patient revenues and in effect are financed by social security programs. This allowed dramatic increases in physician salaries, averaging 25 per cent more in 1973 than in 1968. During this period, and increasingly, the house medical staffs sought collective bargaining agreements; they obtained negotiated settlements in 9 per cent of the teaching hospitals by 1972, and were most successful in government facilities (123). It is conceivable that such unionizing would not have been effective in higher wages if hospitals could not turn to social security health programs to finance their house staffs (which had traditionally had very low pay).

In the early 1970s increasing efforts were also made by some self-employed physicians to form labor unions. This was called "dual organization" by the AMA and opposed because it would prove to be divisive to the needs of the profession to deal effectively with government in a unified way (124). Such local union activity may increase as various forms of group practice, nonprepaid and prepaid variants, vie for consumer and health insurance dollars.

Another example of how a health facility's need for resources may affect its decisions internally is apparent in the hospitals that have provided child day care programs for their personnel. In 1970 more than half of such hospitals were located in the South, where nurses are in shortest supply; there were fewest in the Northeast and West, where nurses are most plentiful. Most of the programs were run by the nursing departments and used by nurses (61 per cent). In effect, the bargaining between hospitals and nursing staffs gave to hospitals that had difficulty getting nursing personnel a means, through child day care, to recruit and retain nurses; it gave to nurses and other women with child care responsibilities (95 per cent of the users were women) the opportunity to work. In the regions of the country where hospitals could more readily obtain personnel, women were not as successful in negotiating day care programs (125).

Finally, a national decision under consideration in the 93rd Congress could measurably alter the bargaining capacity of salaried hospital personnel. This is an amendment to the Taft–Hartley Act which would bring hospitals under the authority of the National Labor Relations Board. The American Hospital Association opposed it, having gotten hospitals exempted since 1947. The American Nurses Association, intern and residents groups, and labor organizations supported the amendment (126).

In the last decade, nurses and other salaried personnel have increasingly organized to seek formal negotiated agreements, using collective action, to bargain for resources within health care facilities. Because of the great social and economic differences between credentialed and other nursing personnel, R.N.s have tended to bargain through their state nursing associations while other personnel have joined labor unions. This, in turn, has sometimes resulted in competition, sometimes in collaboration. The lowest-paid groups of personnel have had salary increases as a bargaining priority. They have also stressed working conditions, however. This means, in effect, attaining some degree of impact, a voice, in the decision making which affects them, which means in turn how organizational resources beyond earnings are to be distributed (127).

Changing Patterns and Bargaining Potential

Changes in the organization of the delivery of health services will also affect the possibilities for relationships between groups of personnel inside health care facilities. Noted earlier was the potential for new decision-making patterns, for informal or formal negotiated arrangements, in HMOs. Further, as health services return, however slowly, to community settings, to ambulatory care centers, to homes, the now-dominant bargaining position of health personnel, their control of decisions for consumers, is likely to change. For they will not be in their own territory. Circumstances are more likely to require them to act as advisors, if not guests.

International Comparisons

Having a nationalized health services and/or financing system does not of course do away with decision making that results from bargaining for resources among interested parties. What it does, however, is to place such bargaining on a basis of more evenly distributed resources, with publically accountable policy making and the use of alternatives confined to that policy; with formalized bargaining processes more open to public scrutiny; with administrative organization as the tool to effectively implement decisions and monitor outcomes, as well as having the capacity to use fiscal and other forms of control to shape the options of all consumers-as-citizens for access to the health care system and to relate the system to the needs of population groups; and it has the potential at least to relate health services policy to social, educational, and environmental policy.

Limits on Bargaining

Under these conditions, no single group or a few groups can have consistent, overpowering undue influence based on their control of large numbers of facilities, services, or funds. Recent decisions in the Scandanavian countries and Great Britain are evidence that the public interest can take precedence when it conflicts with those of certain groups (128).

Denmark, for example, in 1973, did away with private health insurance funds and placed that responsibility in local governments' elected councils (129). Sweden instituted changes in physician payments so as to benefit lower-income patients and provide incentives for younger, primary care physicians (130). In the 1974 reorganization of the British National Health Service the separate administrative networks for hospital, physician, and community health services were integrated at local, regional, and national levels. This was to allow for a focus on the needs of populations in their communities in determining the allocation of resources, rather than the needs for resources of particular types of health care providers, principally hospitals, hospital-based specialists, and others concerned with technological solutions to health care (131). In addition, somewhat wider decisional authority became possible at the local level by district management teams (responsible for 150,000–250,000 people and a general hospital); included on this six-member team are an administrator, community nurse, finance officer, and three physicians each from hospital (specialist), community (GP), or government (the district community physician) (132).

In the view of some critics, the public interest might have been better served if various interest groups had not been as influential in determining the final shape of the British NHS (133). For example, community needs for personal services might have been better served if social and health services had been integrated, or health care might have been potentially more effective if occupational health had been integrated with other health services—as is the case in Sweden and eastern Europe. School health services did, however, become part of the basic health services system (134).

The influence of health professional associations in all phases of health policy and program remains strong. The determination of earnings, however, whether through salaries or the setting of fee schedules, is a negotiated, but open and regularized procedure. Agreement is reached on a national level, such as in England and Sweden, or on a regional level, as for physicians in the Federal Republic of Germany; bargaining is between government or other insurors and the occupational group, which is often in a coalition with other related occupational groups (135). This has resulted in some interesting alliances. For example, in England the British Medical Association, the Medical Practitioners Union, and the Trade Union Council all supported a strike for higher wages by hospital ancillary personnel (136).

The voice of consumers has been given a more explicit place through recent and proposed changes in the health systems of England, Denmark, Sweden, and Canada. This is in agreement with a 1973 recommendation by the World Health Organization intended for all developed and underdeveloped countries (137).

The bargaining position of consumers-as-citizens was improved in these countries by placing final responsibility for health services in elected officials. Further, in the local administration of services, in England for example, community health councils representing private and public interests were given authority to inspect premises and records, make recommendations, and require the publication of reports and actions taken by area health authorities. As a resource for the consumer-as-citizen, an office of ombudsman became part of each health district, a subunit of the areas (138).

Denmark has recently set up boards, composed of citizens chosen by consumer groups and lawyers appointed by the Ministry of Social Affairs. Each board is empowered to investigate and resolve consumer complaints about personal services, including health, welfare, old age, and rehabilitation (139).

Other recent methods for broadening the options available to consumers-as-patients include the Swedish approach to health education, which integrates body knowledge, self-care, and the use of health and other social services in the primary education system; through the public media; and continues adult learning lifelong through a system of flexible educational opportunities. In addition, although patient information in Stockholm is collected in a central computer, the privacy of individuals has been protected by an elaborate coding system which allows access under specific circumstances only; it is particularly stringent concerning psychiatric, venereal disease, and gynecologic records (140). A final example, in England, is the increasing practice of informing patients of their diagnosis in terminal illness, as important step toward allowing them choice as to how to live out the remainder of their lives (141).

Summary

The access of various social groups to the full range of health services and of the health occupations, their options for effective choices, and the relevance of that health care network to what mainstream and outcast groups need result from interorganizational decisions, increasingly taken at the national and governmental level. These decisions—and so the pattern and distribution of services—are in effect the outcome of the bargaining for resources—funds, facilities, personnel, decisional authority—among those groups which have material interests in health care. They have access to decision-making processes at any number of points in the cycle, from policy making (defining the problem, formulating alternative solutions, setting criteria for selection), through implementation (defining administrative regulations), to monitoring and other feedback activities that could affect changes in policy. Such effective access stems from their capacity, financially and as health care-related groups, to organize and gather and disseminate information to the right people at the right time and in the right ways.

All of this shapes the outcome of decisions about health care—organization and financing, delivery, personnel, distribution, and control. The crucial decisions about controls include what types of monitoring will be used—fiscal or nonfiscal, voluntary or mandatory, aimed at consumers or providers, with a planning-for-access focus or cost-control emphasis, using area-wide or individual and institutional methods, administered with or without consumers, and by which health care providers, or some combination and integration of these options.

In contrast, those most affected by these decisions about the shape of the health care system and how it will be controlled, the consumers, have least effective access to decision-making processes. This is in spite of the fact that such decisions set the future options available to them for having a voice concerning their health care, as citizens and as patients.

Similarly, the decisions taken between health care organizations set the range of the possible for the bargaining for resources that goes on between various occupational groups inside health service facilities and agencies.

Any of these decisions concerning the shape and components of health care, as well as the adequacy of the decision-making processes which brought them about, may be the focus of evaluation. That is the type of decision making that is discussed next.

chapter 9

Evaluating Health Care

In the broadest sense, the evaluation of health care is an assessment of prior decisions that were made concerning the organization and financing of health care, if not the processes by which those decisions were made. To judge whether or not those decisions were "good," and how good they were, depends of course on what evaluators determine as the purpose of health care, and the ways and criteria they use to measure the "goodness" of health care. If, for example, the aim of health care is to assure and maintain or improve the health of populations—a seemingly obvious goal—then the focus for evaluating health care must be the health level of populations. If, however, the implicit or explicit goal of health care is to be the provision of health services, evenly accessible and usable for all, and relevant to population needs for services—something of an ideal health services system—then the measure of this goal would include, among other things, the health of the people who use the system. The distinction here is the focus on the *health* of an entire population and what needs to be done to assure it, in contrast to a focus on a system of *health services,* including the people who use it.

Decisions concerning the evaluation of health care are becoming increasingly important as the delivery of health care is becoming more influenced by national and governmental policy. The focus, criteria, and methods of evaluation, as well as who the evaluators are, will have greater potential for more pervasive changes in health care policy and practices than in the past.

Health care in the United States has virtually always and predominantly been evaluated in terms of the provision of personal health services. Further, it has not usually been done at a national level partly because the tools were lacking. With the implementation of Medicare, nationwide comparable data can now be collected and computerized. At local levels, evaluation had rarely concerned the total network of health services. Now beginning efforts at this are being made by the comprehensive health planning agencies. However, evaluation has focused more often on individual programs, or types of programs, such as hospitals, health centers, or occasionally health schools; or on services, such as maternity, geriatric, or rehabilitation services.

Input Measures

In this type of delivery-unit evaluation, whether of a program or service, the determination of its "goodness" or quality was based on, most often, what went into the unit, input measures. These included the credentials of the facility and personnel—their certification or accreditation status, the licensure, degree of specialization, and academic standing of their personnel—as well as their amounts of specialized equipment (1).

Process Measures and Their Use

A second type of criteria, concerning what went on within the delivery unit, the process measures, are becoming more used. This type includes utilization review in hospitals and nursing home or home care programs, and other forms of peer review; it measures quality by comparing program practices with either "customary" practices or statistical norms for providing service to patients with given diagnoses (2). These most commonly have been limited to such figures as numerical summaries of persons using certain services, numbers of visits to or by certain personnel, and dollars expended. For example, of the 60 per cent of community mental health centers who engaged in some form of evaluation, the vast majority used statistics describing the numbers, types, and residence of clients using their services or related services—not the effects of those services. [A minority only included citizen or community attitudes or patients' complaints in evaluating their programs (3).]

At a national level, rates of utilization have been helpful in monitoring and evaluating Medicare when those rates could be compared among regions or groups of patients. For example, comparing the use of hospital services by region and racial group, it was found that although the South had the highest rate per 1,000 enrolled elders, whites were using those services almost two thirds more often than other races, most of whom were blacks, in 1968 (4). Similarly, such data showed that across the country white persons used more services than blacks or other races, with close to a 50 per cent difference in inhospital services, and an even greater difference in physician and other medical services. There was much *less* difference in the use of services among the elders who died. That is, when blacks were ill enough to die, they had easier access to Medicare-paid services than if they were able to survive (5).

Other such data have been used to assess the proportion of elders who bought Supplementary Medical (nonhospital) Insurance, Part B Medicare, in addition to their entitlement to Hospital Insurance, Part A. Measured over time, 1967–1971, the overall proportion increased from 91.6 to 95.5 per cent. These data could also be compared according to age, sex, race, urban–rural, and regional groupings. It showed, for example, that other than white races were increasingly buying Part B (6). Similar data will in time likewise reveal whether the 1972 increases in cost sharing by consumers of Medicare–Medicaid will change the numbers purchasing these services.

Such process measures of national health care financing programs, in other words, can be used to assess the financial access of at least certain social groups, the elders and disabled, to health services, and to suggest regional variations due to a geographic lack of services, and/or racial discrimination which impedes access. This latter charge was recently brought by the American Public Health Association to the House Subcommittee on Civil Rights against HEW's Civil Rights enforcement authorities (7).

The emphases and efficacy of services can also be detected in part through other comparative groupings of Medicare measures of process. For example, 1969 figures showed that in the Northeast, although rates for hospitalized elders, according to age and sickness groups were near the national average, more surgery was performed on them, their stay in the hospital was longer, and the hospitals were reimbursed more per patient than in any of the other three U.S. regions: South, North Central, or West (8). Other utilization data comparing services and expenditures showed, contrary to expressed policy, that increasing amounts of funds were going to hospital services in contrast to home care programs, and that even though all services, inpatient, ambulatory, and home care, decreased in number per 1,000 enrollees, the reimbursement per enrollee increased, especially between 1970 and 1971. Reimbursement increased most for hospital services (9).

Such information can help evaluate both over- and underutilization of services and help establish whether controls that decrease the use of hospital beds necessarily reduce hospital charges and/or foster more appropriate ambulatory and home care, at least for the population groups covered by Medicare–Medicaid (10).

Other process measures have been used to compare on a local level the costs per patient of one form of health delivery unit over another (11), or of the economy of some types of personnel over others (12). At the broadest level, cost information has been used to project the costs in public expenditures of proposed national health insurance bills, and further to assess their total costs, both public and private—that is, the proportion not visible in public accounts (13).

Outcome Measures

A third type of criteria used to determine the quality of health services is through results, the outcome measures, most often related to what happened to individual patients clinically. These have rarely been used to relate forms of health services delivery, for example, to *groups* of patients and their changes in health status (14). Used in a narrower sense, within individual institutions, this method has revealed the development of infections obtained inhospital, variations in postoperative death rates that were non-disease-related, patterned errors in diagnosis, treatment, and prognosis (15); and, in some social rehabilitative programs, actual impairment of persons' capacity to live within their limitations (16).

ACCEPTABILITY AS OUTCOME

Another kind of "result" is the acceptability of the service to the users. Most consumers-as-patients have been found to be satisfied with health services perhaps 9 times out of 10. Some of this acceptance, however, may reflect a dearth of alternative sources of health services, a lack of awareness of what is possible, uninformed judgment about some facets of their services, or simply their vulnerability in profession-dominated facilities. In any case, although consumer satisfaction is a necessary part of the evaluation equation, it is not sufficient, for it does not say anything about the opinions and service requirements of *non*users (17).

PROCESS AND OUTCOME

Occasionally, evaluation efforts have related the *process* of services rendered to *outcome* in benefits to consumers-as-patients. For example, such an assessment of family planning clinics showed that it was indeed more economical and efficient to hire adjunct workers other-than health professionals—resulting in more patient services and more direct time to patients. By relating clinic process to patient outcomes, they learned that more staff time for patients *in clinics* did not help those patients who wanted continued birth control services as much as staff time spent in later, *out-of-clinic* follow-up contacts with patients, thereby assuring the aim of infertility (18).

On a larger scale, a citywide study in New York recently sought to evaluate prenatal services in terms of the outcome, measured by the infants' mortality rates. It found that among the 142,000 births, deaths were higher in the first year of life of those whose mothers had inadequate prenatal care; those mothers were predominantly poor and black or Puerto Rican. These minority-group mothers had more risks, defined as socio-demographic and medical–obstetric. The study concluded that, taking such risks into account, health services resources were grossly misallocated, since a preponderance should be directed at those with highest risk, that is, the poor and women of nonwhite races (19).

This evaluation focused on the relationship of prenatal services to infant mortality, in contrast to the nationwide U.S. study, discussed in Chapter 2, which focused on the relationship of the conditions of living to infant deaths. The U.S. study found that socioeconomic conditions were the prime determinants of death in the first year of life, even when other important factors concerning obstetrical health were taken into account (20).

The distinction here is that the New York study, focusing on services, concluded that a reallocation of services would reduce infant deaths among families-at-risk, a reasonable conclusion. The U.S. study, focusing on the health of the national population and the conditions of life, implies that infant mortality would decrease most effectively if the socioeconomic conditions of the poor and minorities were improved. The New York study recommendation, reallocation of services, would help remedy the health and services deficit caused by the underlying socioeconomic deficit of poor and minority women, but cannot change the fundamental deficit. In contrast, the solution implied by the U.S. study would reach the underlying cause of unhealthy women, mothers, and babies; it would change the socioeconomic environment in which they live and also improve their capacity for ready access to health services.

Thus, under prevalent ways of assessing health care, with the focus on personal health services, the conclusions—more access to better personal health services—at best will allow the poor and other outcast groups better health than the poor and outcast who cannot get those services, but not as good health as they could have if they were not poor or otherwise socially outcast; that is, not as high a level of health as there would be if health were the focus of concern rather than the provision of health services being the focus of concern.

The Context of Evaluation

This then illustrates the importance, if not the crucial nature, of decision making related to evaluation—how the posing of the questions, the *focus* of assessment can limit the kinds of conclusions that are possible. Most service programs, however, have not been designed so as to make even program evaluation possible, that is, accountable in terms of the health status of consumers-as-patients for the expenditure of public or other funds, much less to allow evaluation in terms of the health of the surrounding community population (21).

A design for evaluation of health care that would be more accountable to the public interest—the measure of benefits in health derived from resources invested—would assess the contribution of services toward health but also point toward other nonpersonal health services measures that may be necessary, including health care conceived in its broader ecological sense and other social and economic requirements for health. In this way health services evaluation could lend support to broader basic, social measures, without which personal health services at best can only be remedial and have an unnecessarily temporary effect. The context of evaluation thus can limit its worth to immediate program purposes or allow wider social usefulness.

In other words, a program may be evaluated by assessing the health of its consumers-as-patients and how well its processes—the access it grants, the emphasis of its services and their relationship to patients' needs, their efficiency—contributed to their health outcomes. Or a program may be adjudged by assessing the health of the community around it and how its program processes contribute to that population's health. Each approach would produce different conclusions.

Suppose, for example, that a Home Health Agency in an aging community were providing Medicare services in as nearly perfect a manner as human institutions allow. All elders who needed skilled nursing and related health services had ready access to the agency's preventive, curative, restorative, and rehabilitative services; the services were rendered humanely and efficiently, to the full satisfaction of the elders. Following patients' rehabilitation, services were ended until another request for health services was made. However, for the elders without illness episodes, whose limitations are merely those related to aging and presumably concommitant chronic disease, the agency can provide none of the services needed, whether food shopping and preparation, transportation, home repair, or other requirements for preventing illness episodes. Such services would be far beyond the agency's preventive, personal health services.

How shall this situation be evaluated? Viewing the agency, it is performing its services very well. Viewing persons-in-the-community, the population, the consumers-as-citizens, inhome services to them are not adequate. Their access to personal services is limited; available services are not emphasizing what they need most of the time. This is not uncommon, not only because of traditional agency distinctions between health and social and educational services, but also because funding is granted for specific services to specific agencies rather than for a network of services based on population makeup (22). Other age and social segments of the community might raise similar questions concerning how appropriate, how "good," agency-oriented rather than population-oriented services are or can be.

Further, on a wider scale, a "typical" or "average" U.S. community may have its entire system of personal health services organized and financed to provide access to all social groups, and may emphasize most needed services—such as enough primary care practitioners to deal with the most frequent reasons for physician visits (colds, arthritis, sore throats, bronchitis, mild neuroses); and inpatient services geared to most-needed acute services (digestive disorders, accidents, respiratory and circulatory illness); rehabilitation programs for the most common disabling diseases (of muscle and bone, heart and circulatory, and nervous systems); plus concurrent health education and screening programs (23). Nevertheless, it is likely that its adults will continue to suffer discomfort, disability, and untimely deaths from the chief causes—cardiac disease, cancer, and accidents—as will its infants die from congenital anomalies, asphaxia, and immaturity (24). This description is not so much a prediction as a statement of fact, derived from the experience of middle-income populations, discussed in Chapter 2.

In such communities there would be some further decrease in limitations of activity and unnecessary death if health and other personal services were integrated (well beyond current practices of interagency referrals), and if this network of personal services were tied to even the traditional nonpersonal, or environmental health services—the monitoring of sanitation and sewage, housing safety, water, food, and eating places. That is, even when a community may have what is assessed as a "good" network of health and other personal services, their people will continue to have the ill effects of environmental pollution, auto and other technologically related diseases (including accidents), obesity from lack of exercise, the physical and psychic stress of rapid pace, competitive pressures, and noise, from the superabundant choices of potentially toxic, or nonnutritive, or high-fat foods, and of potentially debilitating cigarettes, drugs, and alcohol.

In "atypical" communities, where relatively more people are poor or of ethnic stock or women or elders or children, the same network of services would have relatively greater impact, because ill health is both more prevalent and often of types more amenable to individual treatment. How "good" it could be in preventing ill health, however, would be limited because it could not control the environmental conditions—physical and socioeconomic—that produce contemporary disease.

The Focus on Populations-in-Communities

Thus a system of health care, if it were to be evaluated in terms of the health of populations, could not get high marks without being a system of personal health services, within a network of other personal services, properly accessible, related to population requirements, and effective for consumers-as-patients/clients; nor without ties to environmental controls over ecological and socioeconomic conditions that generate illness, and to the system or means for lifelong learning necessary to make persons aware of these conditions and how to deal with them (Figure 9–1).

Toward a Broader Concept

Recent proposals have been made to alter the evaluation of health care in the United States. One is to develop a national independent regulatory commission for controlling the quality of personal health services, measured in the outcomes of the health of populations and other criteria. It would carry out monitoring and surveillance of federally funded delivery systems, which would in turn be exempted from other federal quality regulation. It would not be tied to the allocation of resources or to cost control tasks, but would have strong sanctions, including publication of its findings. It would engage in research to develop standards for relating the process of rendering services to outcomes in health and would unite

Figure 9–1   Evaluating Personal Health Services, United States

	Alternative Focal Points	
	The health care system (and/or its components): <ul><li>financing,</li><li>organization (e. g. personnel; training and services facilities; services; controls; evaluation),</li><li>consumers-as-patients (users of services: 20–30% of population in one year)</li></ul>	Populations-in-communities (and/or their subgroups): <ul><li>sex,</li><li>age,</li><li>ethnicity,</li><li>income,</li><li>residence,</li><li>consumers-as-citizens (potential users of health services, 70–80% of population in one year)</li></ul>

CRITERIA
Inputs

Amount, type, sources of revenue, and allocation of resources.

Processes

Access (financial, geographic, temporal, procedural) to services, occupations, decision-making in relation to social groups.

Emphasis (inhospital/in community; specialist/primary care; segmented/integrated) in relation to most needed types of services.

Efficacy: Effectiveness of emphasis (choice of technology and resources). Competent application of resources (individual and organization). Cost-effectiveness.

Outcomes

Levels of health (rates)
Fertility and child-spacing
Growth and development
Disease
Limitation of activity (disability)
Untimely deaths (longevity)
Acceptability

Reassessment of inputs and processes

Can outcomes be improved by:
- Changes in amount, type, source, or allocation of resources?
- Changes in provision of health services?
- Alternative or additional non-health personal services (e.g., social, education)?
- Environmental changes (ecological, socioeconomic)?
- At what cost?
- How acceptable to informed consumers?

with the information arm of governmental health care, the National Center for Health Statistics (NCHS) (25).

In a separate but related proposal, an evaluation of NCHS itself recommended a national system of health accounts to allow for better evaluation, as well as planning and administration of health programs. These accounts would relate resources to health outcomes, would tie general population data, such as census data, to health and other program statistics, and would relate populations' health to environmental pollutants (26). Such a system would provide the tools to evaluate health and the relative contribution of environmental conditions and services to it. This would then allow a reassessment of how resources should be allocated, in what amounts, of what types, to best assure the health of populations, that is, of people living in communities (Figure 9–1).

Reallocations

The question of reallocating resources from personal to environmental programs in order to produce the greatest impact on health improvement has been raised in this and other countries. Diagnosis, treatment, and rehabilitation have been labeled "disease care," while primarily environmental measures, beyond the traditional patterns, have been called "health care" (27).

Investing more resources for raising the ecological quality of the environment, as has apparently begun through recent legislation (28), will not necessarily spread the costs and benefits equitably among various social groups. Although it is true that the poor bear a disproportionately larger burden of environmental degradation (29)—and so would benefit from improvements—they will now, as recently reported, also pay a heavier share of the high costs of pollution controls. At the same time, equal recognition has not been given to the socioeconomically determined aspect of their environment which most immediately affects their health and the diseases they have (30).

National Priorities

This leads to consideration of a far broader context for evaluating the care of the health of populations. That is the relationship between concern for the health of people and its place in national priorities, most visibly measured by the allocation and distribution of resources—in other words, how much these priorities contribute to, how much they detract from, the health of all the people and of particular social groups. Further questions, which can be asked of any health program or system (Figure 9–1) or national policy beyond the amount of resources that support health, include: Where is the burden of financing and where the preponderance of benefits, direct and indirect? Are allocations related to the means that can most effectively give the greatest improvements in health where they are most needed?

To illustrate this perspective of health care in the context of national priorities, the U.S. GNP may be taken as a measure of national resources, over $1 trillion in 1971. Assuming conservatively that consumers-as-

Gross national product (GNP)
$1046.8 (100.0%)

All governments share (federal, state, local)
$233.0 (22.2%)

Total government expenditures
$233.0 (100.0%)

State/local: $21.6 — 10.2%
Federal: $211.4 — 89.8%

Federal government expenditure
$211.4 (100.0%)

Defense	$77.7	36.7%
Other	$54.9	36.1%
Human services	$78.8	37.2%

Human services (100.00%)
$78.8

Personal $22.1 — 28.0%
Environmental $56.7 — 72.0%

Human services as proportion of total federal expenditures

	Total	100.0%
Other		62.8%
Human services		37.2
Environmental		27.0
Ecological		0.05
Socioeconomic		26.95
Personal		10.2
Social		0.6
Educational		2.8
Health		6.8

Environmental services $56.7 (100.0%)

Ecological	$1.1	2.0%
Pollution Cont'd.	($.70)	
Agricultural land and water	($.35)	
Socioeconomic	$55.6	98.0%
Retirement, social security	$55.6	
	($46.3)	
Public assistance	($ 7.8)	
Rural housing public facilities	($.34)	
Low, moderate income housing assistance	($1.24)	

Personal services $22.1 (100%)

Social, individual services	$ 1.6	8%
Education and manpower training	$ 6.0	31%
elementary and secondary	($ 3.2)	
Vocational	($ 0.4)	
Manpower	($ 2.4)	
Health	$14.5	61%
Research and development	($ 2.2)	
Services, financing	($12.0)	
Prevention, control	($ 0.3)	

a Of total state and local expenditures in 1970, 52.1% were for comparable human services (20.3%, environment; 25.3%, education; 6.5%, health).

b Does not include $9.8 billion for veterans' income, education, or health programs.

Data source: U. S. Bureau of Census, *Statistical Abstract of the United States 1972* (Washington, D. C.: Government Printing Office, 1972).

Figure 9–2   Evaluating Health Care, United States

Illustrative Schema for Determining Core-of-Health Priorities: Estimate of Human Services Expenditures by Government, 1971 (billions) citizens have a right, or at least a potentially effective right, to control only that part of the GNP that is spent by government (about 22 per cent of the trillion dollars), we may focus on the federal government expenditures (about 90 per cent of all local, state, and national government expenditures) (31) (Figure 9–2).

Only a rough estimate of the emphasis of federal allocations is readily possible, given the customary gross categories listing expenditures. However, such an analysis shows that about 37 per cent is spent for human services, the same as for military defense.

Ecological and Socioeconomic Of those human services, most (70 per cent) relate to ecological or socioeconomic aspects of the environment and make up about one fourth (27 per cent) of total federal expenditures. Virtually all of these environmental payments are for socioeconomic concerns, the vast proportion (90 per cent) going for retirement benefits, the remainder for public assistance payments, and a small amount for low- to moderate-income urban and rural housing.

Health and Other Of the personal human services, making up one tenth of the entire federal allocations, more than half (61 per cent) go to health services (mostly to the financing and provision of services, a small amount for development and research, and a tiny fraction for prevention and control of health problems). Other personal services include elementary and secondary education and manpower training, and the smallest allocation for social and individual services.

Pluses and Minuses In order for such a breakdown of federal government resources to accurately reflect the priorities of decision makers regarding the care of health, sums might be added which, like public transportation, might assist people to obtain the essentials for health. Likewise, sums might be subtracted where programs detract from health, such as the $36 million in federal expenditures used to promote the tobacco industry, domestically and abroad, including agricultural land programs in the United States. This is but a fraction of an estimated $35 billion in medical treatment and lost wages resulting from human misuse of the environment (32). Other deficits might include the negative effects on health of certain health and social programs, by their direct or indirect effects on particular social groups.

In any case, the point is clear. To evaluate health care by focusing on a system of personal health services will not, indeed, cannot bring about the greatest gains possible in health, even when traditionally defined environmental health services are included. Evaluating health care by focusing on people's health, populations-in-community, population groups in the national setting, could raise new questions about how best to improve health and could place personal health services in proper perspective within the health-determining socioeconomic and ecological facets of the environment. Questions about the amounts, sources, allocation, and distribution of resources could be raised, both at the national budgetary level and within human services expenditures. Rationally, the care of health would imply greater emphasis on reshaping the conditions that most affect health and relatively and selectively less, but done in a planned and coordinated manner, on means that can only temporarily remedy the ill health which those conditions breed. In effect, serious consideration of the contemporary meaning of the prevention of disease would require environmental changes concerning the distribution and control of resources. This is necessarily far beyond traditionally conceived patterns of preventive health services aimed at, for example, the health teaching of patients or potential patients, or at monitoring narrowly defined contagious disease-breeding places.

If we were to raise our vision higher and evaluate the health of the world's populations, similar questions would arise as to amounts of resources and how they should be distributed to give the greatest benefit in health, especially to the most-ill populations in the underdeveloped, outcast nations.

International Comparisons

The socioeconomic and ecological programs of most affluent countries have implicit a focus on the health of their populations as the measure of their care of health. Their human services programs, earlier described (33), of which a national health services system is part, allow synergistic, or mutually reinforcing, benefits in health; they are to varying degrees nationally integrated or coordinated, tying environment and personal services, health, and other programs to population changes, allowing the possibility of planned reallocation of resources. Those national decisions that have most emphasized the critical health-supporting aspects of environment have apparently produced the highest levels of health (34).

FOCUS ON POPULATIONS

In these circumstances the systems of personal health services have the possibility of being shaped to allow their greatest contribution to health. Thus health services development has proceeded and been evaluated according to how much access social groups have to these services, and how closely related the services are to population requirements for them. Such considerations allowed, for example, a decision in England not to develop cardiac transplantation services within the National Health Service, since the expenditure of public resources for the potential gains in health were not considered justifiable; in other words, the inevitable diversion of resources from other more needed and usable services was not in the public interest (35).

In Scotland, the evaluation of their NHS birth control programs was another instance of program assessment based on populations-in-communities. Focusing on the high infant deaths among urban babies in the mid-1960s along with other data, the NHS began the free use of birth control clinics followed by opening the program to unmarried women, eventually adding voluntary sterilization and abortion procedures. The result was a clear drop in infant mortality as well as a decline in the birth rates. As might be expected, however, the outcomes did not improve as much in the poorer cities as in the more affluent (36).

At a broader level, evaluating the total system of personal health services, England and Wales among other countries used process measures to assess changes in use of services. They found, for example, a marked shift in the use of services, before and after NHS implementation, from higher- to lower-income groups, especially among those without health insurance previously. In other words, in this instance of focusing on the services system, access was a prime criterion for its evaluation (37).

Another, recent example of a before-and-after evaluation of a universal (total population coverage) national health insurance system (NHI) was in Quebec, Canada. Certain process and outcome measures were taken before (1969), and a year after (1971), the program was implemented in the general population and among physicians. Using criteria such as access and acceptability the evaluation showed that although the actual number of visits to physicians per person was unchanged, there were marked increases in the use of physician services by the poor, the less educated, ethnic minorities, and by those with medical symptoms. Physicians worked fewer hours, although their overall number and composition did not change; they had more direct contact with patients in their offices, and less through home or hospital visits or by telephone calls. Although they believed more people sought their advice unnecessarily after NHI than before, they also thought that fewer people who needed medical care delayed seeking it under NHI. Over three out of four physicians said medical treatment was the same or improved under NHI; 70 per cent of the general population agreed with this, and 9 out of 10 who actually used the services were satisfied, about the same proportion as prior to NHI. Those who were dissatisfied were from higher-income groups, whose waiting time to see physicians had increased from 6 to 11 days, compared with their experience before NHI (38).

Reallocation of Resources

The evaluation of the care of health by focusing on populations and the impact of whole systems of services on population subgroups allows a reassessment of resource allocation. That is not to say that reassessment is alway done, or that it affects decisions about resource distribution, or even that sufficient and accurate evaluation is always made. As the previous chapter noted, even in planned, national health systems, decisions are negotiated and not necessarily based on definitive evaluation and research (39).

As in the United States, however, there seems to be growing recognition that definitive population-based and program-related information is needed to at least contribute to the decisions concerning the reallocation and redistribution of resources (40). To this end, in the early 1970s in England, for example, a unit within the NHS was created for research and development. One of its main purposes was to ensure the application of findings to policy making. Evaluation and research on services and health care delivery was to be contracted out under an advisory council composed of representatives of various health professions and social sciences (41).

Implicit in international comparisons in the care of health is of course the evaluation of national approaches to health care. A recent study, for example, compared surgical rates in Canada and England–Wales. Using rates standardized for each age and sex group, it showed higher rates, by 2 or more times, for elective surgery in Canada, although rates were similar for acute conditions requiring surgery. The outcomes were no different for patients with cancer or varicose veins treated by surgery in Canada than by nonsurgical means in England–Wales. The study then concluded that surgical rates were related to the higher numbers of surgeons and acute hospital beds in Canada and the fee-for-service incentive for payment to Canadian surgeons, in contrast to English surgeons, who are salaried (42).

Although some still doubt that international comparisons can be validly made (43), there is growing evidence that given the proper perspective and using common criteria, this can be done (44). International collaboration, now an increasing necessity for dealing with national and international problems, also has the potential for helping to reassess national decisions concerning health care.

Summary

Health care practitioners have often, as most individuals do of themselves, evaluated health services in terms of their individual good intentions, their *purpose* of providing good health care and of wanting good health for their patients and communities. However, as much as, if not more than, ever before, health care must be evaluated in terms of the *effects* of collective decisions and actions.

These effects can be evaluated by focusing on the system of services or on one or more of its components, in terms of those who use the services. That is, how accessible are its resources and how appropriate and effective are they for improving the health of consumers-as-patients in general and of subgroups, the outcast populations, in particular? Such evaluation must show the interrelationships between parts of the system and between system and consumers, in order to be usable in reassessing the allocation of resources within the system of services.

At a broader level, the effects of care-of-health decisions, by focusing on populations-in-communities and their health, can point not only to needed changes in the system of health services but also to other environmental—socioeconomic and ecological—measures which would be supportive of the health of populations and thereby allow personal health services to be most effective. Such a perspective could guide reallocation decisions concerning national resources to assure priority to health-supporting rather than health-detracting measures.

Such evaluation processes could only become possible with organized input from consumers-as-citizens and health personnel who were informed and critically conscious of the environmental and personal services requirements for the health of populations and of outcast groups in particular.

Finally, the decisions about changing the personal health services system so as to make it most accessible and effective, given the limitations within which it must exist, and a note on how it might change those limitations, are the subject of the next, and concluding, chapter.

chapter 10

Reshaping the Alternatives for Health Care

The early 1970s have already seen more and broader proposals for changing the system of personal health services than since almost a half-century ago, when a national health care program was first planned, or since the World War I era, when U.S. physicians proposed a national health insurance program (1).

The outcome of contemporary proposals as worked out in the 1970s will become the critical social fact in shaping the range of choices for health services of populations-in-communities in this country for another generation. Most of these plans have been embodied in legislative bills in Congress. Many bills have reflected the interests of the provider groups sponsoring them—whether insurers, institutions, or professional associations—thereby assuring the widest possible decision-making options and advantages to the sponsors, as discussed earlier.

The provisions in these bills have been and may continue to be under consideration or reconsideration for years to come. The following pages will now estimate the effects of alternative provisions within these bills on the people, the potential users of services, especially those in major outcast groups—the poor, the geographically isolated, ethnic minorities, women, elders—who consistently have had limited access to health services, to the health occupations, and to the decision making that shapes their options.

Then, following a brief look at some of the missing alternatives in these legislative proposals, we shall discuss prospects for changing the alternatives for health care.

Legislative Provisions That Affect Access to Health Services, Occupations, and Decision Making

Although most health care has traditionally been shaped by the absence of government policy, the last twenty years or so have brought a marked reversal, with the growing influence of national enactments setting the range of options for local governmental and nongovernmental decisions.

Formal Paths

Some of the informal ways of affecting national decisions were described in Chapter 8. The formal, major sources of national legislation are relatively straightforward. In the federal executive arm are the Office of the President and its White House advisors on domestic affairs, the Office of Management and Budget, and the Office of the Secretary of Health, Education, and Welfare, as well as various HEW agencies. The other source is the Congress, in which legislation is drafted by various combinations of elected officials, their staffs, and the staffs of interested outside parties.

Legislative proposals from any source have a Congressional sponsor who introduces the bill, which is then numbered and entered into the committee structure of either the Senate or House of Representatives. All bills are available without charge to the public once they are introduced (2).

In the complex Congressional network, the most important committees in each chamber with respect to health care are those which authorize new or revise older health services or health-related programs, such as HMOs or health personnel training; those which concern the financing of health services, such as Medicare or national health insurance; and those which appropriate the amount of funds that will actually be available to implement programs once they have been authorized.

In the Senate, health care authorization is the province of the Committee on Labor and Public Welfare, with its Subcommittee on Health and another on Alcohol and Narcotics. Its counterpart in the House is the Interstate and Foreign Commerce Committee, with its Subcommittee on Public Health and Environment. Each chamber has its health-related appropriations subcommittee and others related to the oversight of health matters. The House committee covering financing is Ways and Means. In the Senate, it is the Senate Finance Committee (Figure 10–1).

Recent proposals to reorganize the committee structure of the House would have important effects on health legislation. Possible changes include having separate committees on Appropriations, on the Budget, on Commerce and Health—to have jurisdiction over the nontax aspects of

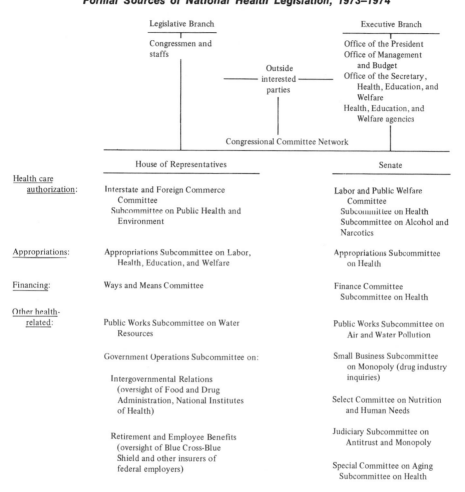

Figure 10–1   Reshaping Alternatives for Health Care, United States

Formal Sources of National Health Legislation, 1973–1974

	Legislative Branch		Executive Branch
	Congressmen and staffs		Office of the President Office of Management and Budget Office of the Secretary, Health, Education, and Welfare Health, Education, and Welfare agencies
		Outside interested parties	

Congressional Committee Network

	House of Representatives	Senate
Health care authorization:	Interstate and Foreign Commerce Committee Subcommittee on Public Health and Environment	Labor and Public Welfare Committee Subcommittee on Health Subcommittee on Alcohol and Narcotics
Appropriations:	Appropriations Subcommittee on Labor, Health, Education, and Welfare	Appropriations Subcommittee on Health
Financing:	Ways and Means Committee	Finance Committee Subcommittee on Health
Other health-related:	Public Works Subcommittee on Water Resources Government Operations Subcommittee on: Intergovernmental Relations (oversight of Food and Drug Administration, National Institutes of Health) Retirement and Employee Benefits (oversight of Blue Cross-Blue Shield and other insurers of federal employers)	Public Works Subcommittee on Air and Water Pollution Small Business Subcommittee on Monopoly (drug industry inquiries) Select Committee on Nutrition and Human Needs Judiciary Subcommittee on Antitrust and Monopoly Special Committee on Aging Subcommittee on Health

health insurance and other services-related programs—on Energy and Environment, and on Ways and Means—to cover financing and taxes, including social security (3). By altering committee jurisdictions, the shape of legislation that is finally voted on in the House (the most complex bills, especially financing, are usually voted on without amendments) would, as now, result from the priorities of committee chairpersons and members. Separating services from financing could allow more attention to organization and planning. Separating health services from environmental programs could further divorce the necessary ties between these concerns.

It is probably fair to say that most health-related Congressional legislation is the result of the work of the staffs of these committees, of the Congressional representatives, and of other interested parties, occurring throughout the policy-making spectrum of posing the issues, the alternative approaches, and narrowing the path to definitive legislation. Much of this occurs prior to and around the public subcommittee hearings usually held during the process of committee deliberations on the disposition of proposals.

Legislative Proposals and Their Effects

Although there were as many as 15–20 Congressional proposals introduced in the early 1970s related to establishing a national health program, most of their provisions fall into a relatively few categories, each of which represents an alternative approach to a given issue. How these various approaches to health care issues are likely to affect certain social groups, especially the outcast, will now be examined. This analysis rests on and summarizes in effect the implications of earlier discussions about access to the health services network by populations-in-communities, that is, by various social groups living in diverse geographic areas (4).

Provisions Affecting Access to Services

FINANCIAL ACCESS

Legislative provisions affecting access to personal health services concern directly or indirectly the financing, organization, and distribution of services. In order to improve access for those who now have it least, proposed measures were directed at making the array of most-needed services available financially and geographically, but with considerable variation in their potential effects.

Economic Participation Most of the proposals emphasized financing, that is, a national health insurance plan. These included basically three approaches: (1) a mandatory plan in which all active people would participate economically, whether employers, employees, or self-employed, although no one would be required to use the services so financed; (2) a mandatory plan for the employers of most workers, requiring them to offer a comprehensive health insurance plan to their employees and to pay for the greatest part of it; (3) a voluntary approach by which, through tax-deduction incentives to individuals and employers, people would buy minimum basic health insurance (Table 10–1).

Population Coverage and Channels for Funds   The mandatory approach would provide financial protection for the total population with a single channel for collection and allocation of funds. The other approaches selectively cover one or more categories of people, such as half- or full-time employees, nongovernmental workers, the unemployed, the poor or near-poor, families with dependent children, single-parent families, the catastrophically ill, the medically uninsurable, the temporarily disabled, those eligible for social security, and elders. Related to the number of covered groups, the channels for funds under these plans are multiple, including combinations of public and private entities at national, regional, state, and local levels.

Some Consequences   There is little doubt that any of these approaches would mean short-term gains for at least some groups, such as the medically high risk, those fully employed in large industries, and the working poor. These and other groups would be assured that a minimum in health benefits would be at least financially available through payment on their behalf in whole or part.

However, the similarity in effects for these approaches ends there. In all except the mandatory universal coverage approach, many social groups would remain or become "uncovered," without financial access to services, especially those who are poorest and who live in the poorest, rural states. This means, in effect, disproportionately large numbers of ethnic minorities, women, and elders.

This unevenness of effect is for several reasons. Under voluntary plans, persons simply may delay or may not apply for the particular program for which they may be eligible—due to lack of information or to the negligible nature of their tax advantages; to the time-consuming complexity of having multiple programs in each state or region; or they may refuse to submit to means tests or grant the insurer access to internal revenue files, as some plans require. Further, some employee groups may refuse health benefits in exchange for other bargainable economic and wage benefits; or, in weakly unionized and non-worker-organized workplaces, employees may not be able to bargain effectively for a comprehensive insurance plan under the voluntary approach; or, under the employer-mandatory approach, they may not be able to effectively report noncompliance by employers who refuse to offer a full plan or to pay the required three fourths of the premium. With multiple programs, supplemental coverage is likely to be different state by state, the fewest benefits being available in the poorest regions.

Selective coverage has the obvious deficiency of allowing some people to "fall through the cracks." The especially vulnerable groups are part-

Table 10-1 Reshaping Alternatives for Health Care, United States

National Legislative Proposals for Comprehensive Personal Health Services, Provisions Affecting Access of Major Outcast Populations, 1973–1974

Provisions	Effects on Major Outcast Groups (low-income, rural: especially minority, women, elders)
Access to Services	
Financial	
Economic participation	
Mandatory	Assures contributions from all except lowest income earners, thus demanding less from those with least.
Mandatory for certain employees	Employees, especially those with low job security, may fear reporting noncompliance by employer.
Voluntary with tax incentives	Lack of information may delay application; other priorities may be more critical; tax incentives are negligible for low and middle incomes; time-consuming paperwork and means tests may be deterrents; employees may not be able to bargain for a comprehensive plan, or, especially in weak or nonunion workplaces where pay is low, may accept wage benefits instead.
Population coverage	
Universal	Makes all coverage automatic, all benefits equal.
Selective (e.g., half- or full-time employees, unemployed, poor, elders, catastrophically ill, medically uninsurable, families with dependent children)	Part-time, seasonal, agricultural, domestic workers (most being low-income, minority, women) would be excluded administratively due to shifting status, or would have to seek out special plans.
Channels for funds	
Single	Administration would be more understandable, quicker, less costly.

Multiple	Application procedures, time lag, benefits will differ state by state, with poorest and most rural having least.
Financing methods Social insurance and public revenues Social insurance, public revenues, insurance premiums, and direct consumer payments	Public revenues (income taxes) allow financing to be shared among all income groups as equitably as currently possible; social insurance (payroll taxes) places a greater burden on lower-income earners; insurance premiums, as a flat payment, are more regressive; direct consumer payments are most regressive, placing the greatest burden on low-income persons (i.e., women, minorities, elders); since tax deductions are allowable under employer plans and for other health payments, the revenue lost to government would be made up in income taxes with a larger share falling to lower-income groups.
Insurer(s) Federal agency	Would make possible the most equitable standards for financing, allocations, and benefits based on need, at least overall administrative cost.
Regional public/private carrier, federal–private fiscal intermediary, and federal–state–private fiscal intermediary	Almost inevitable differences in the burdens of financing, allocations, benefit standards, administrative rules, and higher overall administrative costs would mean some groups would be deficit, most likely the outcasts.
Private insurance carriers, federal–private fiscal intermediary and federal–state–private fiscal intermediary	
Payment bases Community rating	Payments would be made for services based on health care requirements of particular populations-in-communities.
Experience rating	Higher premiums would result for those groups which require the most health services (e.g., the poor, women, elders), and may therefore deter some employers from hiring such people.

Provisions	*Effects on Major Outcast Groups* *(low-income, rural: especially minority, women, eiders)*
Payment methods	
Capitation/salary incentives	Needed primary ambulatory and lower-cost care services would be increased; unnecessary surgery (now most often done on women) would be discouraged; more conservative and possibly safer treatment and preventive services would be encouraged.
Fee-for-service predominance	Would allow continued higher-cost, inpatient, and elaborate forms of treatment.
Fiscal controls	
Provider emphasis (no deductibles or copayments, practitioner risk sharing; prospective budgeting; national ceiling)	Without direct costs to deter lower-income people who have delayed seeking services, plus stronger provider incentives for rendering services on basis of need, costs are more likely to reflect the real value of health services.
Consumer emphasis (deductibles, copayments; practitioner fees at "reasonable cost," rate control commissions)	Direct consumer payments would deter the poor, who are in most need of service, from seeking health care; loose provider controls have not, and especially on an uneven state-by-state basis cannot, contain costs, ultimately borne by consumers.
Range of services	
Benefits pattern	
Narrow/catastrophic	Will deter use of uncovered services; will place greater burdens on low-income families who must spend 10–15% of income before becoming eligible.
Comprehensive	Will encourage early use of health services, including dental and eye, hearing, foot problems, which most often go untreated among lower-income groups.
Practitioners covered	
By task	Would expand availability of primary services, to be given by competent practitioners.
By title	Would restrict availability of primary services only to those with formal titles.

278

Principal site of service Home/community	With broad, primary care coverage, would encourage the development and use of primary services, now least accessible to low-income, and others who have barriers of time, transportation, work-loss costs, child care, etc.
Institutional	Would aggravate current inequities in available services.
Organization of delivery HMO incentives to providers and consumers (nonprofit, minimum benefits, open enrollment, low copayments; subsidy for poor, 24-hour service; ties to inpatient and home services; community or "nonprofit provider group" sponsorship, etc.)	More likely to provide single-site primary care to outcast groups and areas, with fewer deterrents to lower-income groups, and encouragement to service-committed providers seeking to render community-related care.
HMO incentives to providers (for-profit, flexible benefits, closed enrollment, moderate copayments; consumer input optional, etc.)	Most likely to locate in urban and affluent areas.
No direct mention	Would aggravate current disjointed multiple-site services, thereby deterring least-mobile groups, such as working women, those with young children, the isolated, elders, low-income.
Geographic Distribution *Ad hoc* incentives to (re)locate in scarcity areas Incentives and national organized oversight	Would improve access for outcast groups to a limited but uneven extent.

Provisions	Effects on Major Outcast Groups (low-income, rural: especially minority, women, elders)
By advisory council	Recommendations would call attention to inequities, but implementation would not be assured.
By policy-implementing board	Could tie resources supply to allocation and distribution related to the requirements of populations-in-communities.
No direct mention	Would aggravate current maldistribution, most affecting outcast groups.
Access to the Health Occupations Entry, emphasis, and movement within and/or between groups *Ad hoc* incentives To increase supply (recruitment, training from low-income groups; remedial, retraining; stipends; insurance coverage of nonphysician services; increased enrollments) To deemphasize specialization (priority funding of first-year students, diminished training time, training for ambulatory, primary care, health management, team personnel; HMO funding for training and/or employ of nonphysician personnel) To change the conditions of practice (HMO development, nondiscrimination against competent professionals; national minimum training standards and competency criteria)	Greater numbers, especially of more primary and ambulatory personnel, working in less rigid and hierarchical settings would mean some improved access for outcasts into certain occupations and some voice in work conditions; this would not necessarily alter sex-typed occupations, income–race patterns, or allow much movement within or between occupations based on practitioner competency.

Incentives and national organized oversight	
By an advisory body (for guidelines, recommendations)	Might call attention to but could not assure programs to change patterns.
By a board to implement personnel policy (related to regional requirements and planning)	Could relate training to service needs and devise competency criteria which would allow movement within and between occupations.
No direct mention	Would aggravate current patterns of pyramids within and between occupations, keeping low-income, minorities, and women at lower levels.
Access to Decision Making At the delivery level	
HMOs defined as comprehensive direct service organizations	Would encourage direct practitioner–consumer collaboration.
HMOs defined as financial and scattered-site service institutions	Would limit both practitioner and consumer participation in development and operation.
Controls	
National coordination of a system of controls relating quality and cost	Standards would be evenly applicable, with right of appeal.
Strengthening of noncoordinated regulatory agencies with cost-control emphasis	State-by-state regulation would be uneven, subjecting some to different standards; cost emphasis would place greatest burden on low-income and most ill.
Evaluation	
National oversight with research-based standard setting and segregating quality assessment from cost-control enforcement	Can help assure sound planning and monitoring of the organizational and technical effectiveness of services based on requirements of populations-in-communities.

Provisions	Effects on Major Outcast Groups (low-income, rural: especially minority, women, elders)
Undefined methods for national standard setting and quality assessment implicit in cost control	Could allow undue influence in standard setting and allow costs to override importance of quality as needed and effective services.
Consumer participation	
Organized inclusion (national to local levels with representative involvement)	Assures options for input at all organizational levels and through much of decision-making cycle by outcast groups, with legal right of appeal.
Inclusion at providers' discretion (national and area levels)	Cannot assure consumer right of significant input, nor of access by all groups, including outcasts.
No mention	Would intensify current direction, patterns, and perspective of health care.

Sources: S. 3, Sen. Kennedy (H.R. 22, Rep. Griffiths), "Health Security, 1973."

S. 1100, Sen. McIntyre (H.R. 5200, Rep. Burleson), "National Health Care, 1973."

H.R. 1, Rep. Ullman, "National Health Care Services Reorganization and Financing, 1973."

S. 1623, Sen. Bennett, "National Health Insurance Standards, 1971."

S. 2756, Sen. Scott, "Health Rights, 1973."

S. 444, Sen. Hansen (H.R. 2222, Reps. Broyhill and Fulton), "National Health Care Insurance (Medicredit), 1973."

S. 2513 Sens. Long and Ribicoff, "Catastrophic Health Insurance and Medical Assistance Reform, 1973."

S. 2790, Sen. Packwood (H.R. 12684, Rep. Mills), "Comprehensive Health Insurance, 1974."

S. 3286, Sen. Kennedy (H.R. 13870, Rep. Mills) "Comprehensive National Health Insurance, 1974."

time, seasonal, agricultural, and domestic workers, and the temporarily unemployed. They would be shifted from one category to another, each time having to follow different procedures, receiving different benefits, all of which may unduly thwart their motivation to obtain primary, preventive health care and early treatment. Thus, without a single-system universal plan, the poor and those in poor regions, those most likely to be or become ill, are likely to have the least financial assurance of sustained and equally available health services.

Financing Methods, Insurers, and Basis for Payments Other important issues related to a national health insurance plan concern the burden of supporting its program(s). Proposed methods of financing are basically (1) a combination of social insurance (employer–employee–self-employed) taxes and public revenues (with tax relief for persons over 60), and (2) a combination of social insurance and public revenues (for financing the poor and elder-related programs) plus private insurance premiums and direct consumer payments for services (for the nonpoor and nonaged). In the first approach a federal agency would be the insurer and would base the payments for services on the needs of socio–economic–geographic groups, populations-in-communities. Under the second approach, the insurers would be (a) combinations of regionally designated public or private insurance carriers, plus the federal government using private companies as fiscal intermediaries (as under Medicare) and federal–state programs with private fiscal intermediaries (as under Medicaid); or (b) a combination of private insurance carriers (the current pattern), a federal program with private fiscal intermediaries, and federal–state programs with similar intermediaries (for either low-income or supplemental insurance programs). These multiple-insurer approaches would establish premiums based generally on the experience ratings of given insurers for given groups, as is now commonly done.

Methods of Payment and Fiscal Cost Controls Some plans give priority to and incentives for newer methods of payment, which, as earlier discussions showed, clearly affect costs and patterns of services. Thus some proposals encourage capitation or physician-salary methods whereas others do not, allowing fee-for-service to remain predominant.

All plans include fiscal controls over costs. They tend, however, to place greater emphasis on either (1) the consumer or (2) on the providers. Consumer emphasis is done by, for example, requiring such cost-sharing devices as deductibles and copayments, with looser controls on providers, such as allowing fee setting at a "reasonable cost" (equal to the 75th percentile of the prior year's levels) or via insurance or hospital rate-setting commissions within each state.

The alternative emphasis, on controlling provider-generated costs, provides for no deductibles or copayments by consumers, risk sharing by practitioners (through capitation methods), salary incentives, prior-year budgeting subject to approval for hospitals, and a national statutory health budgetary ceiling along with contingency reserves.

Effects: Economic   Public revenue financing is the most equitable fiscal means for spreading the burden of financing human services, since progressive income taxes in theory require more from those with higher incomes. Social insurance, consisting of employer–employee payroll taxes, is regressive, especially when a flat rate is required, as is commonly done under social security. Thus low wage earners and small employers are required to contribute greater proportions of their earnings than those with high incomes. Similarly, insurance premiums are regressive and inequitable since they are essentially a flat rate payment charged alike to low- and high-income individuals and employers.

Further, under the financing methods which propose the use of premiums, these are tax deductible, but to a negligible degree for low- and moderate-income individuals, yet in sizable amounts for employers. Since tax deductions amount to a loss of public revenues, that loss must then be made up in income taxes, which in practice fall disproportionately on low- to moderate-income groups. In effect, these taxpayers would be subsidizing large employer insurance plans, and doing so through a complex and administratively costly route. Alternatively, or in addition, employers could make up for required high insurance premiums through limiting wage increases or raising the prices of their products—in contrast to narrowing their profit margins. Thus insurance premiums and direct consumer payments for services, which are also a flat charge unrelated to need or capacity to pay, are the more inequitable approach to financing, placing a greater burden on lower-income groups.

The use of experience ratings as the basis for setting premiums also brings an added burden to those with medical problems, requiring higher premiums of them or of their employers. This further provides a disincentive for employers to hire such vulnerable groups as the disabled and elders, among others.

Finally, the more unevenly balanced is the burden of financing in relation to economic capacity to pay, program proposals such as those calling for multiple programs and administrative duplication, coverage of high- but not low-cost services, and/or the inclusion of private profits— all of which will add to costs—will result in less equity and access to services for those who most need health care.

Effects on Services   To the extent that newer methods of payment such as capitation are encouraged, there is likely to be an increase in the supply of lower-cost primary, ambulatory care, and, as available data seems to indicate, a decrease in unnecessary and expensive services. This is likely to include a drop in unneeded surgery, much of which is done on women, and to encourage more conservative and safer treatment for the sickest patients, most being the poor and the aged (5).

As studies indicate, however, the use of deductibles and copayments will be an uneven deterrent to the overuse of services, most affecting the poor and their use of services to prevent and treat illness early.

ACCESS TO THE RANGE OF NEEDED SERVICES

Beyond the indirect effects which alternative methods of payment, whether capitation or fee-for-service, are likely to have on shifting services toward outpatient, necessary, and conservative modes of treatment, the financing proposals would have additional direct effects on the array of available services.

Benefits Pattern and Scope   The plans vary in their standard required benefits pattern, some focusing on a narrow and others on a comprehensive range of services. The narrowest are the catastrophic illness plans, which cover only severe illness episodes and take effect only after families have spent a sizable part of their income on medical care in a given year. Other plans exclude certain services, such as dental or emergency treatment during travel; or place time limits on certain services, such as days in hospital or visits to physicians. Their use of copayments and deductibles in addition would tend to restrict the use of the services to which such cost sharing is applied.

The most comprehensive plan covers full payment for all routine preventive, health maintenance, curative, emergency, and restorative services, with limitations under certain conditions on dental, mental health, and nursing home care. Quite clearly, the services for which full payment can be made will be the most likely to be made available by providers and sought by consumers.

Practitioners Covered   Similarly, those plans which cover payments for certain services—rather than for services rendered only by certain practitioners (for example, primary care services rendered by competent practitioners who may be other than physicians)—will encourage a greater supply of those services so covered (in this example, primary care).

Principal Site of Services   The financing proposals will have a further effect on the range of health services depending upon their emphasis, explicit or implicit, as to the principal site for the provision of services. At one end of the spectrum is the provision of services in homes, not only before and after necessary institutional care, but extending, on a demonstration basis, to long-term or permanent inhome services to the chronically ill and elders. This would include all necessary services, whether conventionally health-related or not. In contrast to this home and community focus are the plans in which coverage emphasizes inpatient services, with home care as undefined or narrow aftercare.

Organization of Delivery   Other provisions affecting the availability of community-based services pertain to the organization of delivery systems. Plans have (1) avoided any direct effort to affect health services delivery, or (2) have aimed at altering delivery by encouraging HMO development through principally (a) incentives to providers, or (b) a combination of provider and consumer incentives. The provider-focused incentives amount to fostering a good business investment, such as allowing HMOs to organize as for-profit corporations, with flexible benefit packages, moderate copayments, closed enrollments, optional consumer input, FMC (foundations for medical care) delivery patterns, and by requiring employers to offer an HMO option in providing their employees with a health insurance plan.

The provider–consumer incentives, likewise fostered by the availability of federal grants and loans, would develop not-for-profit HMOs, establish a minimum benefits requirement, allow only low copayments but subsidize copayments for low-income or high-risk persons, require direct delivery of services for all except dental and mental health, 24-hour-service, formal ties to inpatient and home care services, transition funds for allowing neighborhood health centers, and community mental health programs to develop fully as comprehensive HMOs, and sponsorship by community groups or by "nonprofit provider groups" (which would encompass an array of health workers).

Some Effects   At a minimum, all the legislative proposals would have the effect of establishing a national floor for health services, so that the poor in some states would be eligible for more services than they now receive. Under some plans, however, other poor families may have less coverage than currently. To the extent that the plans do not require, or restrict, or exclude coverage of ambulatory, preventive, and primary care services, this is likely to limit the supply and use of such services. Such a result would more heavily affect women and young children, and would delay the use of services by the poor; this is most apparent under the catastrophic plans (6). Without coverage for payment for outpatient drugs, under cost-control methods, the chronically ill, particularly elders, would continue to have heavy direct expenses. Those plans which do not directly deal with the organized delivery of services, or do not require ties between the sites of services—inpatient–ambulatory–home—will very likely aggravate current disjointed multiple-site patterns. This would place greater burdens on those who now experience such cost barriers as transportation, time, child-tending, and other priorities to obtain health services. Fostering one-stop HMOs on a profit-making basis is likely only to bring their development in relatively affluent areas, and thus would be of little help to low-income populations even when financial barriers to services are removed.

Ad Hoc Incentives The legislative proposals as related to the geographic distribution of services vary again from (1) an avoidance of the issue, to (2) providing *ad hoc* incentives to relocate in scarcity areas, to (3) additional provisions for organized redistribution of services. The *ad hoc* incentives include larger development and operating grants to HMOs in scarcity areas, funds for transportation and communication linkages for organized rural services, student loan forgiveness for health care students who agree to work in shortage areas, traineeships in return for five years of service, and a guaranteed above-average income for health professionals who work in such areas.

Organized Oversight Provisions concerning the organized oversight of redistribution center on a national board or council, varying in its potential for impact. It would be given basically (a) an advisory capacity, restricted either to counseling the use of currently available resources, or to studying problems and recommending changes; or (b) it would have a statutory mandate to implement means of balancing health facilities and personnel in relation to the changing requirements of populations-in-communities.

Effects on Outcasts Those provisions which directly deal with the uneven geographic access to services are likely at a minimum to result in a greater public accountability with respect to this issue. National oversight of this problem is not likely to be very effective in redistributing health services without authority to tie the supply of resources to the distribution of resources. Clearly, an explicit national policy of even distribution related to population requirements, with the mechanism to implement such policy, would have the greatest favorable impact on those who live in poor and isolated areas, who in turn are disproportionately more the low-income, minorities, elders, and women.

Provisions Affecting Access to the Health Occupations

The provisions in the national legislative proposals concerning access to the health occupations vary along lines similar to many of the services-related provisions. That is, by (1) omitting direct involvement with the issue, (2) offering *ad hoc* incentives affecting entry to and emphasis within the health occupations, or (3) providing additionally for a national organizational structure with potential to both coordinate the incentives and tie health training to the requirements for the delivery of health services.

Some *ad hoc* provisions that would help open entry into the health field are those increasing the supply of personnel through recruitment and training of persons from low-income groups, remedial training, retraining of older workers, scholarships and stipends, the earlier noted incentive of insurance coverage for the services of nonphysicians, and funds for schools that increase their enrollments. Further, entry would become easier for those currently restricted through measures that deemphasize specialization and provide incentives for training in primary care and for ambulatory care personnel. Such provisions include priority funding for first-year students and for schools that diminish training time and stress most-needed primary personnel training programs, training funds for HMOs both to train and/or fully employ nonphysician health personnel, reimbursement to HMOs for the clinical education of health professionals trained under other auspices, and funding for training health care management personnel and team training of physicians. This lessening of the emphasis on specialization could be a deterrent to the growing hierarchies within the health occupations.

Finally, are the measures affecting the site and conditions of health care practice, such as HMO development, with salaried or other means to limit topearners; nondiscrimination against competent professionals; national minimum standards for the training of allied personnel; and, following licensure in a single state, compliance with national competency criteria to allow practice in any state. This would be likely to allow greater freedom of movement within, if not among, the health occupations.

The additional provisions for national structures to be concerned in part with oversight of health personnel policy fall again into two basic types: (a) a council that can make recommendations and set up guidelines regarding entry to and mobility within the health occupations—but without a capacity to implement changes; (b) a board that can set priorities for the recruitment and education of needed personnel on a regional basis, in consultation with area planning and professional groups, and, as well, implement policy through a health resources development fund tied to the health insurance trust fund.

This latter approach has at least the potential for relating the training of personnel to the kinds necessary to deliver most-needed health services. Taken further, it could also seek the most economical and fluid methods to train competent practitioners, capable of the flexibility and breadth necessary to work in communities, in ambulatory care settings, in homes, among diverse population groups, in communication with consumers, and jointly with other personnel. It could also assure them opportunity for both cumulative and alternative areas of learning.

Possible Effects The obvious beneficiaries of such training patterns, beyond the users and payors of health services, would be those groups of health personnel who have been limited because of current emphases on specialization and formal credentialing, which have created pyramids among and within the occupations. This means again, of course, low-income persons, minorities, and women.

In other words, even though access to the health field may become somewhat easier because of provisions for more, and for less specialized, personnel, this alone will not change the income–sex–race-related composition of the occupations. For that, provision must also be made for reorganizing the professionally segregated pattern of training.

Provisions Affecting Access to Decision Making

All the proposals for national health insurance plans contain provisions relating directly and indirectly to decision making at various levels, local to national. These provisions amount to whether or not patterns of decision making will be changed very much.

AT THE DELIVERY LEVEL

At the community level, the point of delivery of health services, the provisions that define the health maintenance organization become important for determining control over the delivery of services. Mainly these provisions define HMOs either as (1) an organization that *directly* provides most of its services to a geographically defined population, thereby also limiting its size, or as (2) as organization that may *arrange for* the rendering of services to a group of people. The latter definition would allow an HMO to be a very large organization, would permit services and the people to be served to be scattered geographically (thereby allowing it to be less effectively accountable to its group of consumers). Perhaps most important under definition (2) is that financial institutions, insurance companies, banks, or other profit makers could qualify as HMOs; they would then contract for the delivery of certain health services with various practitioners and would basically control the delivery system so designed.

Further, whether or not an HMO is a self-contained unit—providing direct comprehensive services in a single ambulatory care setting—will have an effect on the decision-making patterns that are possible *within* health delivery settings. Scattered-site services would tend to perpetuate current pyramids of power between occupation groups and make less likely an enhanced bargaining capacity for most nonphysician health personnel.

CONTROLS

State Regulation   Provisions concerning controls over health services tend to fall into two categories: (1) the strengthening of current non-coordinated regulatory agencies or (2) the national coordination of a system of controls. The regulatory agency approach emphasizes state-level commissions for cost controls on state insurance plans for the poor, review of professional practice, HMO regulation, and, at the delivery level, a continuation of utilization review, and other forms of peer review, and hospital accreditation.

National Coordination   The approach that emphasizes national co-ordination concerns the setting of guidelines or standards with or without the leverage for effective enforcement. Standard-setting provisions call for minimum benefit packages and premium parameters in order for insurance companies to qualify as fiscal intermediaries or "approved plans"; professional competence criteria; participation standards for hospitals and HMOs to receive federal capitation or other funds, such as nondiscrimination against health personnel or consumers; and utilizing basic lists of generic drugs and maintaining common record and reporting systems. Further provisions concern national ties to state and area services and facilities planning, as well as personnel planning as noted above, with the authority to refuse funds for unneeded or ineffective services; and all results would be published.

EVALUATION

Criteria   The criteria against which controls would be instituted vary again, with most (1) emphasizing cost controls implicit in the regulatory agency approach most often, and others (2) including quality indices such as local population need based on health levels, acceptability to consumers, and health outcomes of the users of services.

Standard Setting and Quality Assurance Provisions concerning decision making also differ as to the process by which standards for controls should be set and the relation of cost to quality controls. In other words, their evaluation systems, as well as criteria, differ. They tend either to (1) divorce standard setting from study or research and at the same time make control over quality implicit with cost control; or, by contrast, (2) establish a means for basing standards on research (as well as for funding such research, as on health care outcomes), but separating standard setting concerning quality from the enforcement of cost controls. The intent here is to safeguard quality, defined as the competent provision of needed services to high-risk populations-in-communities, when this may entail relatively higher costs.

A CONSUMER VOICE

As to whether consumers should have a voice in health care decision making, the proposals present something of a continuum, from (1) no consumer input, to (2) having consumer involvement at the discretion of providers, to (3) mandatory inclusion of consumers in an organized way.

Sites Where consumers are to have some voice, provisions differ as to where and how this would be done. Most emphasize the national level, either allowing or requiring consumers up to a majority on an advisory body. Others go further, calling for consumers on regional and/or area planning and policy-making levels, in "equitable" numbers, or as a majority representative of the population served.

One proposal goes still further, to the HMO as the unit for delivering services. There, the policy-making body would include a one-third consumer component as a requirement for HMO participation in the national health insurance program. There would also be funds available for training such consumer representatives. For the consumer-as-patient provision is made to supply information as to the alternatives available for obtaining health services, how best to use the services, and how to contribute to self-health. Grievance procedures would be established in HMOs; and area-wide consumer-majority boards, having informational and fiscal responsibilities, could also perform as ombudsmen.

Effects Throughout the spectrum of provisions about decision-making processes, wherever national provider-aimed standards become enforceable is likely to mean some improvement in services for populations-in-communities, or at least set up their right to appeal poor standards of service. This would be especially important for those groups which have been least favored.

Because of the weaknesses of the regulatory agency approach to controls, particularly when uncoordinated and sited at state levels, it is likely to be ineffective in controlling costs or quality and to continue to be dominated by providers. This will have consequences for consumers in economic terms and in the evenness of effective health services across the country. Again, the financial burden and health service deficits will weigh heaviest on lower-income, rural, elders, and other outcast groups.

Further, if cost controls become paramount, without other criteria to measure the allocation and distribution of health care resources, it is the outcast who will suffer most. Being more vulnerable to illness, their need for and the costs of their health care are higher than their more-favored counterparts. This prospect becomes particularly plausible should financial and profit-making organizations further increase their capacity to shape health services delivery, as, among other provisions, a loose definition of HMO would allow.

Finally, it is not likely that consumers, especially those from outcast groups, would have any significant voice in devising health service patterns under a new national health program, unless their voice was mandated and safe-guarded by open and organized means. At least as important as area and national policy making is their effective participation at the level of the delivery of services. This is likely to have the most meaning and interest to them, having more immediacy to everyday concerns. At all levels, however, training for such participation, aimed at establishing a critical consciousness, would be essential for consumers and for most providers as well.

Clearly the array of provisions represented in Congressional proposals would in their adoption mean wide differences in the options available under a revised system of health services and in the possibilities for further changing such a system. However well-intentioned *ad hoc* incentives for changes may be, when they are implemented in a nonorganized and non-planned manner, without links to known population–geographic requirements, their effects can only be haphazard, sometimes fortuitous, creating oases, but often breeding more problems. Without organized ties—between policy–planning–allocations, between health services and populations-in-communities, between health training and health services, between resources put in and evaluation of effects on health—there is little chance that a national health program will improve access to health care for outcast groups. Indeed, without such links a national program may create new outcasts, if only by placing a greater and growing burden of financing on the majority of working people.

The problems involved in developing a national program that assures an effective right to health care grow year by year. They are far more complex today than a generation or two ago when most affluent countries were developing such programs. Not only are private interests vastly more influential, but also other *ad hoc* governmental health service-related programs are increasingly multiplying, as earlier chapters have described.

Any effective national program would have to take these private and public bureaucracies into account, and yet few legislative proposals show clearly how this would be done. Other separate attempts to consolidate federal programs are being made, in the areas of planning and control, of personnel training, of financing, but such attempts have not themselves been interrelated.

Further, virtually no effort has been made to relate such environmental policy as may exist to health services policy, or to assess their relative impact on health, in costs and gains. Yet, environmental protection programs are being legislated, and policy is being formulated affecting energy use, food production, housing, land use, mass transit, and workplace environments—all quite isolated from changes in personal health services.

Another omission in proposed national health programs is a tie with policy affecting personal socioeconomic circumstances, principally the incomes of people, which, as always, are more directly essential to health among the outcast groups.

A final major tie that is lacking concerns the system of education, in terms of either youthful or lifelong learning. Without awareness of what is necessary for health—all of what is needed for consumers-as-citizens and consumers-as-patients (beyond the traditional admonitions about hygiene, and into the realm of organization, decision making, and the socioeconomic and ecologic environments)—the effective use of personal health services, much less their effective development, is not likely.

WEIGHING COSTS AND BENEFITS

Without such organized links and the means to assess the relative impact of programs, national policy making and budgetary allocations would seem impossible if indeed the health of the population were a priority. Customarily, the economic costs of the proposed health programs have been evaluated in terms of (1) new federal dollars required, consisting of tax losses and new approprations; (2) new costs, that is, charges (paid by private or public sources) for services which are "induced"—which would not otherwise have been used except for the new program (this is about a 25–40 per cent increase, the highest increase being for dental and eye services); (3) the transfer of expenditures to a federal agency of funds that would otherwise have been spent by state and local governments; and (4) the transfer of payments from the private sector (from what would be otherwise paid in insurance premiums and direct consumer expenses) to a federal health agency. Thus calculated, the difference in total cost of the proposed programs varied from an additional $2–9 billion beyond what would have been spent without any new programs in fiscal year 1974 (105.4 Bil.), according to a Congressional study (7).

What is further needed to assess even the economic impact of such legislation is some estimate of the relative economic benefits to various social groups—in terms of costs of services or payments received of the $105–114 billion that would be expended—and the proportions each group would contribute to the total. In other words, public accounting should include the relative economic benefits and costs to outcast groups in particular, with or without a new national health program.

Finally, it is necessary to also estimate the relative costs and gains in health of populations-in-communities to estimate whether the new billions, or indeed the current billions spent for health services, might not be more effective if allocated to certain other programs which, for example, would improve the socioeconomic environment of the poor or the breathing space of communities. Careful comparisons with other countries could help in this assessment.

Again, however, such assessment by government and private organizations, much less for effective public discussion and debate, is virtually impossible without explicit and planned interlinking structures, without exposure to public scrutiny, and without a trained awareness by the public of alternatives and their possible consequences. Otherwise an awareness of sorts comes only after the looming of "crises," which in turn tend to produce only *ad hoc* action.

Removing the Constraints on Personal Health Care

In sum, this discussion says that a system of personal health services, in order to be most effective in contributing to health, must be viewed in its planning and development within the context of health-allowing, health-depriving social and physical realities, in particular the socioeconomic and ecological environments of social groups as they exist in communities. Ideally, plans would begin by viewing the picture of the limited health in communities, and from there build the socioeconomic and ecological programs, and the personal human services, which could best improve health.

Without changes in the context in which personal health services exist, medical care, even at its best, will continue only to try to repair the damage done by the environments of populations, of outcast groups, and of more favored social groups as well.

Consumers-as-Citizens

However unlikely are the prospects for altering the conditions under which various populations-in-communities exist—given sociopolitical realities—the most likely source and possibly last hope for such impetus is the organized consumer-as-citizen. Rather ironically, even among those professionals who have been most vocal about "consumer participation," there has been little organized effort to educate and involve consumers in the issues at stake in designing a national health program. Perhaps as a consequence, the array of alternatives represented in the legislative proposals of the early 1970s by no means include an entire spectrum of options—no group, for example, has proposed a national health service, what is usually considered "socialized medicine."

CONSUMER–CITIZENS AS SOCIAL GROUPS

"Consumers-as-citizens" are not, of course, a single social group. Their identities and concerns are tied to their economic life, where they live, their sex, age, and ethnicity. Those who are likely to be more aware of how their circumstances have limited their choices are those in outcast groups. Outcasts also stand to gain most from substantial social changes. Thus the most likely candidates for developing a critical consciousness concerning the conditions for health, with respect to changes in the environment and in a system of personal health services, are outcast groups —those who live in inner-city and rural areas, the poor and near-poor, women, elders, and ethnic minorities, among others.

Priorities Almost by definition, however, outcasts have other urgent priorities. The issues at stake in national health and related legislation are far removed from necessities which they must face almost daily. Thus, gaining the attention of such groups of consumers would have to be done not only at a grass roots level, in everyday surroundings, but would also have to mesh with each group's priorities.

Organized Strategies In order to warrant their involvement, health-related issues would have to be tied to the concerns around which many such groups are already organized. In many respects, groups of racial minorities, women, and elders have long been concerned about their limited options for educational and personal services, employment, and other areas of decision making. Proposals that shape their options in health-related matters could readily be joined to these concerns.

Beyond such organizational forums are possibilities for intergroup alliances, seminars, workshops, or formal courses offered along a spectrum of age groups under educational or other community-group auspices. Beyond the local level, of course, are necessary ties to informational channels and feedback to and from policy makers, particularly to the elected officials whose committees shape health and health services-related legislation. At all levels, from national to the local community, the public media, particularly television, have vast potential for public education, so often cited and so little effected. Education-as-awareness should be possible not only through documentary programming—expensive and perhaps inevitably focused to a narrow range of views as it is—but also through informal television discussion and debate among the broadest spectrum of participants, with viewer feedback. Issues could be aired, problems defined, alternatives explored, processes examined, and possible consequences for various social groups made clear.

Again, as unlikely as such critical consciousness and responsiveness is, it seems the best hope for any organized effort to alter personal health services and the context in which they exist, to devise changes so that outcast groups as well as their more-favored counterparts can have health-bringing options. Without public awareness of the very different consequences of numerous proposals all of which are labeled "national health insurance," there is likely to be little consumer response to Congressional moves. Without definitive public response, Congressional approaches are likely to follow familiar paths, with the result that changes will not alter current prerogatives very much, outcasts will gain little, and the health of the American majority is not likely to improve.

PROFESSIONALS AS COLLABORATORS

Creating such a truly democratic responsiveness would meet with many impediments, beyond finding sources for the funds that would be needed. Among them is the fact that health professionals—who are assumed to be experts on health—are often unaware, or narrowly aware as a result of their training and other reasons, of the big picture, of the context in which they work. In effect, they are more concerned about health services than about health.

Further, most health care providers are part of large groups and associations. Thus group decisions and organizational priorities are likely to take precedence over personal doubts, to stifle questions, to close options to new ways. And soon the newer—and sometimes more open—health personnel accept the same constraints and rewards as their mentors. Personal intention to do good and perform well takes or retains priority over the critical examination of the effects of collective actions. Were it otherwise, organized health professionals would probably have significant policy-making influence toward support for the health-deriving social changes that would make personal health services more effective.

Individual Strategies   Health care practitioners may and do, of course, make wider individual commitments and take personal risks in terms of their economic or job-related aspirations. They have worked as collaborators with various consumer groups, have criticized the effects of traditional health services patterns, and have tried to establish a critical consciousness in the education of health care students. And they thereby have often received the disdain and ostracism of their colleagues. Such individuals often work alone.

Others have joined in small groups with like-minded colleagues. These have attempted to build community-based services and to influence decisions within the established professional associations, urging them to go beyond vested interest concerns or to occasionally develop ties with outcast social groups. However, without sustained financing such oases soon vanish or at best do not and cannot have wider effects. As earlier chapters have suggested, health professionals as a group are not likely to change unless major changes occur in their patterns of education and in the organization of their work settings.

A tragedy, and one not confined to the health field, is that the dissentors, if not quieted, leave their field as options close for them. In many ways their loss means that the "growing edge" of health care is blunted. To the extent that they exist and persist they become the best hope for making a new caring-for-health system workable.

Summary

Many important changes that affect health and personal health services will occur in this decade. The shape of the changes, intimately tied to the processes that set out the range of alternatives, will have very different consequences, especially for outcast groups. They may or may not go very far in providing for broad health-confering social changes or in granting access for outcasts to personal health services, to the health occupations, and to related decision making. However far they go, their well-intended effects will be better accomplished if people—consumers and providers—are prepared for them. The best preparation would be to understand the problems of bringing about health and to have a part in devising health-supporting systems. Second best is to at least be aware of what is happening. Thus is the case for a critical consciousness—in health care providers, in health care consumers, and, if the dual barriers of professional aloofness and consumer apathy could be overcome, for professional–consumer joint learning and collaboration.

The "final answer" to the problems of caring-for-health is of course not to find solutions that produce no problems—all answers bring more problems. Rather it is to find solutions that do not create more problems for people just because they belong to certain social groups—because they are women, or ethnics, or elders, or children, or poor. In human terms, the ideal answers will be those which bring problems of similar sorts to all social groups. Thus all will have a stake in seeking continuing answers, will share frustrations and intermittent satisfactions. All groups would have access (which they may nevertheless shun) to health-supporting patterns of living.

Taken to the global level, the same must be said, both for moral reasons and because access for outcasts has become necessary for human survival. Today, only the affluent nations have the economic and technological *potential,* in a word the power, to alter the options for health and life in the peoples of the outcast countries. Should that potential not be mobilized and used in an internationally coordinated and concerted effort to change their outcast status, to create the socioeconomic and ecological conditions for humane existence, the result can only mean their widespread misery and death in the shorter term. In the longer term—given the inextricable and ever-increasing ties between human and natural worlds, between affluent and poor world sectors, between human environments and human health—it will mean the loss of humane living among us all.

Images of Access

In order for populations-in-communities, for consumers-as-patients and consumers-as-citizens to have real choices, to make real decisions about their lives, they must have access to the decision making which shapes their environment and the services they receive. At the same time, decisions taken far beyond their immediate world, at national and state levels, set the limits and possibilities for their input and impact, with or without their knowledge, and whether or not they are interested or able to organize an informed voice should they be given the opportunity to speak.

The three images that follow relate instances of how higher-level governmental priorities affect local choice-giving possibilities, as in India, and how in certain settings individuals and organized groups can begin to have a voice in shaping the conditions for their life and health, as in Amsterdam and Edinburgh.

vi For Rural Isolates, Orissa, India

The fountainhead of God has been frozen in time in the sikhara stone sculptural form crowning unique ten-century-ago temples in Orissa, the large state south of West Bengal. Mountains and desert meet palm trees and plantain at its eastern coast on the Bay of Bengal. It is one of the most rural—only 6 per cent of the people live in cities—and least developed areas in India. It still has large numbers of Untouchables: Gandhi's term was, *harijans* "children of God." Although their outcast status has been outlawed, they keep to their own quarter in the villages. Another large and less-favored group among Orissa's people are the *adibashi*, literally "people of ancient times," indigenous tribal persons of non-Hindu, non-Muslim origin. These 4 million people remain isolated even from the cross-roads of rural life.

A major problem in providing health care to the countryside is that professional workers—coming mainly from affluent backgrounds and education in the city—do not want to work in rural isolation, an environment "foreign" to them. One physician, describing why he did not like to work among the poor, said: "They don't respect my qualifications . . . don't understand that I'm doing them a favor . . . don't follow my advice . . . *expect* to be given free treatment. . . ." These views are shared by medical students, who, like their Western counterparts, are seeking more specialized education. India's urban areas have about one physician for each 7,000 people. The rural areas have one for about 50,000–60,000 people.

Even public health nurses, often on congenial terms with village folk, soon return to the city. The nurses have either a four-year college education after eleven years of basic schooling, or three years of hospital training, six months of midwifery, and ten or more months of training in community health. A Master's degree in this field may soon become part of their educational possibilities.

Points of view in India seem sharply divided as to what to do about training health workers in sufficient numbers and having them work in all areas of the country. One side says that physicians should be encouraged to specialize, that nurses should have a college degree, and that there should be two public health nurses at each Primary Health Centre rather than one, as currently planned for but not yet attainable.

The other side wants to emphasize general practice among physicians, maintain hospital schools for hospital nurses (where training is based on the care of the sick), and do away with public health nurses in community health centers (whose training is initially in the care of the sick). Instead, they would set up rural schools of medicine to train physicians from the villages, and train more alterprofessionals such as *dais,* the village midwives, in the short term; then, increasingly, they would train auxiliary nurse midwives (whose training is in basic nursing care, first aid, maternity and child care, and family planning) from the villages.

The State of Orissa, with all its difficulties, is doing what others have only talked about. It is revamping its system of community health workers in the direction of alterprofessionals. Public health nurses are no longer budgeted for the Primary Health Centres. In their places are Lady Health Visitors, hired at a lesser salary (salary ranges for all types of personnel in government programs are set by the central government of India). These women, however, need not, and increasingly will not, have the conventional Health Visitor training (two and one-half years for nursing–midwifery–community health at Lady Health Visitor Schools; Orissa has only one of these twenty-one schools). Those who are now hired as Lady Health Visitors are, rather, "new" nurses, that is, those with the common three-year hospital school education—to which have been added in all schools six weeks of living and working in village health centers— and six months of midwifery, plus, following graduation, three months of community health training and supervised fieldwork. These "new" nurses then receive, as health visitors, about a 25 per cent increase in salary. Thus the savings from the fewer higher-wage positions, usually held by higher-income urbanites, is being dispersed to the larger numbers in lesser-paid positions.

Health visitors in turn supervise the Auxiliary Nurse Midwives, commonly known as ANMs, the community health worker now being trained in largest numbers. The ANMs are in many ways the central and pivotal health workers, closest to the villagers. Six months of their first year of training—done in ANM Training Schools—involves the care of the hospitalized sick and first aid. The second year of midwifery includes three months of community-based work and birth control teaching under the tutelege of nurses and health visitors.

One such young graduate lives and works at a new maternal and child health subcenter almost literally under the shadow of the famed Temple of the Sun at Konarak near the eastern shore. Three months ago she completed the ANM course in the district where her parents live; they are not far away in miles but too many hours distant in travel time for her to continue to live with them. This is her home ground. She does not feel isolated as urban-bred personnel might if they had to live there without any means of transportation.

Because she has had ten years of basic education, she could, after some experience as an ANM, enter a school of nursing and in only two and one half years (instead of three and one half) become a "new" nurse, raising her basic wage from $12 per month (about what her father earns as a farmer) to $18 for beginning "new" nurses, or even to $22 if she chose to take the additional three-month training in order to qualify as a Lady Health Visitor.

Her living quarters are two rooms in the mud-dung subcenter, not more than about 12 by 18 feet altogether. One room is a kind of office where she talks to women about their children's health and nutrition, about their pregnancies, about birth control. Her district covers thirty-seven villages, about 13,000 people. Last month she was able to walk to thirteen villages, all within a five-mile radius, and convinced 16 women to accept the IUD birth control device.

The IUDs were then inserted by her supervisor, the Lady Health Visitor from the Primary Health Centre. She comes each month or so with other birth control workers to hold a mobile "Loop (IUD) Camp." These circulating Camps have helped give Orissa a higher rate of "births prevented" than for India as a whole, about 14 per cent better, and about 20 per cent higher than the state to the South, better-educated and wealthier Tamil Nadu.

Although the ANM talks to some of the mothers about health, she has no vitamins to give them or immunizations. Most pregnant women go to the village midwife, an untrained *dai*. About 8 of 10 births in rural areas are attended by *dais,* as are at least half the births in urban areas. There are no other workers at the subcenter; there is no state money to hire them. When there is money, a village *dai* might be persuaded to work with the young ANM for about $3 per month, plus $0.15–0.50 for each person she can convince to use the IUD or be sterilized.

At another subcenter about eight miles from the Primary Health Centre, an ANM lives with her husband in a single room. She is older and has the minimum basic education required for ANM training, seven years. After six years there, and as an older woman, the village mothers readily turn to her. She has found that by gathering a few women in one of their huts, perhaps once a week, she can persuade them to convince their husbands to get vasectomies—in this way forty men agreed to sterilization last year, and another fifty-five agreed through more direct means, mainly the Male Family Planning Fieldworkers from the Primary Health Centre.

These male fieldworkers and two female workers of the same sort visit the subcenter about once a week to intensify the birth control program. In this way, virtually all mothers are visited shortly after childbirth by the ANM and women fieldworkers. The fieldworkers have had one month of concentrated training in family planning methods and education. Now, under the revised training system, if they have had ten years of basic education they may, and are being encouraged to, enter ANM training, thus going from a specialized to a more general type of community health work.

Seventeen ANM Training Centers are located throughout the state and are therefore accessible to prospective students. Most of the graduates, about 90 per cent, are placed in state family planning programs; a very small proportion seek nongovernment work, about 2 per cent. Since most of the new trainees come from schools that are supported by family planning funds, they almost invariably regard birth control as the focus of their work, in contrast to ANMs trained many years ago, or those in other states, or Lady Health Visitors, who tend to view maternity care as the most important part of their job.

This combination of fieldwork and rotating Loop Camps, plus the availability of vasectomies, has helped make for a lowered birth rate in this district, about 30 per 1,000 population. The birth rate for India is about 42.

The basic reason for this concentrated birth control program and reshuffling of community health worker training—as well as for the relative weakness of maternity and child care programs—is that funds for family planning are offered in large amounts by the central government to the states, for services and for training fieldworkers and ANMs. Maternal and child care monies come from state coffers. Thus Orissa, in need of development funds for training, services, and employment opportunities—economically limited as it is—availed itself of national funds. With that leverage it was able in less than six years to reorganize training, more than doubling the number of ANM schools, and to implement a relatively effective birth control program. Central government family planning funds granted to Orissa are now 32 times more than the Orissa state-allotted funds budgeted for maternity–child health services. The eventual aim is to integrate the services in maternal–child care and family planning, but for financial and other reasons, at present that exists mainly on paper (1).

vii   For Surinam Blacks, Amsterdam

There are rumblings, a man-made stirring, in the underpinnings of Amsterdam, capital of the Lowlands, a city reclaimed from the sea. Within its foundations a subway is being built that will connect it with its new satellite town rising to the southeast, Bijlmer Meer.

As a country with the highest population density in the world, the Netherlands has a housing problem. One means for alleviating it was begun in 1968. It is Bijlmer Meer, a residential satellite for Amsterdam. After the polder—the grassy wetland that virtually covers the country—was dried and leveled, one of the first buildings to go up in the new town was the Community Center. It is set in a square among the beginnings of shopping, eating, and service facilities, crossed with walkways and lawn. This is the core of complexes of cinder-block apartment dwellings, eventually to house 120,000 people, now in varying stages of construction. Each set of buildings will be separated by grassland and waterways, and joined by bikeways—no cars allowed.

After three years, 18,000 people are living here, with 1,000 new renters arriving each month. About one fourth of the people who live here, and about half the school-age children, are black. They are immigrants from what was once the colony of Dutch Guiana in South America and is now Surinam. In a sense, the Surinam blacks are coming to claim reparations for the labor their fathers gave to the Dutch masters.

The Community Center at Bijlmer Meer is perhaps an acknowledgment by the Dutch government that reparations are due. The Center's reason-for-being, simply put, is to help the residents of Bijlmer Meer make of it whatever they want it to be.

One of the Center's chief workers, who tries, often day and night, to make this happen, is Marijke, a single woman in her late thirties with long, straight hair and big, round glasses. She was once a trained nurse but found that too regimented. Then she became a teacher of young children but found formal educational institutions too confining. Now she is a self-made, and self-learning, community organizer.

According to Marijke, the Center has become a crossroads, at least for the younger residents, in spite of the fact that the Center's budget is limited. The low, flexible facility is alive daytime and evenings with young people, mostly blacks. The music, craft, and painting rooms, the children's playroom, the theater–dance–recreation hall, the coffee house, all are free for use by resident individuals or groups, regulated only by self-imposed rules of cleaning up afterward. Tutoring of Dutch, or other specific requests, is set up by the Center's staff. The flow between the Dutch and Surinams is obviously helpful to immigrant youngsters, who must know the Dutch language when they enter school at age 6.

One of the social facts that makes Bijlmer Meer both fascinating and difficult, says Marijke, is the great diversity between inhabitants. Although the apartments were originally intended as low-rent housing, the costs of construction have now required a higher rent, beginning at about 270

Dutch guilders per month, or $90. This means that renters must earn a minimum of about $6,000 per year, a figure set by the Amsterdam housing authority—the agency that is also financing the construction through loans to nonprofit housing corporations, *Woning Bouw Verening.* So, compared to housing in central Amsterdam at about $30–50 per month, Bijlmer Meer is expensive. (However, plans are under way to equalize urban and suburban rents to avoid segregated housing patterns based on income.)

The mix of people in the apartment blocks thus tends to be families of middle-income or more and—as a matter of policy preference—rather affluent but often segregated people, such as homosexuals. In addition are the low-income families, predominantly the Surinams, for whom the government provides rent subsidies.

According to Marijke, a low-income person receives about $300 per month through supplementation of earnings by the broad and efficient Netherlands Social Security System. This is further added to for families by Children's Allowances, which range in quarterly payments from $50 to $90. A well-organized national health program gives additional security to the people of The Netherlands, regardless of their income or point of origin.

Such differences in income and life style, in language and culture, pose problems to Marijke as a group organizer. Currently, the common denominator around which adults are coming together is the question of how the apartment buildings should be governed and used. The consensus thus far seems to be that each block should decide on its own form of rule making or lack of rule making.

One thing that has and will encourage tenants to work together is the fact that the ground floors of the housing units, the "collective rooms," have been left vacant and unplanned. It is up to the tenants to do with these large spaces what they will. One unit, predominantly housing Surinams, set up a bar–coffee house atmosphere with space for music and theatrical entertainment; others have art and recreation areas. Another building has a cooperative day nursery—a service that will be in increasing demand as more married women seek jobs to help pay the high rents.

Although there is no direct separation of the Surinams and Dutch on the basis of color or income, a kind of *de facto* segregation may occur. This is a possibility because the nonprofit housing corporations, each of which is constructing its own block of apartments, were historically organized according to the religious, class, or occupational group of the members, and were responsible for finding housing for their members. Thus, insofar as these societies have predominantly white or black members, the housing units which they provide will reflect that membership.

There are signs in some of the buildings that the tenants do not regard their living quarters as their own, that they perhaps feel "foreign": broken and boarded windows, and unused hollow-sounding space.

Social workers and visiting nurses assigned to the Community Center (in Holland there are three-of-a-kind auspices for most community services: Catholic, Protestant, and nonreligious, all nevertheless government-subsidized) admit to being somewhat at a loss as to where to begin. Neither their training nor life experience has put them into natural contact with Surinam people. They feel like foreigners among the foreign immigrant blacks. They ask the question of the outsider among outcasts: how to connect in order to provide the services they have to offer. They turn to Marijke for her untutored expertise gleaned from day-by-day encounters.

In nightime discussions over *genever,* the Dutch gin apertif, at one of the little canal-side eating places in old Amsterdam, Marijke says she can offer no clear-cut answers. She tells them in effect to forget their formal training and the artificial boundaries it places on what they should and should not do. Work with people on things they want to work on. Learn, and keep learning from everyday situations. Learn to understand the language and style of the outcasts, but expect to remain an outsider. Be human. Make mistakes, learn from your mistakes. Allow others to do the same.

Marijke is working in a country that has one of the longest years-of-life and lowest infant death rates in the world. She is working in a setting where outcasts are entitled to basic living essentials: housing of the same quality as that of others; an income floor that does not have to be depleted through payment for housing or health care; in time, rapid transit to the work and social facilities of the central city; and an essentially pollution-free environment. Within that framework, her own flexible style makes possible further connections with the outcasts in those things that they regard important. Whether or not all this is sufficient to bring the diverse people of Bijlmer Meer into a mix that will allow their differences to enrich each other is a matter for the future to show(2).

viii   For Working-Class Tenants, Edinburgh

The aged elegance and stone walkways of the "Royal Mile" lead to the estate of Edinburgh's royal household, set on green hills in the heart of the city. Another road, tarred and often littered with broken glass, gives access to a section of public housing, perennially gray and flat, in an outlying fringe. Fishmongers and poulterers, bakers and green grocers line its narrow sidewalks—yet they do not seem to have the flare and crispness of the shops in the older, classically historic part of the city. Children seem rather lightly dressed for the frosty mist of December. Their fathers earn about 15–20 per cent less than most workingmen.

This is Craigmillar, one of two low-income areas in Edinburgh. As the center of government and home of the monarchy, this city has a smaller task of dealing with its unskilled and low-paid workers than does its industrial sister, Glasgow.

Craigmillar, hidden from full view of the main road, has little beyond its rows of housing. The primary school has a stoney playfield, and an old house, now the Community Center, has muddy surroundings. The people say that little planning was done to make Craigmillar a living, as well as a housing, area. They have recently decided to see that it does become a place for living.

In the early 1960s, with the encouragement of the city fathers, an *ad hoc* group, the Craigmillar Festival Society, was formed to arrange an annual talent festival, and so to revive the spirit of the tenants in Craigmillar. By the end of the decade, the Society was working on a year-round basis, trying to deal with the complaints of the people. By the end of the 1960s they had received a three-year grant from the City under a new national Urban Aid Program.

With about a $7,500 budget, they hired a part-time social worker and engaged staff workers from the local Church of Scotland to coordinate relations with various health and welfare agencies. They thus shortly established a day nursery and a number of other children's programs. For the elders—many pensioners live in the housing units—they formed social groups as well as trained neighborhood workers. These workers are Craigmillar residents who visit the elders on an individual basis and work with them in group activities. They are paid about $625 per year.

The Society also arranged for the training of Neighborhood Aides. This has become in effect a local version of the Home Help Service, a national program for rendering inhome services tied to the National Health Service. A family member is paid by the Local Health Authority when he or she must leave employment to take care of an ill or dependent family member.

One of the prime movers behind this community building is Helen Crummy, one of the tenants. Now, as Organizing Secretary, she is paid about $1,800 for what she had long been doing without pay. She says that in the early years, the Society quickly realized that talking about community spirit was meaningless when people did not have the things they needed in order to, in effect, fill their spirit.

But today, having put together a number of needed community

services, Craigmillar people say this is not yet enough. Recently they had heard that a highway was being planned that would split Craigmillar. This threat was then the impetus for the new Craigmillar Pilot Scheme.

What the tenants are proposing to city officials is that they become part of the decision-making processes for the planning of housing, facilities and services, transportation, and other aspects of the Craigmillar environment, including the esthetic.

On a damp December night a final meeting was held at the Community Center before the last draft of the proposal was written. Helen Crummy made sure that a variety of tenants' representatives were present, as well as a number of outside influentials, including their Member of Parliament, a judge, a physician, the school's headmaster, and the local clergy. Away from the sounds of young people meeting in the recreation room, and around several pots of tea and biscuits, served by a man and a woman, the tenant representatives reported on the responses to the Pilot Scheme by their "constituents," the youth, the elders, the workers, the women.

Alice, in boots, a minidress, and long, dyed hair—she is a Neighborhood Worker and a mother—pointed out a potential danger to the Society were it to be officially connected with the city: it could become coopted. For instance, she said in a thick brogue, a city official had asked her to announce to the tenants that a housing rehabilitation program was soon to begin. If she and the other Neighborhood Workers were to do that, they would become agents of the city, making city programs seem pallatible and positive. But, in reality, the rehabilitation program was promised years ago, so the government was only going to do what it should have done a long time ago; *that* is the crucial fact that she and the others should be conveying to the people.

One of Mrs. Findlay's concerns, speaking for the old-age pensioners, was that whatever the decision-making procedures agreed to between the city and Craigmillar, they be definitive and conclusive, so that there be no stalemates. After all, the elders were no more interested or able to wait years and years for the eating and social area they wanted in their housing units than the young people who wanted recreation facilities or the housewives who were tired of looking out on bleak and barren terrain.

A trade union member, Jim Grinder, added that it would always be important for Craigmillar to first work out its own differences and set its own priorities so that it could present a united front to city planners.

Under Helen's guidance, the meeting moves quickly. No one attempts to monopolize. She would not allow it. All present their views fully, all with clarity, some most articulate through their words, others through the communication of their feelings. A wide range of ages, experiences, formal education, income, and status are represented. The diversity contributes to a common cause, to acquire enough power to have a voice, to make choices, about their community. As such, Craigmillar is unique in Scotland, if not in Great Britain.

A decade ago, Edinburgh officials with all good intentions wanted simply to bolster the spirits of the tenants in Craigmillar. Now, those who were to be organized have become the organizers, those who are outcast are together working to open and enter the decision-making network that sets their options for living (3).

Notes

Chapter 1—Rich and Poor Nations: The Widening Gap

1. International Planned Parenthood Federation, *Family Planning on Five Continents* (London: IPPF, 1972); International Commission for the Development of Education, *Learning To Be* (Paris: UNESCO, 1972), 28.

2. L. Brown, *World Without Borders* (New York: Random House, 1972), 25.

3. Ibid.; Food and Agricultural Organization Report, *The Times* (London), June 7, 1973; for full description of the effects of environment worldwide, see World Health Organization, *Health Hazards of the Human Environment* (Geneva: WHO, 1972); A. Berg, *The Nutrition Factor: Its Role in National Development* (Washington, D.C.: The Brookings Institution, 1973).

4. Brown, op. cit., 43.

5. International Commission for the Development of Education, op. cit., 94.

6. Brown, op. cit., 73; D. Jellife and E. Jellife, "The Urban Avalanche and Child Nutrition." *J. Amer. Diet. Assoc.* 57:114 (1970).

7. Ibid.

8. For example, I. Berg, *Education and Jobs* (New York: Praeger, 1970); I. Illich, *Deschooling Society* (New York: Harper & Row, 1970); P. Freire, *Pedagogy of the Oppressed* (New York: Herder and Herder, 1971); M. Craft, *Social Class, Family and Education* (London: Longman, 1970); International Commission for the Development of Education, op. cit.

9. W. Handwerker, "Technology and Household Configuration in Urban Africa: The Bassa of Monrovia." *Amer. Sociol. Rev.* 38:182–97 (Apr. 1973).

10. International Commission for the Development of Education, op. cit., 287.

11. Ibid.

12. Committee for Economic Development, *Assisting Development in Low-Income Countries: Priorities for U.S. Government Policy* (New York: CED, 1969), 65; for another moderate view of MNCs, see L. Turner, *Multinational Companies and the Third World* (New York: Hill and Wang, 1973).

13. Brown, op. cit., 217.

14. Ibid., 220.

15. International Commission for the Development of Education, op. cit., 244.

16. G. Myrdal, *The Challenge of World Poverty* (New York: Random House, 1970), 285.

17. Ibid.

18. Committee for Economic Development, op. cit.

19. H. Singer, "Outlook for the Poor World." *New Internationalist* 5 (July 1973); G. Borgstrom, *Focal Points: A Global Food Strategy* (New York: Macmillan, 1973).

20. Committee for Economic Development, op. cit.

21. Ibid.; Borgstrom, op. cit.

22. For example, see discussions in Brown, op. cit.; International Commission for the Development of Education, op. cit.; Myrdal, op. cit.; writings of Ivan Illich; issues of *New Internationalist;* proceedings from the 12th World Conference of the Society for International Development, Ottawa, Canada, May 1971; *Limits of Growth: The Club of Rome's Projection on the Predicament of Mankind* (New York: Potomac Associates, 1972); United Nations Environmental Program Report, 1973; Study Commission on Environmental Aspects of a National Materials Policy, *Man, Materials, and Environment* (Washington, D.C.: National Academy of Science and National Academy of Engineering, 1973); W. Nordhaus and J. Tobin, "Is Growth Obsolete?" in *Economic Research: Retrospect and Prospect* (New York: National Bureau of Economic Research, 1973); *Population and the Future: Report of the Commission on Population and the American Future* (Washington, D.C.: Government Printing Office, 1972); Organization for Economic Cooperation and Development Council, *Social Indicators Newsletter,* July 1973; U.S. Senate Committee on Foreign Relations, *Foreign Economic Assistance, 1973.* Hearings, June 26–27, 1973 (Washington, D.C.: Government Printing Office, 1973), Sen. Fulbright, 39–43.

23. Myrdal, op. cit., 291; International Commission for the Development of Education, op. cit., 258.

24. Ibid.; *New Internationalist,* May–July 1973.

25. World Health Organization, "Organizational Study on 'Methods of

Promoting the Development of Basic Health Services': Report of the Working Group" (Geneva: WHO, Jan. 16, 1973).

26. National Center for Health Statistics, *Height and Weight of Children in the U.S., India, and the UAR* (Washington, D.C.: Department of Health, Education, and Welfare, Sept. 1970).

27. Pan American Health Organization, *Goals in the Charter of Punta del Este: Facts on Health Progress* (Washington, D.C.: World Health Organization, July 1969), 9, 12; R. Puffer and C. Serrano, "The Role of Nutritional Deficiency in Mortality: Findings of the Inter-American Investigation of Mortality in Childhood." *Bol. Ofic. Sanit. Panamer.* (English Ed.) 7:22 (1973).

28. J. Bryant, *Health and the Developing World* (Ithaca, N.Y.: Cornell University Press, 1969), 39; World Health Organization, op. cit.

29. R. Freedman (ed.), *Population: The Vital Revolution* (New York: Doubleday, 1964), 1–12.

30. Brown, op. cit., 135–42.

31. Ibid.

32. Public Health Service, *Protecting the Health of Eighty Million Americans, A National Goal for Occupational Health* (New York: National Advisory Environmental Health Commission, 1965). For further discussion and illustration of these relationships, see Myrdal, op. cit., Chap. 5; Bryant, op. cit., 98–112; W. Galenson and G. Pyatt, *The Quality of Labor and Economic Development in Certain Countries* (Geneva: International Labor Organization, 1964); J. Kelly and J. Scanlon, *Decayed, Missing and Filled Teeth Among Children* (Washington, D.C.: Government Printing Office, 1971); National Center for Health Statistics, *Current Estimates from the Health Interview Survey, United States, 1971* (Rockville, Md.: Department of Health, Education, and Welfare, Feb. 1973).

33. C. Taylor and M. Hall, "Health, Population, and Economic Development." *Science* 157:651–57 (Aug. 11, 1967).

34. R. Elliot et al., "U.S. Population Growth and Family Planning: A Review of the Literature." *Family Planning Perspectives* 2 (Suppl.), Oct. 1970; see also L. Orleans, *Every Fifth Child: The Population of China* (Stanford, Calif.: Stanford University Press, 1972).

35. Myrdal, op. cit., Chap. 5.

36. *India's Family Planning Program: A Brief Analysis* (New Delhi: Ford Foundation, 1970); B. Weinraub, "New Delhi," *New York Times,* Aug. 5, 1973.

37. See Note 22 for references.

Chapter 2—Poor and Rich Nations: Similarities

1. World Health Organization, "Organizational Study on 'Methods of Promoting the Development of Basic Health Services': Report of the

Working Group" (Geneva: WHO, Jan. 16, 1973); International Commission for the Development of Education, *Learning To Be* (Paris: UNESCO, 1972), 72ff.

2. Proceedings from the 12th World Conference of the Society for International Development, Ottawa, Canada, May 1971.

3. K. Nair, "The Green Revolution in South Asia." University of Michigan lecture, July 23, 1970.

4. G. Myrdal, *The Challenge of World Poverty* (New York: Random House, 1970), 80–100; Nair, op. cit., and in *The Lonely Furrow: Farming in the U.S., Japan, and India* (Ann Arbor, Mich.: University of Michigan Press, 1969); see also F. Frankel, *India Green Revolution: Economic Gains and Political Costs* (Princeton, N.J.: Princeton University Press, 1971); G. Overstreet, "Village Politics and Development: India," in J. Christoph (ed.), *Cases in Comparative Politics* (Boston: Little, Brown, 1965).

5. J. Petras and R. LaPorte, *Cultivating Revolution: The United States and Agrarian Reform in Latin America* (New York: Random House, 1971); Myrdal, op. cit., 452ff.; C. Furtado, *Obstacles to Development in Latin America* [New York: Doubleday (Anchor), 1970], 150.

6. Myrdal, op. cit., 450–60, 80–100; L. Brown, *World Without Borders* (New York: Random House, 1972), 59, 78.

7. H. Magdoff, *The Age of Imperialism: The Economic Aspects of U.S. Foreign Policy* (London: Modern Readers Paperbacks, 1968).

8. Pan American Health Organization, *Goals in the Charter of Punta del Este: Facts on Health Progress* (Washington, D.C.: World Health Organization, July 1969).

9. Myrdal, op. cit., 404, Chap. 13.

10. Social Security Administration, *Social Security Programs Throughout the World, 1971* (Washington, D.C.: Government Printing Office, 1972).

11. Brown, op. cit., 47.

12. Great Britain Central Statistical Office, *Social Trends* No. 3, 1972 (London: Her Majesty's Stationery Office, 1973), 10, 86.

13. Associated Press Report, *Toronto Globe and Mail,* Aug. 8, 1972.

14. Social Security Administration, op. cit., iii; The Swedish Institute, "The Economy of the Swedish Family" (Stockholm: The Institute, 1971); D. Schewe et al., *Survey of Social Security in the Federal Republic of Germany* (Bonn: Federal Ministry for Labor and Social Affairs, 1972); P. Fisher, "Social Reports of the German Federal Republic 1970–71." *Social Security Bull.* 35:16–29 (July 1972).

15. U.S. Department of Health, Education, and Welfare, *Toward a Social Report* (Ann Arbor, Mich.: University of Michigan Press, 1970), 44; U.S. Bureau of Census, *Statistical Abstract of the United States 1972* (Washington, D.C.: Government Printing Office, 1972), 324; Women's

Bureau, *Facts on Women Workers of Minority Races* (Washington, D.C.: Department of Labor, 1972).

16. Department of Labor study reported in the *New York Times,* Dec. 31, 1972; between 1968 and 1971, the proportion of Americans who were poor dropped slightly, from 12.8 to 12.5 per cent, but the actual number of poor individuals increased from 25.4 million to 25.6 million [J. Kasun, "U.S. Poverty in World Perspective." *Current History* 64:247–52 (June 1973)].

17. Financial reports, *Boston Globe,* June 17, 1973, and July 24, 1973.

18. Great Britain Central Statistical Office, op. cit.; Great Britain Department of Health and Social Security, *Annual Report 1971* (London: Her Majesty's Stationery Office, 1972); *The European Economic Community* (June 1973).

19. U.S. Bureau of Census, op. cit., 323; Office of Research and Statistics, *Social Security Farm Statistics, 1966* (Washington, D.C.: Social Security Administration, 1971). See Table 2–4 for a more detailed breakdown.

20. Appalachian Regional Commission, *Appalachia* (Washington, D.C.: ARC, 1969); U.S. Bureau of Census, op. cit., 334; R. Morrill and E. Wohlenberg, *The Geography of Poverty in the United States* (New York: McGraw-Hill, 1971).

21. Committee for Economic Development, *Education for the Disadvantaged* (New York: CED, 1971), App. A.

22. Economic Research Service, *U.S. Population Mobility and Distribution: Charts on Recent Trends* (Washington, D.C.: U.S. Department of Agriculture, Dec. 1969).

23. *The European Economic Community* (June 1973).

24. B. Stein, *On Relief: The Economic of Poverty and Public Welfare* (New York: Basic Books, 1971), 141; J. Kelley, "Causal Chain Models for the Socioeconomic Career." *Amer. Sociol. Rev.* 38:481–93 (Aug. 1973).

25. International Commission for the Development of Education, op. cit., 73.

26. Ibid.; Myrdal, op. cit., Chap. 6; M. Craft, *Social Class, Family, and Education* (London: Longman, 1970), 4–7; R. Tilford and R. Preece, *Federal Germany: Political and Social Order* (London: Dufour, 1969), 59–70; C. Silver, "Women in France." *Amer. J. Sociol.* 78:836–51 (Jan. 1973); M. Rutkevich (ed.), *The Career Plans of Youth* (New York: International Arts and Sciences Press, 1969); U.S. Bureau of Census, *Current Population Reports, Special Studies* (Ser. P-23 No. 40 (Jan. 1972), 20.

27. M. Craft. op. cit., 49–71; Educational Testing Service, *Report of CSS Panel on Financing Poor and Minority Students, U.S.* (Princeton, N.J., 1968); Department of Health, Education, and Welfare, op. cit., 19–22; International Commission for the Development of Education, op. cit., xxviii.

28. Craft, op. cit., 6, 7; M. Archer and S. Giner (eds.), *Contemporary Europe: Class, Status, and Power* (New York: St. Martin's Press, 1971).

29. International Commission for the Development of Education, op. cit., 37, 282, 285; Myrdal, op. cit., 167–76; W. Scott, "Cross-National Studies of the Impact of Levels of Living on Economic Growth." *Internat. J. Health Serv.* 1, No. 3:225–32 (1971).

30. International Commission for the Development of Education, ibid.; Myrdal, ibid.

31. International Commission for the Development of Education, op. cit., 70–71; Myrdal, op. cit., 195; Carnegie Commission on Higher Education, *The More Effective Use of Resources* (United States) 1972.

32. Scott, op. cit.; J. Bryant, *Health and the Developing World* (Ithaca, N.Y.: Cornell University Press, 1969), 92, 201, 321; Myrdal, op. cit., 181; Proceedings of the Society for International Development, op. cit.; B. Jacobson and J. Kendriek, "Education and Mobility: From Achievement to Ascription." *Amer. Sociol. Rev.* 38:439–60 (Aug. 1973); A. Berg, *The Nutrition Factor: Its Role in National Development* (Washington, D.C.: The Brookings Institution, 1973), 16; P. Freire, *Pedagogy of the Oppressed* (New York: Herder and Herder, 1971); International Commission for the Development of Education, op. cit., 230–33.

33. I. Berg, *Education and Jobs* (New York: Praeger, 1970); B. Greenberg, "Review of the Literature Relating to the Use of Nonprofessionals in Education, 1942–67" [New York: New Careers Development Center, Nov. 1967 (mimeo)]; T. Corcoran, "The Coming Slums of Higher Education?" *Change* 30–35 (Sept. 1972); R. Baldwin, "Down with the Degree Structure!" *Change* 50–55 (Mar. 1973); D. Hoyt, "The Relationship Between College Grades and Adult Achievement" (Washington, D.C.: American Council on Testing Research Reports, 1965).

34. Baldwin, op. cit.; Craft, op. cit., 49–71; R. Hauser and D. Featherman, "Trends in the Occupational Mobility of U.S. Men, 1962–1970." *Amer. Sociol. Rev.* 38:302–10 (June 1973); M. Milner, *Illusion of Equality* (San Franciso: Jossey-Bass, 1972).

35. L. Sharpe, *Education and Employment: The Early Careers of College Graduates* (Baltimore, Md.: Johns Hopkins Press, 1970); F. Crossland, *Minority Access to College* (New York: Schocken Books, 1971); W. Hansen and B. Weisbrod, *Benefits, Costs and Finance of Higher Education* (Chicago: Markham, 1969); K. Kelsall et al., *Graduates: The Sociology of an Elite* (London: Methuen, 1972).

36. U.S. Census Report, *Boston Globe,* July 23, 1973; P. Cross, "The New Learners." *Change* 31–32 (Feb. 1973); W. Taylor, *Hanging Together: Equality in an Urban Nation* (New York: Simon and Schuster, 1971); Department of Health, Education, and Welfare, op. cit.; P. Sexton, *Education and Income* (New York: Viking Press, 1964).

36a. Many studies are now available. For example, A. Jaffe and W. Adams, *American Higher Education in Transition* (New York: Columbia University Press, 1969), 100; W. Schafer and C. Olexa, *Tracking and Opportunity* (Scranton: Chandler, 1971), 87; R. Birnbaum and J. Goldman, "The Graduates: Follow-up Study of New York City High School Graduates of 1970" (New York: City University of New York Center for Social Research, 1971); B. Clark, "The 'Cooling-Out' Function of Higher Education." *Amer. J. Sociol.* 65 (May 1960); J. Karabel, "Community Colleges and Social Stratification." *Harvard Educational Review* (Nov. 1972).

37. Stein, op. cit., 141.

38. International Commission for the Development of Education, op. cit., 94.

39. E. Bonacich, "A Theory of Ethnic Antagonism: The Split Labor Market." *Amer. Sociol. Rev.* 37:547–59 (Oct. 1972).

40. Ibid.

41. P. Baran and P. Sweezy, "Monopoly Capitalism and Race Relations," in D. Mermelstein (ed.), *Economics: Mainstream Readings and Radical Critiques* (New York: Random House, 1970), 310ff.

42. U.S. Women's Bureau, *Careers for Women in the 1970s* (Washington, D.C.: Department of Labor, 1973).

43. S. Levitan, *Programs in Aid of the Poor for the 1970s* (Baltimore, Md.: Johns Hopkins Press, 1969), 58; T. Mayer, "Position and Progress of Black America," in Mermelstein, op. cit., 297–308; J. Leggett and C. Cervinka, "Countdown Labor Statistics Revisited." *Society* 10:99–103. (Nov. Dec. 1972, July 1973); Morrill and Wohlenberg, op. cit., 18.

44. G. Bowker, *Education of Coloured Immigrants* (New York: Humanities Press, 1968), 35–36; W. Daniel, *Racial Discrimination in England* (London: Penguin, 1968), 13.

45. Indian Health Service, "Demographic and Socio-cultural Characteristics: Off-Reservation Service Population, Sells Service Unit" (Tucson, Ariz.: Public Health Service, Dec. 1968); Mayer, op. cit., 300.

46. L. Suter and H. Miller, "Incomes of Men and Career Women." *Amer. J. Sociol.* 78:962–74 (Jan. 1973).

47. See Images of Access, i, iv, vi.

48. E. Boserup, *Woman's Role in Economic Development* (New York: St. Martin's Press, 1970); C. Harinasuta, "The Need for Clinical Assistants in Thailand." *Lancet* 1298–1300 (June 9, 1973).

49. Myrdal, op. cit., Chap. 6.

50. Great Britain Central Statistical Office, op. cit.; Social Security Administration, "Relative Importance of Income Sources of the Aged." *Res. Stat. Note* 11 (May 29, 1973); Morrill and Wohlenberg, op. cit., 18; see App. Table 18a.

51. See Images of Access, v.

52. J. Powers, *The New Proletarians* (London: British Council of Churches, 1972); see App. Table 18a, and Images of Access, ii, vii.

53. D. Schewe et al., op. cit., 38.

54. J. Powers, "The Third World in Paris." *New Internationalist* 5:24 (July 1973); Brown, op. cit., 63.

55. Great Britain Office of Population Census and Surveys, *Registrar General's Statistical Review of England and Wales 1971*, Part II (London: Her Majesty's Stationery Office, 1972); see also D. Hiro, *Black British, White British* (New York: Monthly Review Press, 1972).

56. Powers, *Proletarians*, op. cit.; O. Gish, "Immigrant Physician." *New Internationalist* 2:18–21 (Mar. 1974).

57. U.S. Immigration and Naturalization Service, *Annual Report 1971* (Washington, D.C.: INS, 1972).

58. Bonacich, op. cit.

59. For example, S. Steiner, *La Raza* (New York: Harper & Row, 1970); Daniel, op. cit.; Bowker, op. cit.; Powers, *Proletarians*, op. cit.

60. Brown, op. cit., 63; R. Ash, *Social Movements in America* (Chicago: Markham, 1972), 15–20; Powers, *Proletarians*, op. cit.

61. *Sunday Times* (London), June 24, 1973.

62. Senate Committee on the Judiciary, *Report on Equal Rights for Men and Women Amendment* (Washington, D.C., Mar. 14, 1972); L. Dewey, "Women in Labor Unions." *Monthly Labor Rev.* 42–48 (Feb. 1971).

63. J. Bernard, *Women and the Public Interest* (Chicago: Aldine, 1971), 123; J. Hedges, "Women Workers and Manpower Demands in the 1970s." *Monthly Labor Rev.* 19–29 (June 1970).

64. Office of Research and Statistics, op. cit.

65. Economic Research Service, op. cit., 7.

66. V. Oppenheimer, "Demographic Influence on Female Employment." *Amer. J. Sociol.* 78 (Jan. 1973); Women's Bureau, "Women Workers in Regional Areas, 1971" (Washington, D.C.: Department of Labor, June 1972), 6; U.S. Senate Special Committee on Aging, *The Multiple Hazards of Age and Race: The Situation of Aged Blacks in the United States* (Washington, D.C.: Government Printing Office, 1971), 13, 51.

67. See App. Tables 7 and 8; see also E. Martinez and G. López y Rivas (eds.), *The Chicanos* (New York: Monthly Review Press, 1973).

67a. Something of an exception to this seems to occur among black women who actually attain full-time positions within certain professions. For example, of the minorities in medicine, 9.6 per cent were women; of white in medicine, 7 per cent were women; this is similar also in law, for reasons suggested by C. Epstein, "Successful Black Professional Women." *Amer. J. Sociol.* 78:912–35 (Jan. 1973).

68. National Center for Health Statistics, *Infant Mortality Rates: Socioeconomic Factors, U.S.* (Washington, D.C.: Department of Health, Education, and Welfare, Mar. 1972).

69. Ibid.

70. Great Britain Central Statistical Office, op. cit.

71. F. Bamford, "Immigrant Mother and Her Child." *Brit. Med. J.* 1:267–80 (Jan. 30, 1971).

72. National Center for Health Statistics, *Report of the International Conference on the Perinatal and Infant Mortality Problem of the United States* (Washington, D.C.: Department of Health, Education, and Welfare, June 1966).

73. National Center for Health Statistics, *Infant Mortality Rates,* op. cit.

74. H. Chase, "The Position of the United States in International Comparisons of Health Status." *Amer. J. Public Health* 581–89 (Apr. 1972).

75. National Center for Health Statistics, *Trends in "Prematurity," United States, 1950–67* (Washington, D.C.: Department of Health, Education, and Welfare, Jan. 1972).

76. Ibid., 28.

77. National Center for Health Statistics, *Infant Mortality Rates,* op. cit., 39; Smithells and Spindell, "Prenatal Influences and Prenatal Diagnosis." *Brit. Med. J.* 4:105–108 (July–Sept. 1971).

78. Chase, op. cit.

79. National Center for Health Statistics, *Infant Mortality Rates,* op. cit., 9; Pan American Health Organization, op. cit., 9.

80. National Center for Disease Control, *Highlights of the 10-State Nutrition, 1968–70* (Atlanta: Department of Health, Education, and Welfare, 1972).

81. National Center for Health Statistics, *Medical Care, Health Status, and Family Income* (Washington, D.C.: Department of Health, Education, and Welfare, 1964); M. Lerner, "Social Differences in Physical Health," in R. Kosa et al., *Poverty and Health: A Sociological Analysis* (Cambridge, Mass.: Harvard University Press, 1969), 69–112.

82. *U.S. Congressional Record* 118:H9679 (Oct. 11, 1972); National Center for Health Statistics, *Limitation of Activity Due to Chronic Conditions, United States, 1969 and 1970* (Rockville, Md.: Department of Health, Education, and Welfare, Apr. 1973).

82a. National Center for Health Statistics, *Mortality Trends: Age, Color, and Sex, United States, 1950–69* (Rockville, Md.: Department of Health, Education, and Welfare, Nov. 1973).

83. Bamford, op. cit.; Great Britain Central Statistical Office, op. cit., 20–30.

84. L. Corsa et al., "Population Stabilization in the United States" [Ann Arbor, Mich.: University of Michigan School of Public Health, Oct. 1970 (mimeo)].

85. U.S. Commission on Population and the American Future, op. cit.

86. Corsa, op. cit.; National Center for Health Statistics, "Summary Report. Final Natality Statistics 1969." *Monthly Vital Stat. Rept.* 22 (Oct. 2, 1973).

86a. O. Anderson, *Health Care: Can There Be Equity?* (New York: Wiley, 1972), 245.

87. National Center for Health Statistics, June 27, 1973, and Nov. 1973, op. cit. For detailed analysis see National Center for Health Statistics, *Mortality Trends: Age, Color, and Sex, United States, 1950–69* (Rockville, Md.: Department of Health, Education, and Welfare, Nov. 1973) and *Mortality Trends for Leading Causes of Death, United States, 1950–69* (Rockville, Md.: Department of Health, Education, and Welfare, Mar. 1974).

88. Regional Office for Europe, *Risk of Disease and Disability* (Copenhagen: World Health Organization, 1972), 3; Regional Office for Europe, *Public Health Practice* (Copenhagen: World Health Organization, 1972); National Center for Health Statistics, *Recent Retardation of Mortality Trends in Japan* (Washington, D.C.: Department of Health, Education, and Welfare, 1968).

89. National Center for Health Statistics, *Mortality Trends in Czechoslovakia, 1930–1967* (Washington, D.C.: Department of Health, Education, and Welfare, 1969).

90. H. Tyroler and J. Cassel, "Health Consequences of Culture Change: Effect of Urbanization on Coronary Heart Mortality in Rural Residents of North Carolina." *J. Chronic Dis.* 17:167–77 (1964).

91. C. Cook, "Energy: Planning for the Future." *Amer. Scientist* 61:61–65 (Jan.–Feb. 1973).

92. J. Cassel, "Planning for Public Health: The Case for Prevention." Paper presented at Invitational Conference on Revising Nursing Education for Public Health, Washington, D.C., May 22–25, 1973 (mimeo).

93. J. Arehart-Treichel, "Slow Agents of Death." *Science News* 103:245 (Apr. 14, 1973); see also A. Chase, *The Biological Imperatives: Health, Politics and Human Survival* (New York: Holt, Rinehart and Winston, 1971).

94. National Center for Disease Control, op. cit., 11; U.S. Senate Select Committee on Nutrition and Human Needs, *Nutrition and Diseases 1973.* Hearings, Part II, Apr. 3–May 2, 1973 (Washington, D.C.: Government Printing Office, 1973).

95. J. Jerome, *Death of the Automobile* (New York: W. W. Norton, 1972).

96. J. Gordon et al., *Industrial Safety Statistics: A Re-examination: A Critical Report Prepared for the U.S. Department of Labor* (New York: Praeger, 1971); *President's Report on Occupational Health,* 1972.

97. N. Sachuk, "A Mass Social-Hygienic Investigation of a Very Old Population in Various Areas of the USSR." *J. Gerontology* 25:256–61 (July 1970); Great Britain Central Statistical Office, op. cit.

98. Regional Office for Europe, *Public Health Practice,* op. cit.; National Center for Health Statistics, June 27, 1973, op. cit.; H. Somers, "Profile of Health Care in America." *Perspective* 33–36 (Second Quarter 1973).

99. W. Gore and J. Tudor, "Sex Roles and Mental Illness." *Amer. J. Sociol.* 78:812–35 (Jan. 1973).

100. J. Frank, "The Bewildering World of Psychotherapy." *J. Soc. Issues* 28:27–46 (1972).

101. A. Thomas and S. Sillen, *Racism and Psychiatry* (New York: Brunner/ Mazel, 1972), 57; another example is a recent decision by the American Psychiatric Association to no longer characterize homosexuality as a mental illness (V. Cohn, *Washington Post,* Nov. 6, 1973).

102. W. Ryan, *Blaming the Victim* [New York: Random House (Vintage), 1971].

103. K. Lennane and R. Lennane, "Alleged Psychogenic Disorders in Women —A Possible Manifestation of Sexual Prejudice." *New Eng. J. Med.* 288:288–91 (Feb. 8, 1971).

104. D. Phillips, "Data Collection As a Social Process: Its Implications for 'True Prevalence' Studies of Mental Illness," in E. Friedson and J. Lorber, *Medical Men and Their Work* (Chicago: Aldine, 1972), 453–72.

105. H. Riley, "Hospital-Associated Infections." *Pediatric Clin. North America* 16: 701–34 (Aug. 1969); J. McNerney, "Why Does Medical Care Cost So Much?" *New Eng. J. Med.* 282:1459–64 (June 25, 1970); N. Milio, "Values, Social Class, and Community Health Services." *Nursing Res.* (Winter 1967); and findings of U.S. Senate Committee on Finance Report 92–1230, Sept. 26, 1972, 254–69. Lower life expectancy for women seems related to a combination of Muslim culture and low levels of industrialization with poverty (see Table 1–4). Nigeria has a large Muslim population. However, many Arab Muslim states do not report separate male–female rates for life expectancy, thus making any conclusions tentative.

106. Comptroller General of the United States, *Study of Health Facilities Construction Costs* (Washington, D.C.: Government Printing Office, 1972), 847.

107. K. White et al., "Technology and Health Care." *New Eng. J. Med.* 287:1223–27 (Dec. 14, 1972).

108. P. Sanazaro et al., "Research and Development in Quality Assurance." *New Eng. J. Med.* 287:1125–31 (Nov. 30, 1972).

109. M. Braven and J. Elinson, "The Relationship of a Clinical Examination to Mortality Rates." *Amer. J. Public Health* 62:1501–1505 (Nov. 1972).

110. A. Williams and H. Wechsler, "Interrelationships of Preventive Actions in Health and Other Areas." *Health Serv. Rept.* 87:969–76 (Dec. 1972); see also National Center for Health Services Research and Development, *Utilization of Health Services: Indices and Correlates. A Research Bibliography 1972* (Washington, D.C.: Department of Health, Education, and Welfare, Dec. 1972).

111. The President's Committee on Heart Disease, Cancer and Stroke, *A National Program,* Vol. 1 (Washington, D.C.: Executive Office, Dec. 1964); R. Auster et al., "The Production of Health: An Exploratory Study." *J. Human Resources* (Fall 1969), 430.

112. Study Commission on the Environmental Aspects of a National Ma-

terials Policy, *Man, Materials, and Environment* (Washington, D.C.: National Academy of Science and National Academy of Engineering, 1973).

113. J. Gordon et al., *Indian J. Med. Res.* 51:304 (1963); "New Hope for the Aged." *World Health* (Apr. 1972).

114. National Center for Health Statistics, Apr. 1973, op. cit.

115. W. De Geyndt, "Health Behavior and Health Needs of Urban Indians in Minneapolis." *Health Serv. Rept.* 88:360–66 (Apr. 1973).

116. N. Anderson, "Services to Older Persons." *Evaluation* 1, No. 2: 4–6 (1973).

117. R. Fraser, "Health and General Systems of Financing Health Care." *Med. Care* 10:345–57 (July–Aug., 1972); similar studies, focusing on birthweight (and related deaths for low-birthweight infants) also report the relatively greater importance of environment over medical care for assuring infant life and health [R. Lewis et al., "Relationship Between Birthweight and Selected Social, Environmental and Medical Care Factors." *Amer. J. Pub. Health* 63:973–81 (Nov. 1973); F. Shah and H. Abbey, "Effects of Some Factors on Neonatal and Postneonatal Mortality." *Milbank Mem. Fund Quart.* (Jan. 1971); Milio, op. cit.].

118. R. Klein, "The Political Economy of National Health," in Congressional Research Service, *Resolved: That the Federal Government Enact a Program of Comprehensive Medical Care for All United States Citizens* (Washington, D.C.: Government Printing Office, 1972), 377–88.

119. S. Matek, "Some Key Features in the Emerging Context for Future Health Policy Decisions in America." Paper presented at Invitational Conference for Redesigning Nursing Education for Public Health (Washington, D.C.: May 22–25, 1973); Somers, op. cit.

120. World Health Organization, Jan. 16, 1973, op. cit.

121. International Commission for the Development of Education, op. cit., 242ff.

122. See Images of Access, v, viii.

123. B. Myers, "Health Services Research and Health Policy: Interactions." *Med. Care* 11:352–58 (July–Aug. 1973).

124. N. Milio, "Innovation and Health Care Organizations." *J. Health Soc. Behav.* 12:163–73 (June 1971).

Chapter 3—Distribution of People and Services

1. Social Security Administration, *Social Security Farm Statistics, 1966* (Washington, D.C.: Department of Health, Education, and Welfare, Sept. 1971).

2. S. Altman, *Present and Future Supply of Registered Nurses* (Washington, D.C.: Department of Health, Education, and Welfare, 1972), 28; see

also *Distribution of Health Manpower: An Annotated Bibliography* (New York: National Health Council, 1973).

3. *U.S. Congressional Record* 118:H9679 (Oct. 11, 1972).

4. Congressional Research Service, *Resolved: That the Federal Government Should Enact a Program of Comprehensive Medical Care for All United States Citizens* (Washington, D.C.: Government Printing Office, 1972), 54.

5. P. de Vise, "Persistence of Chicago's Dual Hospital System," in *Slum Medicine: Chicago's Apartheid Health System* (Chicago: Community and Family Study Center, 1969), 20; C. Fernow, "Types of Hospital Appointments Held by Physicians in Various Socioeconomic Areas of New York City." *Med. Care* 10:310–22 (July–Aug. 1972).

6. S. Joroff and V. Navarro, "Medical Manpower: A Multivariate Analysis of the Distribution of Physicians in Urban United States." *Med. Care* 9:428–38 (Sept.–Oct. 1971).

7. Report on Testimony Before the Committee on Labor and Public Welfare, Aug. 16, 1972, S. 3716 (U.S. Senate Report, No. 92–1064).

8. Compare App. Tables 15 and 16. The migration of personnel, most of whom are women, is primarily caused by the influence of husband's job and children's needs. See Altman, op. cit., for a full discussion.

9. Council on Medical Education, "Medical Education in the United States, 1971–72." *J. Amer. Med. Assoc.* 222 (Nov. 20, 1972); Carnegie Commission on Higher Education, *Higher Education and the Nation's Health* (New York: McGraw-Hill, 1970), 81–90.

10. Department of Health, Education, and Welfare, "National Program to Identify Health Services Scarcity Areas." Sept.–Dec. 1972 (unpublished).

11. T. Bice et al., "Economic Class and Use of Physician Services." *Med. Care* 11:287–96 (July–Aug. 1973); see also R. Andersen et al., *Health Service Use: National Trends and Variations 1953–71* (Rockville, Md.: Department of Health, Education, and Welfare, 1972); National Center for Health Services Research and Development, *Utilization of Health Services: Indices and Correlates. A Research Bibliography 1972* (Rockville, Md.: Department of Health, Education, and Welfare, 1972).

12. Ibid.; see also E. Haisinger and D. Hobbs, "Relation of Community Context to Utilization of Health Services in a Rural Area"; and B. Friedman et al., "Influence of Medicaid and Private Health Insurance on Early Diagnosis of Breast Cancer." *Med. Care* 11:485–522 (Nov.–Dec. 1973).

13. E. Saward and M. Greenlick, "Health Policy and the HMO." *Milbank Mem. Fund Quart.* 50:147–77 (Apr. 1972). See also Chap. 2, Notes 108–111.

14. S. Stoiber, Commission for National Health Insurance. *MS. Magazine* June 1973), 117–19; see also Chapters 4 and 9 of the text.

15. R. Morris and E. Harris, "Home Health Services in Massachusetts, 1971: Their Role in the Care of the Long-Term Sick." *Amer. J. Public Health* 62:1088–93 (Aug. 1972); see also D. Baggish with C. Kimball, "Prob-

lems of Transportation to Medical Facilities on an Indian Reservation."
Med. Care 11:501–508 (Nov.–Dec. 1973).

16. R. Wolk and R. Wolk, "Professional Workers' Attitudes Toward the Aged." *J. Amer. Geriatric Soc.* 19:624–39 (July 1971); J. Walsh and R. Elling, "Professionalism and the Poor." *J. Health Soc. Behav.* 9:16–28 (Mar. 1968); L. Fidell, 53rd Annual Convention, Western Psychological Association, Anaheim, Calif. Apr. 10–13, 1973.

17. Great Britain Department of Health and Social Security, *Health and Personal Social Services Statistics 1972* (London: Her Majesty's Stationery Office, 1973).

18. Social Security Administration, "Main Features of Selected National Health Care Systems." *Res. Stat. Note* 9 (May 18, 1973).

Chapter 4—Organization—How Services Are Delivered

1. Comptroller General of the United States, *Study of Health Facilities Construction Costs* (Washington, D.C.: Government Printing Office, 1972), 98, 759, 847; N. Anderson, "Evaluation Overview: Services to Older Persons." *Evaluation* 1, No. 2:4–6 (1973).

2. *Social Security Bull.*, Oct. 1968.

3. Social Security Administration, *Net Income of Hospitals, 1961–69,* Staff Paper 6 (Washington, D.C.: SSA, Dec. 1970); R. Rapoport, "A Candle for St. Greed's." *Harper's* 70–75 (Dec. 1972).

4. Ibid.; National Center for Health Statistics, *Health Resources Statistics 1971* (Washington, D.C.: Department of Health, Education, and Welfare, 1972).

5. Social Security Administration, op. cit.

6. National Center for Health Statistics, "Utilization of Short-Stay Hospitals —Summary of Nonmedical Statistics: 1970." *Monthly Vital Stat. Rept.* 21:9 (Dec. 6, 1972).

7. National Center for Health Statistics, *Inpatient Health Facilities 1969* (Rockville, Md.: Department of Health, Education, and Welfare, Dec. 1972).

8. W. McNerney, "Why Does Medical Care Cost So Much?" *New Eng. J. Med.* 282:1459–65 (June 25, 1970).

9. *Hearings Before the Senate Committee on Labor and Public Welfare,* May 16, 1972, Rept. 92-1064, p. 7; Comptroller General of the United States, op. cit.; *1973 AHA Guide to the Health Care Field* (Chicago: American Hospital Association, 1973).

10. Comptroller General of the United States, op. cit., 847; "Open Heart Surgery." *Perspective* 23–24 (Third Quarter 1972).

11. McNerney, op. cit.; Comptroller General of the United States, op. cit., 811.

12. American Public Health Association, *Nation's Health,* Nov. 1972.

13. National Center for Health Statistics, *Health Facilities,* op. cit.; Comptroller General of the United States, op. cit., 799.

14. National Center for Health Statistics, *Health Facilities,* op. cit.; National Center for Health Statistics, *Services and Activities Offered to Nursing Home Residents, United States, 1968* (Rockville, Md.: Department of Health, Education, and Welfare, 1972); a 1973 HEW survey showed that 59 per cent of SNFs were not meeting fire-safety requirements. *Boston Globe* 205, No. 16 (1974).

15. Comptroller General of the United States, op. cit., 798.

16. Ibid., 783–90.

17. National Center for Health Statistics, *Health Resources Statistics 1971,* op. cit.; Social Security Administration, *Social Security Disability Applicant Statistics, 1968* (Washington, D.C.: Department of Health, Education, and Welfare, 1972); C. Ryder et al., "Home Health Services—Past, Present, and Future." *Amer. J. Public Health* 59:1720–29 (Sept. 1969).

18. National Center for Health Statistics, *Aging Patterns in Medical Care, Illness, and Disability, 1968–69* (Washington, D.C.: Department of Health, Education, and Welfare, 1972); H. Kistin, "Home and Community Provision for the Elderly and Disabled—Program Alternatives" (draft). Brandeis University, Levinson Gerontological Institute, June 1972; see also Chapter 9 of the text.

19. Ibid.

20. U.S. Senate Special Committee on Aging, 93rd Congress, *Home Health Services in the United States, Current Status,* July 1973, and Apr. 1972 (92nd Congress) (Washington, D.C.: Government Printing Office); F. Caro, "Professional Roles in the Maintenance of the Disabled Elderly in the Community: A Forecast." Brandeis University, Levinson Gerontological Institute, Dec. 1972 (unpublished paper); Comptroller General of the United States, op. cit., 789; see also Chapters 6 and 7 of the text.

21. U.S. Senate Hearings, May 16, 1972, op. cit.; Health Care Facilities Service, *Hill-Burton Program Progress Report 1947–1970* (Rockville, Md.: Department of Health, Education, and Welfare, Oct. 1971).

22. National Center for Health Statistics, *Health Resources Statistics,* op. cit.; Comptroller General of the United States, op. cit., 847; A. Somers, *Health Care in Transition* (Chicago: Hospital Research and Educational Trust, 1971), 30.

23. Ibid., 871; G. Gibson, "EMS: A Facet of Ambulatory Care." *Hospitals* 47:59 (May 16, 1973).

24. M. Creditor and D. Nelson, "Regional Medical Programs and the Office of Management and Budget—Parallel Philosophies." *N. Eng. J. Med.* 289:239–42 (Aug. 2, 1973).

25. For example, R. Bergland, "Neurosurgery May Die." *N. Eng. J. Med.* 288:1043–46 (1973); National Center for Health Statistics, *Acute Conditions: Incidence and Associated Disability, United States, July 1970–*

June 1971 (Washington, D.C.: Department of Health, Education, and Welfare, Apr. 1973); "Allied Medical Help with Physicals." *Allied Med. Educ. Newsletter* 8:7 (Aug. 1, 1973); A. Jacobs and J. Gavett, "Case Classification of Ambulatory Care Demand." *Amer. J. Public Health* 63:721–26 (Aug. 1973).

26. Institute of Medicine, *Costs of Education of the Health Professions, Interim Report* (Washington, D.C.: National Academy of Science, Mar. 1973), 21.

27. Comptroller General of the United States, op. cit.; National Center for Health Statistics, *Health Resources Statistics,* op. cit.; R. Kane, "Community Medicine on a Navajo Reservation." *HSMHA Health Repts.* (1971).

28. T. Bodenheimer, "Patterns of American Ambulatory Care." *Inquiry* 7, No. 3:26–37.

29. National Center for Health Statistics, *Health Resources Statistics,* op. cit.

30. Ibid.; Social Security Administration, *Medical Care Expenditures, Prices, and Costs: Background Book* (Washington, D.C.: Government Printing Office, 1973).

31. Comptroller General of the United States, op. cit., 810.

32. Hearings Before the House of Representatives Subcommittee on Public Health and the Environment, *Health Maintenance Organizations 1973,* Mar. 6–7, 1973, Ser. 93-26 (Washington, D.C.: Government Printing Office, 1973); HMO Service, Publ. HSM 73-13009, Department of Health, Education, and Welfare, 1972.

33. Comptroller General of the United States, op. cit., 812.

34. Ibid.

35. R. Egdahl, "Foundations for Medical Care." *N. Eng. J. Med.* 288:491–99 (Mar. 8, 1973).

36. Hearings, H.R., Mar. 6, 1973, op. cit., 162–65.

37. *Health Planning Memorandum* 48 (Aug. 16, 1973); Hearings, H.R., Mar. 6, 1973, op. cit., 80–85.

38. Ibid., 162–65.

39. Ibid.; Comptroller General of the United States, op. cit.; E. Saward and M. Greenlick, "Health Policy and the HMO." *Milbank Mem. Fund Quart.* 50:147–77 (Apr. 1972).

40. Payments were from Office of Economic Opportunity and Medicaid. Hearings, op. cit., 162; G. Sparer and A. Anderson, "Utilization and Cost Experience of Low-Income Families in Four Prepaid Group Practice Plans." *N. Eng. J. Med.* 289:67–72 (July 12, 1973).

41. Hearings, op. cit.

42. See Chapter 3; also R. Weinerman, "Problems and Perspectives of Group Practice," in R. Elling, *National Health Care* (Chicago: Aldine, 1971), 206–23.

43. Hearings, op. cit., 263–64; *Health Law Newsletter* 22 (Feb. 1973).

44. J. Vohs et al., "Critical Issues in HMO Strategy." *N. Eng. J. Med.* 286:1082–86 (May 18, 1972).

45. "Legislation—Reported Testimony, HMOs." *Med. Care Rev.* 29:621–34 (June 1972).

46. N. Milio, *9226 Kercheval: The Storefront That Did Not Burn* (Ann Arbor, Mich.: University of Michigan Press, 1970).

47. "Draft of Prototype Standards for Ambulatory Health Care Centers." Department of Health, Education, and Welfare, Regional Office, June 1972 (mimeo).

48. S. 14, *Health Maintenance Organization and Resources Development Act of 1973* (Sen. Kennedy); Hearings, H.R., Mar. 6–7, 1973, op. cit., 321.

49. Great Britain Central Statistical Office, *Social Trends* No. 3, 1972 (London: Her Majesty's Stationery Office, 1973).

50. *The New York Abortion Story* (New York: Planned Parenthood Federation, 1972).

51. W. Pearse, "The Maternal and Infant Program." *Obstetrics and Gynecology* 35:114–119 (Jan. 1970).

52. N. Wright, "Some Estimates of the Potential Reduction in the U.S. Infant Mortality Rate by Family Planning." *Amer. J. Public Health* 62:1130–34 (Aug. 1972).

53. For example, J. Rosoff, "Legislative and Administrative Responsibilities for Federally-Supported Family Planning Services." *Family Planning Perspectives* 8 (Winter 1973), 39; V. Navarro, "National Health Insurance and the Strategy for Change." Johns Hopkins University, School of Hygiene and Public Health, Nov. 1972 (unpublished).

54. R. Dodds, *Background Papers on Health for the 1970 White House Conference on Children and Youth* (Washington, D.C.: Government Printing Office, 1970), 279–333.

55. G. Landsberg, "Consumers Appraise Storefront Mental Health Services." *Evaluation* 1, No. 2:66–68 (1973).

56. Hearings Before the Senate Health Subcommittee, Aug. 16, 1972, 46, Rept. 92-1064.

57. L. Reed et al., *Health Insurance and Psychiatric Care* (Washington, D.C.: American Psychiatric Association, 1972), 40.

58. S. Low and P. Spindler, *Child Care Arrangements of Working Mothers in the United States* (Washington, D.C.: Departments of Health, Education and Welfare and Labor, 1968); J. Bernard, *Women and the Public Interest* (Chicago: Aldine, 1971), 50–51.

59. A. Toft, *Care of Children and Young People* (Copenhagen: Ministry of Labor and Social Affairs, 1967); L. Dittmann (ed.), *Early Child Care* (New York: Atherton, 1968); *A Brief Report on Child Welfare Services in Japan 1970* (Tokyo: Ministry of Health and Welfare, 1971); M. Field,

Soviet Socialized Medicine (New York: Free Press, 1967); J. Andrews, "Medical Care in Sweden." *J. Amer. Med. Assoc.* 223:1369–75 (Mar. 19, 1973).

60. *The Organization and Administration of Maternal and Child Health Services* (Geneva: World Health Organization, 1969), 27.

61. N. Milio, "Getting Resources for Innovation in Health Care." *J. Nursing Admin.* (May–June 1971).

62. Navarro, op. cit.; see also E. Flook and P. Sanazaro, *Health Services Research and Research and Development in Perspective* (Ann Arbor, Mich.: Health Administration Press, University of Michigan, 1973), 155–58.

63. Comptroller General of the United States, op. cit., 1–75.

64. Ibid., 740–52.

65. Ibid.

66. Ibid.

67. "Emergency Medical Services." *Health Planning Memorandum* 46:5–10 (May 16, 1973); a full examination of how the removal of motor vehicles would improve health is made by A. Chase, *The Biological Imperatives: Health, Politics, and Human Survival* (New York: Holt, Rinehart and Winston, 1971).

68. Andrews, op. cit.

69. "National Health Service." *Med. Care Rev.* 29:1041–47 (Oct. 1972).

70. Great Britain Central Statistical Office, op. cit.

71. *Lancet* (July 14, 1973), 108.

72. H. Kistin, "Home and Community Provision for the Elderly and Disabled—Program Alternatives" (draft). Brandeis University, Levinson Gerontological Institute, June 1972.

73. "Report of the Commission on the Health Center Project to the Conference of Ministers." *Can. Med. J.* (Aug. 19, 1972).

74. J. Query, "Total Push and the Open Total Institution: The Factory Hospital." *J. Appl. Behav. Sci.* 9, Nos. 2/3:294 (1973).

75. *A Brief Report on Child Welfare Services in Japan 1970,* op. cit.

76. Personal interviews, Ministry of Health, New Delhi, India, Jan. 1971.

77. Department of International Health, "Health Care in Nigeria and French West Africa: Reflections of British and French Forms of Colonialism" (lecture, mimeo). Johns Hopkins University School of Hygiene and Public Health, Oct. 5, 1971.

78. V. Navarro, "Health Services in Cuba." *N. Eng. J. Med.* 287:954–59 Nov. 9, 1972); T. Hall, "Peru—The Latin American Style of Health Services" (lecture, mimeo). Johns Hopkins University School of Hygiene and Public Health, Sept. 23, 1971.

1. *Perspective* (Second Quarter 1973), 12, 13.

2. Committee for Economic Development, *Building a National Health Care System* (New York: CED, 1973).

3. "Life and Death and Medicine." *Scientific American* (Sept. 1973), 151; see also Chapter 10 of the text.

4. U.S. Environmental Protection Agency, Expenditures FY 1971–72 (Total Pollution Control Expenditures and Federal-State Funding and Manpower for State Water Quality Agencies); projections for 1972–1981 show average annual expenditures as $10.2 billion for government; $8.4 billion for consumers; $8.8 billion for industry; total: $27.4 billion per year [*Environmental Quality 1973* (Washington, D.C.: Government Printing Office, 1973)]; another set of figures, which does include health training but not pollution control expenditures, is in *The Changing Role of the Public and Private Sectors in Health Care* (New York: National Health Council, 1973), 15.

5. Committee for Economic Development, op. cit., 42; Social Security Administration, *Medical Care Expenditures, Prices, and Costs: Background Book* (Washington, D.C.: Government Printing Office, 1973).

6. Social Security Administration, "Medical Care Price Changes Under the Economic Stabilization Program." *Res. Stat. Note* 8 (May 15, 1973).

7. National Center for Health Statistics, "Personal Out-of-Pocket Medical Expenses, 1970." *Monthly Vital Stat. Rept.* 22 (Apr. 2, 1973).

8. Department of Labor, *Boston Evening Globe,* June 17, 1973.

9. *Sourcebook of Health Insurance Data* (New York: Health Insurance Institute, 1972), 45.

10. Social Security Administration, "Relative Importance of Income Sources of the Aged." *Res. Stat. Note* 11 (May 29, 1973); Social Security Administration, "Preliminary Findings from the Survey of New Beneficiaries," Rept. 10 (June 1973).

11. *Perspective* (Fourth Quarter 1972); *Health Law Newsletter* 25 (May 1973); Social Security Administration, *Medicare: Hospital Insurance for the Aged 1971* (Washington, D.C.: Government Printing Office, 1973), xxv and following.

12. Comptroller General of the United States, *Study of Health Facilities Construction Costs* (Washington, D.C.: Government Printing Office, 1972).

13. *Health Law Newsletter,* op. cit.; Hearings, U.S. House of Representatives, Mar. 6–7, 1973, Rept. 93-26.

14. Ibid.

15. *Perspective,* op. cit.; *Health Law Newsletter,* op. cit.

16. *Social Security Bull.* (May 1972); Social Security Administration, *Res. Stat. Note* 8 (Mar. 27, 1974).

17. Ibid.

18. *Perspective,* op. cit.; R. Andersen et al., *Expenditures for Personal Health Services: National Trends and Variations 1963–70* (Rockville, Md.: Department of Health, Education, and Welfare, Oct. 1973).

19. *Health Law Newsletter,* op. cit.

20. Perspective, op. cit.

21. P.L. 92–603 and *Health Law Newsletter,* op. cit.

22. U.S. House of Representatives, Committee on Ways and Means, "Cost Study of Health Insurance Proposals Introduced in the 92nd Congress" (Washington, D.C.: Government Printing Office, 1972).

24. Comptroller General of the United States, op. cit., 833–43; Social Security Administration, "Impact of Cost-Sharing on Use of Ambulatory Services Under Medicare: Preliminary Findings, 1969." *Health Insurance Stat.,* Oct. 10, 1973.

25. Ibid., 843–45.

26. Ibid.

27. Data from Committee for National Health Insurance, Washington, D.C.; Hearings, House of Representatives, op. cit., 175.

28. Ibid.

29. Health Maintenance Organization Service, "Questions Physicians Are Asking About HMOs" (Washington, D.C.: Department of Health, Education, and Welfare, Dec. 1972), 8. Other methods affecting providers' reimbursement, included in the 1972 Social Security Amendments, include (1) as a condition for participating in Medicare, a written plan, containing an annual operating budget and a three-year projected capital expenditures plan; (2) "reasonable charges" to physicians defined as those which do not exceed the 75th percentile of actual charges for similar services in the geographic area during the previous year. Non-hospital-based and non-group-practice physicians have been increasingly less willing to accept this limitation on their fees for their patients who are covered by Medicaid–Medicare and for whom states are willing to pay the deductible and coinsurance charges. Thus the patient becomes liable for these charges [Social Security Administration, "Assignment Rates for Supplementary Medical Insurance Claims, 1970–72." *Health Insur. Stat.* 46 (June 30, 1973)].

30. H. Somers and A. Somers, *Medicare and the Hospitals* (Washington, D.C.: The Brookings Institution, 1967); Social Security Administration, *Net Income of Hospitals 1961–69* (Washington, D.C.: Department of Health, Education, and Welfare, Dec. 1970); I. S. Falk, "Medical Care in the U.S.A. 1932–72," in *Health and Society, Milbank Mem. Fund Quart.* 51:1–40 (Winter 1973).

31. Institute of Medicine, op. cit., 8; see also S. Berki, "Economic Effects of NHI." *Inquiry* 8:37–55 (June 1971); for 76 per cent of teaching hospitals, patient revenues were their major source of support for house staff in 1972–1973 [Council of Teaching Hospitals, *Survey* (Washington, D.C.: American Association of Medical Colleges, 1973)].

32. *New York Times,* July 14, 1973, 31.

33. R. Dodds, *Background Paper for Health: 1970 White House Conference on Children and Youth* (Washington, D.C.: Government Printing Office. 1971), 279–333; J. Rosoff, "The Future of Federal Support for Family Planning Services." *Family Planning Perspectives* 5:8 (Winter 1973); *The Size and Shape of the Medical Care Dollar 1972* (Washington, D.C.: Department of Health, Education, and Welfare, 1973).

34. Committee on Ways and Means, op. cit., 184; R. Weiss et al., "Trends in Health Insurance Operating Expenses." *N. Eng. J. Med.* 287:638–41 (Sept. 28, 1972); W. Cohen, *Perspective* (Third Quarter 1973).

35. Social Security Administration, *Res. Stat. Note* 19 (Nov. 29, 1972).

36. Bureau of Health Manpower, *Inventory of Federal Programs That Support Health Manpower Training 1970* (Washington, D.C.: Department of Health, Education, and Welfare, 1971.

37. Institute of Medicine, op. cit., 29.

38. Ibid.

39. Ibid., 53.

40. Ibid., 8.

41. R. Magraw et al., "Perspectives from New Schools—The Costs and Financing of Medical Education." *N. Eng. J. Med.* 289:558–62 (Sept. 13, 1973).

42. Ibid.

43. Social Security Administration, *Social Security Programs Throughout the World 1971* (Washington, D.C.: Department of Health, Education, and Welfare, 1972).

44. W. Glaser, *Paying the Doctor: Systems of Remuneration and Their Effects* (Baltimore, Md.: Johns Hopkins University Press, 1970), 286.

45. The Greater Medical Profession, Report of a Symposium Sponsored Jointly by the Royal Society of Medicine and the Josiah Macy, Jr., Foundation (New York: Macy Foundation, 1973), 25; J. Andrews, "Medical Care in Sweden." *J. Amer. Med. Assoc.* 223:1269–75 (Mar. 19, 1973).

46. Glaser, op. cit.

47. B. Shenkin, "Politics and Medical Care in Sweden: The 7 Crowns Reform." *N. Eng. J. Med.* 288:555–59 (Mar. 15, 1973).

48. Social Security Administration, 1972, op. cit.

Images of Access i, ii, iii

1. Based on a field visit to Chanakyapuri and to Mobile Creches office with Mrs. Mahadevan and a review of their records, Feb. 9, 1971. Information on preschools is based on interviews with and papers from Dr. R. Muralidharan, president, Indian Association for Preschool Education, and Research Associate, Department of Educational Psychology and Founda-

tions for Education, National Institute for Education, Jan. 30, 1971, New Delhi. Supplementary information came from Mr. J. Kaul, Director, S.O.S. Children's Village, Haryana.

2. Based on a field visit to Etten-Leur, and discussions with Dr. Mol, Sn., Dr. Franz Mol, Dr. Peter Mol, the staff at Kraamcentrum, De Nobelaer Community Center, and Lebensschool voor Jonge Arbeiders, Oct. 22; and with Antonia Mol, social worker, University of Amsterdam, Oct. 18, 20, and 22, Amsterdam; also "Social Security in The Netherlands" (The Hague: Ministry of Social Affairs, Sept. 1971).

3. Based on a field visit to St. Christopher's Hospice, London, and discussions with founder and director Dr. Cicely Saunders; Jane Lowenstein, volunteer; and other members of the staff and patients, Nov. 11, 1971.

Chapter 6—From Student to Practitioner: Patterns and Effects

1. U.S. Environmental Protection Agency, "Fund for State Air Pollution Control Agencies, FY 1971" and "Funding and Manpower for State Water Quality Agencies, 1971–72" (computed in man-years).

2. American Hospital Association, *1973 Guide to the Health Care Field* (Chicago: AHA, 1973); K. Davis, "Hospital Costs and the Medicare Program," *Social Security Bull.* (Aug. 1973) reports capital expenditures rose faster than labor costs, 1962–1968.

3. Rep. Rogers, "Public and Allied Health Personnel Act of 1973" (H.R. 9341), U.S. House of Representatives; Institute of Medicine, *Study of the Costs of Education for the Health Professions* (Washington, D.C.: National Academy of Science, 1973).

4. L. Smith and A. Crocker, *How Medical Students Finance Their Education* (Washington, D.C.: Department of Health, Education, and Welfare, 1970); J. Walsh and R. Elling, "Professionalism and the Poor." *J. Health Soc. Behav.* 9:16–28 (1968); C. Lopate, *Women in Medicine* (Baltimore: Johns Hopkins University Press, 1968), 75.

5. Smith and Crocker, op. cit.

6. *Boston Globe,* Oct. 7, 1973; "Medical Education in the United States, 1971–72." *J. Amer. Med. Assoc.* 222 (Suppl.):983 (Nov. 20, 1972).

7. U.S. Senate Committee on the Judiciary, *Report on the Equal Rights for Men and Women Amendment,* Washington, D.C., Mar. 14, 1972, Rept. 92-689, 8.

8. Council on Medical Education and Council on Health Manpower, *Physician Manpower and Medical Education* (Chicago: American Medical Association, June 1971), 18; W. Dube et al., "Study of U.S. Medical School Applicants." *J. Med. Educ.* 46:837 (Oct. 1971); T. Dublin, "The Migration of Physicians to the United States." *N. Eng. J. Med.* 286:870–77 (Apr. 20, 1972).

9. Ibid.; *Annual Report 1972* (Philadelphia: Education Council for Foreign Medical Graduates).

10. *J. Amer. Med. Assoc.* 222, op. cit.

11. M. Halberstam, "Foreign Surgical Residents in University-Affiliated Hospitals." *Ann. Surgery* 71:485–500 (Apr. 1970); M. Dasco, "FMG Training in the United States." *Ann. Internal Med.* 68:1105–13 (May 1968).

12. *Amer. Med. News* 14:2 (Nov. 29, 1971).

13. R. Knobel, "Placement of Foreign-trained Physicians in U.S. Medical Residencies." *Med. Care* 11:224–39 (May–June 1973).

14. *J. Amer. Med. Assoc.* 222, op. cit., 992.

15. Council of Teaching Hospitals, *Survey of House Staff Policy 1973* (Washington, D.C.: Association of American Medical Colleges, 1973).

16. M. Pennell and J. Renshaw, "Distribution of Women Physicians 1970." *J. Amer. Med. Women's Assoc.* 27:197–203 (Apr. 1972); Dublin, op. cit.; *Med. Care Rev.* (Dec. 1972), 1234.

17. *J. Amer. Med. Assoc.* 222, op. cit., 1004; *Amer. Med. News* 14 (Nov. 20, 1971).

18. L. Powers et al., "Practice Patterns of Women and Men Physicians." *J. Med. Educ.* 44:481–91 (June 1969).

18a. H. Tilson, "Stability of Physician Employment in Neighborhood Health Centers." *Med. Care* 11:484–500 (Sept.–Oct. 1973).

19. D. Solomon, "Ethnic and Class Differences Among Hospitals as Contingencies in Medical Careers," in E. Friedson and J. Lorber (eds.), *Medical Men and Their Work* (Chicago: Aldine, 1972), 163–73.

20. S. Altman, *Present and Future Supply of Registered Nurses* (Washington, D.C.: Department of Health, Education, and Welfare, 1972), 40–44.

21. L. Knopf, *From Student to RN: A Report of the Nurse Career-Pattern Study, National League for Nursing* (Washington, D.C.: Department of Health, Education, and Welfare, 1972), 68.

22. "Educational Preparation for Nursing—1971." *Nursing Outlook* 20:599–601 (Sept. 1972).

23. In 1970–1971, the number of graduates were 14,750, 22,300, and 9,900 from the two-, three-, and four-year programs, respectively (ibid.).

24. Lecht, op. cit., app.

25. *Interagency Conference on Nursing Statistics Report,* Nov. 23, 1971 (Washington, D.C.: Department of Health, Education, and Welfare, 1972).

26. Department of Finance, "Nurses and California: An Overview of Past and Present and Projections for the Future," State of California (unpublished), Aug. 1972. The Board of Directors of the American Nurses Association stated in 1973 that it may have erred in attempting in 1965 to distinguish "professional" from "technical" nurses on the basis of their training programs; they concluded that in actual practice the differences had not been demonstrated ("ANA Board of Directors Statement on the Role and Status of the Diploma School Graduate." *Amer. J. Nursing,* July 1973).

27. M. Kohnke, "Do Nursing Educators Practice What Is Preached?" *Amer. J. Nursing* 73:1571–75 (Sept. 1973). Another analysis of licensing examinations in New York state showed that graduates of the three- and four-year programs had a similar range of scores in 1968 (A. Sadler et al., *The Physician's Assistant* (New Haven: Yale University School of Medicine, 1972), 66.

28. H. Greenfield with C. Brown, *Allied Health Manpower: Trends and Prospects* (New York: Columbia University Press, 1964), 24–36, 109.

29. Altman, op. cit., 92–95, 108; B. Tate, "Rate of Graduation in Schools of Nursing." *Internat. Nursing Rev.* 15:339–46 (1968).

30. National Center for Health Statistics, *Health Resources Statistics 1971* (Washington, D.C.: Department of Health, Education, and Welfare, 1972).

30a. For a historical perspective, see B. Ehrenreich and D. English, *Witches, Midwives, and Nurses* (Old Westbury, N.Y.: Feminist, 1972).

31. "Life and Death and Medicine." *Scientific American* 229 (Sept. 1973), reporting a Canadian national survey, 1950–1951, pp. 77–82.

32. Ibid., reporting a British study, 1955.

33. Ibid.; *The Greater Medical Profession,* Report of a Symposium Sponsored Jointly by the Royal Medical Society and the Josiah Macy, Jr., Foundation (New York: Macy Foundation, 1973), 47.

34. H. Cross, "Educational Needs as Determined by the Problem-Oriented Medical Record." *J. Maine Med. Assoc.* 61:49–54 (Mar. 1970). "Life and Death and Medicine," op. cit., reporting a 1958 British study, pp. 27–30, and a Cleveland study 1948–1958, pp. 77–82.

35. National Center for Health Statistics, *Acute Conditions: Incidence and Associated Disability, United States, July 1970–June 1971* (Washington, D.C.: Department of Health, Education, and Welfare, 1973), Tables A, C.

36. A. Jacobs and J. Gavett, "Case Classification of Ambulatory Care Demand." *Amer. J. Public Health* 63:721–26 (Aug. 1973).

37. *Greater Medical Profession,* op. cit., 206; C. Sheps, "The Influence of Consumer Sponsorship on Medical Services." *Milbank Mem. Fund Quart.* 50:41–69 (Oct. 1972), Part II, 48, 56.

38. "Life and Death and Medicine," op. cit., 30.

39. Bureau of Public Health Economics, *Medical Care Chartbook* (Ann Arbor, Mich.: University of Michigan School of Public Health, 1972), E-21.

40. F. Caro, "Professional Roles in the Maintenance of the Disabled Elderly in the Community: A Forecast" (mimeo). Brandeis University, Levinson Gerontological Institute, Dec. 1972; Walsh and Elling, op. cit.

40a. R. Bergland, "Neurosurgery May Die." *N. Eng. J. Med.* 288:1043–46 (1973).

41. G. Rosen, "Changing Attitudes of the Medical Profession to Specializa-

tion," in E. Friedson and J. Lorber, *Medical Men and Their Work* (Chicago: Aldine, 1972), 103–12.

42. J. Weiss, "Socioeconomic and Technological Factors in Trends of Physicians to Specialize." *HSMHA Health Rept.* 86:46–51 (Jan. 1971); American Medical Association, *1972 Profile* and *J. Amer. Med. Assoc.* 222, op. cit., 1004.

43. M. Field, "Health Personnel in the Soviet Union." *Amer. J. Public Health* 56:1904–20 (Nov. 1966).

44. T. Ingles, "An American Nurse Visits the USSR." *Amer. J. Nursing* 70:754–62 (Apr. 1970).

45. R. Badgley, "Studies in Planning Health Manpower." *J. Health Soc. Behav.* 12:4–10 (Mar. 1971).

46. S. Hall, "Availability of Health Services and Personnel to School-Age Children According to Income Groups in Nigeria and the United States." Boston University School of Nursing Seminar on Issues in International and U.S. Health Care, Apr. 1973; C. Harinsuta, "The Need for Clinical Assistants in Thailand." *Lancet* 1298–1300 (June 9, 1973).

47. M. Jeffreys et al., "Comparison of Men and Women in Medical Training." *Lancet* 2:1381–83 (June 26, 1965); J. Shuval, "Sex Role Differentiation in the Professions: The Case of Israeli Dentists." *J. Health Soc. Behav.* 11:236–44 (Sept. 1970).

48. N. Milio, " 'Outcast' Clients and Human Services Workers: Questions of Access and Equity" (unpublished research), Boston University, 1973; see also Badgley, op. cit.   •

49. G. MacLachlin, *Problems and Progress in Medical Care* (London: Oxford University Press, 1971), 159.

50. Personal communication, Great Britain Department of Health and Social Security, June 1973.

51. Office of Research and Statistics, Department of Health and Social Security, *Social Trends 1972* (London: Her Majesty's Stationery Office, 1973).

52. R. Nelson-Jones and D. Fish, "Social Characteristics of Applicants to Canadian Medical Schools." *J. Med. Educ.* 45:918–28 (Nov. 1970).

53. de Kock van Leeuwen, "Some Social and Emotional Aspects of Health Manpower Training," in Regional Office for Europe, *Methods of Estimating Health Manpower* (Copenhagen: World Health Organization, 1969), 110–19; The Swedish Institute, "Organization of Medical Care in Sweden" (Stockholm: The Institute, Dec. 1971); J. Ben-David,

Chapter 7—Solutions and Their Problems

1. Division of Allied Medical Education, "Allied Medical Education Research Review, Spring 1973" (Chicago: American Medical Association, 1973).

2. *New Members of the Physician Health Team: Physician's Assistants* (Washington, D.C.: National Academy of Science, 1970); also described in R. Hoekleman, "Pediatric Nurse Practitioner." *N.Y. State J. Med.* 72:1991–2000 (Aug. 1, 1972).

3. S. Berki, "The Economics of New Types of Health Personnel." Macy Conference on Intermediate-Level Health Personnel, Williamsburg, Va., Nov. 11–14, 1972 (mimeo).

4. A. Yankauer et al., "Pediatric Practice in the United States with Special Attention to Utilization of Allied Health Worker Services." *Pediatrics* 45:259–92, Part II, Suppl. (Mar. 1970), 266, 275.

5. Ibid., 263–64, 275.

6. Berki, op. cit., 18–19.

7. Yankauer, op. cit., 266.

8. Ibid., 280.

9. "Physician's Assistants: A Socioeconomic Report of the Bureau of Research and Planning, California Medical Association." *Calif. Med.* 112: 73–76 (Apr. 1970); A. Bergman et al., "Time-Motion Study of Practicing Pediatricians." *Pediatrics* 38:254–63 (1966).

10. M. Todd and D. Foy, "Current Status of the Physician's Assistant and Related Issues." *J. Amer. Med. Assoc.* 220:1714–20 (June 16, 1972); A. Jacobs and J. Gavett, "Case Classification of Ambulatory Care Demand." *Amer. J. Public Health* 63:721–26 (Aug. 1973).

11. B. Brody and J. Stokes, "Use of Professional Time by Internists and General Practitioners in Group and Solo Practice." *Ann. Internal Med.* 73: 741–49 (Nov. 1970).

12. E. Shanas, "Measuring the Home Health Needs of the Aged in Five Countries." *J. Gerontology* 26–39 (Jan. 1970).

13. S. Smale, "Activities of Nurses and Physicians in Ambulatory Care." *Nursing Clin. North America* 6:489–98 (Sept. 1971).

14. A. Yankauer et al., "The Practice of Nursing in Pediatric Offices—Challenge and Opportunity." *N. Eng. J. Med.* 282:843–47 (Apr. 9, 1970).

15. W. Hoff, "Resolving the Health Manpower Crisis—A Systems Approach to Utilizing Personnel." *Amer. J. Public Health* 61:2491–2504 (Dec. 1971).

16. P. Paterson and A. Bergman, "Time–Motion Study of Six Pediatric Office Assistants." *N. Eng. J. Med.* 281:771–74 (Oct. 2, 1969).

17. J. Cauffman et al., "Community Health Aides: How Effective Are They?" *Amer. J. Public Health* 60:1904–09 (Oct. 1970).

18. *Summary of Training Programs: Physician Support Personnel* (Washington, D.C.: Department of Health, Education, and Welfare, June 1972); C. Medeiros, "Physician Assistants and Related Allied Health Professionals: An Analysis of Basic Issues and Current Literature" [Community Health, Inc., New York, July 1972 (unpublished paper)]; personal communications, Medex program, University of Washington, Feb. 1973; and

Physician Assistant Program, Stanford University Medical Center, Dec. 1972; B. Schutt, "Frontier's Family Nurse." *Amer. J. Nursing* 72:903–09 (May 1972).

19. G. Rosen, "The Physician Assistant and the Provision of Care." *Amer. J. Public Health* (Jan. 1973).

20. Medex Program, op. cit.; *Summary of Training Programs,* op. cit.; Department of Health, Education, and Welfare, *Health Resources News* 1 (Sept. 1973).

21. Hoekleman, op. cit.

22. Personal communication, Albert Einstein Medical College, Bronx, N.Y.; J. Morton, "Experiences with a Maternity and Infant Care Project." *Amer. J. Obstetrics Gynecology* 107:362–68 (June 1, 1970).

23. W. Willis, "Nurse-Midwifery in the United States" (mimeo). Massachusetts Department of Public Health, Boston, 1973.

24. National Center for Family Planning Services, "Non-physician Professionals Being Trained to Provide Family Planning Care." *Family Planning Digest* 2:1–6 (July 1973); R. Willson, "Health Care for Women: Present Deficiencies and Future Needs." *Obstetrics and Gynecology* 36:178 (1970).

25. R. Smith, "Medex." *Lancet* (July 14, 1973); *The Greater Medical Profession* (New York: Macy Foundation, 1973), 162.

26. J. Shulman and C. Wood, "Experience of a Nurse Practitioner in a General Medical Clinic." *J. Amer. Med. Assoc.* 219:1453–61 (Mar. 13, 1972); C. Lewis and B. Resnik, "Activities, Events and Outcomes in Ambulatory Patient Care." *N. Eng. J. Med.* 280:645–49 (Mar. 20, 1969); Albert Einstein Medical Center, op. cit.

27. K. Kaku, et al., "Comparison of Health Appraisals by Nurses and Physicians." *Public Health Rept.* 85:1042–46.

28. L. Harris et al., "Nurse-Midwifery in New York City." *Amer. J. Public Health* 61:64–77 (Jan. 1971); J. Fairweather and A. Kifolo, "Improvement of Patient Care in a Solo Ob.-Gyn. Practice by Using an R.N.-Physician's Assistant." *Amer. J. Public Health* 361–63 (Mar. 1972); National Center for Family Planning Services, op. cit.

29. *Secretary's Commission on Medical Malpractice Report,* No. OS 73-88 (Washington, D.C.: Department of Health, Education, and Welfare, 1973).

30. *Greater Medical Profession,* op. cit., 153–54.

31. R. Scheffler and O. Stinson, "Physician Assistants: A Report on Earnings." *Phys. Assoc.* (Apr.–May 1973).

32. Personal communication, Medex, op. cit.

33. R. Scheffler and O. Stinson, "Characteristics of Physician's Assistants: A Focus on Specialty" (working paper). Health Services Research Center, University of North Carolina, Chapel Hill, 1973; R. Scheffler, "Relation-

ship Between Medical Education and Statewide Per Capita Distribution of Physicians." *J. Med. Educ.* 46:995–98 (Nov. 1971).

34. Scheffler and Stinson, working paper, op. cit.

35. Yankauer et al. (Mar. 1972), op. cit.

36. Sadler et al., op. cit., 37; personal communication, Council, Idaho, Oct. 1972.

37. Berki, op. cit.

38. Yankauer *et al.* (Mar. 1972), op. cit.; Albert Einstein Medical Center, *op. cit.*

39. Yankauer et al. (Mar. 1972 and Mar. 1970), op. cit.; H. Silver and B. Duncan, "Time–Motion Study of Pediatric Nurse Practitioners: Comparison with 'Regular' Office Nurses and Pediatricians." *Med. Care* 79:331–36 (Aug. 1971).

40. National Center for Family Planning Services, op. cit.

41. A. Yankauer et al., "Physician Productivity in the Delivery of Ambulatory Care." *Med. Care* 35–46 (Jan.–Feb. 1970).

42. Willson, op. cit.; Todd and Foy, op. cit., 1717.

43. Personal communication, Medex, op. cit.; Scheffler and Stinson, working paper, 1973, op. cit.; *Summary of Training Programs,* op. cit.

43a. Todd and Foy, op. cit.; Committee on Allied Health Personnel, *Allied Health Personnel: A Report on Their Use in the Military Services As a Model for Use in Non-military Health Care Programs* (Washington, D.C.: National Academy of Science, 1969), 12–14.

43b. *Allied Med. Educ. Newsletter* 8:7 (Aug. 1, 1973).

44. Personal communication, Medex, op. cit.; Scheffler and Stinson, working paper, 1973, op. cit.; *Summary of Training Programs,* op. cit.

45. Scheffler and Stinson, *Phys. Assoc.,* op. cit.

46. Sadler et al., op. cit., 28–37; Albert Einstein Medical Center, op. cit.; F. Lohring, "The Marshfield Clinic P.A. Concept." *Group Practice* (July 1969).

47. Department of Health, Education, and Welfare, Extending the Scope of Nursing Practice. A Report of the Secretary's Committee to Study Extended Roles for Nurses (1971) excerpted in *Intern. Nursing Rev.* 19: 219–37, 1972, and *J. Amer. Med. Assoc.* 220:1231–37 (May 29, 1972); Hoekleman, op. cit.

48. Todd and Foy, op. cit., 1717; at the AMA Annual Convention, New York, June 24–28, 1973, "Outgoing AMA President, C. A. Hoffman, M.D., told the AMA House of Delegates: "I see a tendency—a dangerous tendency, in my judgment—to resort to second-line personnel—particularly physician's assistants—as the remedy for underserved areas. We of the AMA endorse larger roles and broader responsibilities for nurses and other allied personnel . . . provided the duties are well defined and the physicians' authority is maintained. The role of physician's assistants must be clearly defined and its limitations clearly understood.

Properly placed and properly employed, they can play an effective role in doing what their name implies—assisting the physician. But they must be content with that role. In any event, we must oppose absolutely any attempt to make physician's assistants physician substitutes. And we must reject completely any program that would cast them in that role" [*Allied Med. Educ. Newsletter* 8:7 (Aug. 1, 1973)].

49. *Medical Opinion* survey reported in *Allied Med. Educ. Newsletter* 8:8 (Aug. 1, 1973); Hoekleman, op. cit.; Yankauer et al., Mar. 1970, op. cit.

50. *Conference on Nursing Statistics 1971* (Washington, D.C.: Department of Health, Education, and Welfare, 1972).

51. T. Adamson, "Critique and Description of Physician Assistant Programs." School of Public Health, University of California, Berkeley, Mar. 1970 (unpublished paper), 21; see also quotation in Note 48.

52. Todd and Foy, op. cit.; "Allied Medical Educational Programs." *Allied Med. Educ. Newsletter* 6:11 (May 1, 1973).

53. American Medical Association House of Delegates, in *Amer. Nurse* (July–Aug. 1972).

54. American Medical Association, 156,000 in 1972, a drop of 12,000 from 1970 (*Allied Med. Educ. Newsletter,* Sept. 1, 1973); ANA, about 260,000 in 1971 of 748,000 employed nurses. (See International Council of Nurses, *National Reports of Member Associations 1969.*)

55. "American Nurses Association Views the Emerging 'Physician's Assistant'." *Intern. Nursing Rev.* 19, No. 2:190 (1972).

56. Sadler et al., op. cit., 211; J. Rothberg, "Nurse and Physician Assistant: Issues and Relationships." *Nursing Outlook* 21:154–158 (Mar. 1973).

57. Willis, op. cit., 18–19; J. Record and H. Cohen, "The Introduction of Midwifery in a Prepaid Group Practice." *Amer. J. Public Health* 354–60 (Mar. 1972).

58. See, for example, E. Selmanoff, "Strains in the Nurse–Doctor Relationship." *Nursing Clin. North America* 3:117–127 (Mar. 1968); B. Bates, "Doctor and Nurse: Changing Roles and Relations." *N. Eng. J. Med.* 283 (July 16, 1970); H. Mauksch, "Ideology, Interaction, and Patient Care in Hospitals" (mimeo). Third International Conference on Social Science and Medicine, Aug. 13–19, 1972; R. Corwin and M. Taves, "Nursing and Other Health Professions" in H. Freeman, S. Levine, and L. Reeder (eds.), *Handbook of Medical Sociology* (Englewood Cliffs, N.J.: Prentice-Hall, 1963), 187–211; H. Wise, "The Primary Care Health Team." *Arch. Internal Med.* 130:438–44 (Sept. 1972).

59. R. Alvarez and W. Moore, "Information Flow Within the Professions: Some Selective Comparisons of Law, Medicine, and Nursing," in S. Wheeler (ed.), *On Record: Files and Dossiers in American Life* (New York: Russell Sage Foundation, 1969), 95–139; A. Strauss, *Professions, Work and Careers* (San Francisco: Sociology Press, 1971).

60. H. Wilensky, "The Professionalization of Everyone?" *Amer. J. Sociol.* 70:137–58 (Sept. 1964).

61. Rueschemeyer, op. cit.

62. E. Rayack, *Professional Power and American Medicine: The Economics of the American Medical Association* (New York: World, 1967). For other references, see Chapters 6 and 9 of the text.

63. C. Lopate, *Women in Medicine* (Baltimore, Md.: Johns Hopkins University Press, 1968), 23; C. Lewis, "Experiments in the Delivery of Health Care and Their Impact on Medical Schools." *Arch. Internal. Med.* 127:312–13 (Feb. 1971).

64. For example, H. Becker et al., *Boys in White* (Chicago: University of Chicago Press, 1961); G. Psathas, "The Fate of Idealism in Nursing School." *J. Health Soc. Behav.* 9:52–64 (Mar. 1968); I. Simpson, "Patterns of Socialization into Professions: The Case of Student Nurses." *Soc. Inquiry* 37:47–54 (Winter 1967); B. Sherlock and R. Morris, "The Evolution of a Professional: A Paradigm." *Soc. Inquiry* 37:27–46 (Winter 1967); E. Hughes, *Men and Their Work* (New York: Free Press, 1958); E. Freidson, *Professional Dominance: The Social Structure of Medical Care* (New York: Atherton, 1970); D. Mechanic, "Sociology and Public Health: Perspectives for Application." *Amer. J. Public Health* 146 (Feb. 1972).

65. B. Dana and C. Sheps, "Trends and Issues in Interprofessional Education: Pride, Prejudice, and Progress." *Educ. for Soc. Work* (Fall 1968).

66. N. Milio, " 'Outcast Clients' and Human Services Workers" (unpublished research report), Boston, 1973.

67. See Becker et al., op. cit., and Psathas, op. cit.

68. C. Epstein, *Woman's Place: Options and Limits in Professional Careers* (Berkeley, Calif.: University of California Press, 1970), Chap. 5; C. Lopate, *Women in Medicine, op. cit.;* Alvarez and Moore, op. cit.; H. Vollmer and D. Mills (eds.), *Professionalization* (Englewood Cliffs, N.J.: Prentice-Hall, 1966).

69. J. Walsh and R. Elling, "Professionalism and the Poor." *J. Health Soc. Behav.* 9:16–28 (1968); Rueschemeyer, op. cit.; A. Hollingshead and F. Redlich, *Social Class and Mental Illness* (New York: John Wiley, 1958); N. Lourie, "Impact of Social Change on the Tasks of Mental Health Professionals." *Amer. J. Orthopsych.* 35:43 (Jan. 1965).

70. *Report on Licensure and Related Health Personnel Credentialing* No. HSM 7211 (Washington, D.C.: Department of Health, Education, and Welfare, June 1971) 7–10.

71. R. Akers, "The Professional Association and the Legal Regulation of Practice." *Law Society Rev.* 2 (May 1968).

72. *Report on Licensure,* op. cit., 29; Rayack, op. cit., 5–6; see also C. Gilb, *Hidden Hierarchies: The Professions and Government* (New York: Harper & Row, 1966).

73. *Report on Licensure,* op. cit., 23–29.

74. *Report on Licensure,* op. cit., 136.

75. *Study of Accreditation of Selected Health Educational Programs Commission Report* (Washington, D.C.: National Committee on Accrediting, May 1972), 5–13; Testimony on Allied Health Personnel, Senate Health Subcommittee, May 19–20, 1970.

76. *Report on Licensure,* op. cit., 11–13; beginning 1974, NCA Board of Commissioners reported a reorganization to include, for the first time, 3 public members on its 30-person board [*Allied Med. Educ. Newsletter* 6 (Dec. 1, 1973)].

77. SASHEP, op. cit., 6.

78. *Report on Licensure.* op. cit., 23, 137.

79. Ibid., 15–20, Table 3.

80. B. Agree, "The Threat of Institutional Licensure." *Amer. J. Nursing* 73:1758–63 (Oct. 1973).

81. *Report on Licensure,* op. cit., Table 2; Greenfield and Brown, op. cit., 71, Table 4.1.

82. S. Rosen, "Building Career Ladders in Health Occupations—Opportunities and Obstacles" (mimeo). New Careers Development Center, New York University, 1968; M. Pennell et al., *Accreditation and Certification in Relation to Allied Health Manpower* (Washington, D.C.: Department of Health, Education, and Welfare, 1971).

83. P. Ellwood et al., *Assuring the Quality of Health Care* (Minneapolis: InterStudy, 1973), 29.

84. J. Williamson et al., "Evaluation of Patient Care: An Approach." *J. Amer. Med. Assoc.* 214 (Dec. 14, 1970).

85. M. Kohnke, "Do Nursing Educators Practice What Is Preached?" *Amer. J. Nursing* 73:1571–75 (Sept. 1973).

86. M. Egelston, "Licensure—Effects on Career Mobility." *Amer. J. Public Health* 50–53 (Jan. 1972).

87. Ellwood et al., op. cit., 31.

88. *Allied Med. Educ. Newsletter* (Oct. 1973).

89. W. Dean, "State Legislation for Physician's Assistants: A Review and Analysis." *Health Serv. Rept.* 88:1–12 (Jan. 1973); W. Curran, "Physicians' Assistants: The Question of Legal Responsibility." *Amer. J. Public Health* 60:2400–2401 (Dec. 1970).

90. Legal opinion is that current medical practice acts already allow this delegatory authority to physicians [R. Carlson, *Law Contemp. Prob.* 35:868 (Autumn 1970)].

91. Council on Health Manpower, *Licensure of the Health Occupations* (Chicago: American Medical Association, 1970), 6.

92. Dean, op. cit.

93. *1973 Report of the Secretary's Commission on Medical Malpractice* (Washington, D.C.: Department of Health, Education, and Welfare, 1973); W. Curran, "Legal Responsibility for Actions of Physicians' Assistants." *N. Eng. J. Med.* 286:254 (Feb. 3, 1972).

94. Dean, op. cit.

95. M. Todd, "National Certification of Physicians' Assistants by Uniform Examinations." *J. Amer. Med. Assoc.* 222:563–66 (Oct. 30, 1972); J. Hubbard, "Evaluation, Certification, and Licensure in Medicine: New Directions." *J. Amer. Med. Assoc.* 225:401–06 (July 23, 1973).

96. *Allied Med. Educ. News.* (Oct. 1973).

97. Idaho State Boards of Nursing and of Medicine, "Minimum Standards, Rules, and Regulations for the Expanding Role of the Registered Professional Nurse" (Boise, Idaho, June 1972); "Where Nurses Can Diagnose and Prescribe." *RN* 31 (Aug. 1973); Agree, op. cit.

98. "S. 8274, Amending the Education Law In Relation to the Practice of Nursing." New York Senate–Assembly, Feb. 9, 1972 (passed in 1972).

99. Sadler et al., op. cit., 128.

100. Amendment to the Public Health and the Education Law, effective Apr. 1, 1972, State of New York.

101. "ANA Board Statement on the Role and Status of Diploma School Graduates." *Amer. J. Nursing* (July 1973); C. Kinsella, "Who Is the Clinical Nurse Specialist?" *Hospitals* 72–80 (1973); Bureau Health Manpower Education, *Extending the Scope of Nursing Practice* (Wash., D.C.: Dept. of HEW, PM 2); national changes may eventually be most significant for shaping these perspectives. For example, recent legislation has been proposed in Congress which would provide subsidies to schools of nursing and other organizations and institutions for the training of nurses "to develop training programs, and train nurse practitioners to serve as physician's assistants in extended care facilities." Physician's Assistant is defined as an individual who assists a physician in the performance of certain medical services in the absence of the physician and who is responsible for the medical care in an extended care facility under the continuous supervision of the physician (S. 2496, "Nurse Practitioners Training as Physician's Assistants," introduced Sept. 27, 1973).

102.

| | Changes in Nursing Practice Acts | | | |
	Arizona	Idaho	Washington	New York
Ratio per 100,000 population				
M.D.s	157	99	152	238
R.N.s	366	280	374	408
Physician support	n.a	Yes	No	No

Source: National Center for Health Statistics, *Health Resources Statistics 1971* (Washington, D.C.: Department of Health, Education, and Welfare, 1972).

103. The physician assistants have formed the American College of Physician Associates. Regarding the proliferation of professional status, see R.

Bucher and A. Strauss, "Professions in Process." *Amer. J. Soc.* 66:325–34 (Jan. 1961); F. Goldner and R. Ritti, "Professionalization as Career Immobility." *Amer. J. Sociol.* 72:489–502 (Mar. 1967); "Pediatric Nurse Practitioners Form ANA Council." *Amer. J. Nursing* 73:1972 (Nov. 1973).

104. For example, W. Hoff, "The Role of the Community Health Aide in Public Health Programs." *Public Health Rept.* 84:998–1002 (Nov. 1969); J. Steward and W. Hood, "Using Workers from 'Hard Core' Areas to Increase Immunization Levels." *Public Health Rept.* 85:177–85 (Feb. 1970); J. Frank, "The Bewildering World of Psychotherapy." *J. Soc. Issues* 28:27–46 (1972).

105. Professional Examination Service, *Guidelines for Training Entry Level Personnel: Performing Health Education Functions* for the Society of Professional Health Educators and Public Health Education Section, American Public Health Association (Washington, D.C.: APHA, 1973); "Alaskan Villages Receive Human Services." *HSMHA Health Rept.* 87:121–126 (Feb. 1972).

106. H. Greenfield with C. Brown, *Allied Health Manpower* (New York: Columbia University Press, 1969), 24–34; A. Gartner, "Health Systems and New Careers." *Health Serv. Rept.* 88:128–130 (Feb. 1973); E. Gilpatrick, *Suggestions for Job and Curriculum Ladders in Health Center Ambulatory Care: A Pilot Test* (New York: Research Foundation, City Univ. of New York, 1972), 1–5; "Inservice Training Program." Lincoln Community Mental Health Center Careers Escalation and Training Department, New York, Oct. 1970 (mimeo); Rosen, op. cit.

107. Hoff, op. cit.; Gartner, op. cit.; J. Otis, "Problems and Promise in the Use of Indigenous Personnel." *Welfare in Rev.* 3:12–19 (June 1965); Wise, op. cit.; S. Altman, *Present and Future Supply of Registered Nurses* (Washington, D.C.: Department of Health, Education, and Welfare, 1972), 13, 21; "Final Report of the Subcommittee on Allied Health Professions" (mimeo) Albert Einstein College Medicine, New York, Mar. 25, 1971, 24–27.

108. Ibid.; F. Stein, "New Careers in Family Planning." *Family Planning Perspectives* 1:42–44 (Oct. 1969); N. Hicks, "Health Care Workers Facing Job Uncertainty with Rapid Expansion of Training Programs," *New York Times*, 30 (Mar. 19, 1972); Gartner, op. cit.; Gilpatrick, op. cit.

109. Pennell, op. cit., 12–14; Study of Accreditation of Selected Health Educational Programs, op. cit., 5–13; W. Selden et al., "Health Occupations Credentialing: 3 Views." *Amer. Voc. J.* 48 (Feb. 1973).

110. Rosen, op. cit.; Egelston, op. cit.; Pennell, op. cit.; *Report on Licensure,* op. cit., 73–77.

111. Ibid.; R. Derbyshire, *Medical Licensure and Discipline in the United States* (Baltimore: Johns Hopkins Press, 1969); J. Hubbard, "Evaluation, Certification and Licensure in Medicine: New Directions." *J. Amer. Med.*

Assoc. 225:401–06 (July 23, 1973); M. Hornback, "Measuring Continuing Education." *Amer. J. Nursing* 73:1576–79 (Sept. 1973); W. McNerney, "Why Does Medical Care Cost So Much?" *N. Eng. J. Med.* 282:1459–65 (June 25, 1970).

112. R. Carlson, "Health Manpower Licensing and Emerging Institutional Responsibility for the Quality of Care." *Law and Contemporary Problems* 35:849–78 (Autumn 1970); N. Hershey, "An Alternative to Mandatory Licensure of Health Professionals." *Hospital Progr.* 50:71–74 (Mar. 1969); *Report on Licensure,* op. cit.

113. ANA House of Delegates resolution, *Amer. J. Nursing* 73:1761 (Oct. 1973); Ellwood, op. cit., 30.

114. *Report on Licensure,* op. cit.; Carlson, op. cit.

115. A. Somers, *Health Care in Transition* (Chicago: Hospital Research and Educational Trust, 1971); Council on Health Manpower, op. cit., 6; Agree, op. cit., 1761; *Amer. Nurse* (Oct. 1973).

116. E. Forgotson and R. Roemer, "Government Licensure and Voluntary Standards for Health Personnel and Facilities." *Med. Care* 6:345–54 (Sept.–Oct. 1968).

117. Ellwood, op. cit., 89, 90.

118. Similar proposals have been made for the reorganizing of Canada's health services (see "Report of the Community Health Center Project to the Conference of Health Ministers." *Can. Med. Assoc. J.* 107:362–384 (Aug. 19, 1972).

119. Selden, op. cit.; Ellwood, op. cit., 37.

120. Altman, op. cit., 21, 24; see also Scheffler and Stinson on physician assistants; "Manpower Crisis." *Lancet* 1501 (June 30, 1973).

121. Council on Allied Health Manpower, *Education and Utilization of Allied Health Manpower* (Chicago: American Medical Association, 1972); R. Scheffler, "The Relationship Between Medical Education and Statewide Per Capita Distribution of Physicians." *J. Med. Educ.* 46:995–998 (Nov. 1971); R. Kaplan and S. Leinhardt, "Determinants of Physician Office Location," 401–408 and H. Wechsler, "Choice of Practice Location." *Med. Care* 11:409–15 (Sept.–Oct. 1973).

122. U.S. Congress, H. R. 7724, "National Research Service Awards and Protection of Human Subjects Act of 1973"; *Lancet,* June 30, 1973, op. cit.

123. American Nurses Association, *Amer. Nurse,* Oct. 1973, p. 4; S. Wolfe and R. Badgley, "The Family Doctor 1960–2000 A.D." *Med. Care* 11:363–72 (Sept.–Oct. 1973); G. James, "Primary Care in the U.S.: Present Status and Future Prospects." *J. Internat. Health Serv.* (May 1972), 192.

124. *Med. Care Rev.* 1235 (Dec. 1972); R. Bergland, "Neurosurgery May Die." *N. Eng. J. Med.* 288:1043–46 (1973); an American College of Surgeons panel reported evidence of underemployment among U.S. surgeons (*Hospital Tribune* 7, Nov. 12, 1973).

125. *Lancet,* June 30, 1973, op. cit.

126. G. MacLeod and J. Pruissin, "The Continuing Evolution of HMO's." *N. Eng. J. Med.* 288:439–443 (Mar. 1, 1973); Sheps, op. cit., 56.

127. J. Millis, *A Rational Public Policy for Medical Education and Its Financing* (New York: National Fund for Medical Education, 1971); see also Carnegie Commission on Higher Education, *Higher Education and the Nation's Health* (New York: McGraw-Hill, 1970).

128. See "Comprehensive Health Manpower Training Act of 1971" and "Nurse Training Act of 1971," U.S. Congress; *Med. Care Rev.* 29:973–77 (Oct. 1972).

129. J. Scott, "Federal Support for Nursing Education—1965 to 1972." *Amer. J. Nursing* 72:1855–63 (Oct. 1972); H. Tilson, "Stability of Physician Employment in Neighborhood Health Centers." *Med. Care* 11:384–400 (Sept.–Oct. 1973); *1973 Survey of National Professional Health Association*, Apr. 1973).

130. See Guidelines for Title IX, Education Amendments of 1972, Affirmative Action Programs, Aug. 1972, for Civil Rights Act of 1964 (Office for Civil Rights, Department of Health, Education, and Welfare). About 1–2 per cent of medical school department heads are women (Lopate, op. cit., 23).

131. *Amer. J. Nursing* 72:1794 (Oct. 1972).

132. E. Weinberg and J. Rooney, "The Academic Performance of Women in Medical School." *J. Med. Educ.* 48: 240–47 (Mar. 1973); J. Buchanan, "Selection of Medical Students." *J. Amer. Med. Women's Assoc.* 24:555–60 (July 1972).

133. Council on Medical Education and Council on Health Manpower, *Physician Manpower and Medical Education* (Chicago: American Medical Association, 1971), 23.

134. J. Chapman, "A Common Denominator in the Equation Toward a Medical Education." *J. Amer. Med. Women's Assoc.* 24:561–65 (July 1969).

135. Councils on Medical Education and on Health Manpower, op. cit., 15, 24; this is in spite of the fact that a country such as India, which supplies the largest proportion of FMGs (17.4 per cent) to the United States, has stopped allowing the prerequisite FMG-certification examination to be given on its territory (*Annual Report, 1972,* Education Council for FMGs, Philadelphia).

136. E. Rosinski, "Education and Role of the Physician: A Redefinition." *J. Amer. Med. Assoc.* 222:473–75 (Oct. 23, 1972); S. Proger, "Doctor of Primary Medicine (PMD)." *J. Amer. Med. Assoc.* 220:410–11 (Apr. 19, 1972).

137. R. Magraw et al., "Perspectives from New Schools—The Costs and Financing of Medical Education." *N. Eng. J. Med.* 289:558–62 (Sept. 13, 1973), 562; Institution of Medicine, *Costs of Education of the Health Professions* (Washington, D.C.: National Academy of Science, 1973), 34.

138. D. Yett, "Causes and Consequences of Salary Differentials in Nursing." *Inquiry* 7:78–100 (Mar. 1970); D. Yett, "Lifetime Earnings for Nurses

in Comparison with College Trained Women." *Inquiry* 5:35–70 (Dec. 1968).

139. L. Hauser, "An Appraisal of Physician Manpower Projections." *Inquiry* 7:102–113 (Mar. 1970); "Physician Assistants: A Socioeconomic Report." *Calif. Med.* op. cit.

140. See R. Fein, *The Doctor Shortage: An Economic Diagnosis* (Washington, D.C.: The Brookings Institution, 1967); D. Stetten, "The Physician Shortage—Some of Its Consequences" in *Health Services Working Conference* (Rutherford, N.J.: Fairleigh Dickenson University, Jan. 1970), 41–54; Yankauer et al., Mar. 1970, op. cit., 280–282; A. Robbins, "Allied Health Manpower—Solution or Problem?" *N. Eng. J. Med.* 286:918–923 (Apr. 27, 1972); *Greater Medical Profession,* op. cit., 170–180.

141. H.R. 9341, "Public and Allied Health Personnel Act of 1973," Rep. Rogers.

142. Comprehensive Health Manpower Training Act of 1971; Nursing Training Act of 1971.

143. Wolfe and Badgley, op. cit., 372; Sadler et al., op. cit., 128; "Consultation on Multiprofessional Training of Health Personnel, Nov. 30 to Dec. 4, 1970" (mimeo) Geneva: World Health Organization, 1971); National Commission on Community Health Services, *Health Is a Community Affair* (Cambridge, Mass.: Harvard University Press, 1966) Chap. 12, Position J.

144. Among many examples are W. Kissick, "Health Manpower in Transition." *Milbank Mem. Fund Quart.* 46:53–90 (Jan. 1968); Western Interstate Commission for Higher Education, "Health Manpower: Adapting in the 70's: Education and Training" (prepared for the 1971 National Health Forum, San Francisco, Mar. 14–16, 1971); T. Ingles, "A Proposal for Health Care Education." *Amer. J. Nursing* 68 (Oct. 1968); T. Ingles and M. Montag, "Debate: Ladder Concept in Nursing Education." *Amer. J. Nursing* 71:726–30 (Nov. 1971); T. Ingles, "Mobility in Nursing." *Rhode Island Med. J.* 54:313–15 (June 1971); H. Silver and P. McAtee, "Health Care Practice: An Expanded Profession of Nursing for Men and Women." *Amer. J. Nursing* 72:78–80 (Jan. 1972); Gartner, op. cit.; "Nursing Education in the 70s." *Nursing Outlook* 20:271–2 (Apr. 1972); B. Dana and C. Sheps, "Trends and Issues in Interprofessional Education." *Educ. for Soc. Work* (Fall 1968); R. Kinsinger, "A Core Curriculum for the Health Field." *Nursing Outlook* 15:68 (Feb. 1967); R. Kramer, "A Core Curriculum Approach in Allied Health Education." *J. Practical Nursing* 23:26–33 (Oct. 1973); National Commission on Community Health Services, op. cit., 98; Carnegie Commission, op. cit.; *Institute of Medicine Educating for the Health Team: Report of a Conference October 1972* (Washington, D.C.: National Academy of Science, 1973).

145. *Greater Medical Profession,* op. cit., 193; Dana and Sheps, op. cit.; M. Rockoff, "Interactions Between Medical Students and Nursing Person-

nel." *J. Med. Educ.* 48:725–731 (1973); "Highlights of an Education Plan for a School for Health Professions. Working Document, August, 1973" (mimeo) (San Francisco: University of Pacific Medical Center, 1973); "A Design for Large Scale Training of Subprofessionals" (mimeo) (New York: New York University New Careers Training Laboratory, n.d.); D. Challenor et al., "An Educational Program for Allied Health Personnel." *Amer. J. Public Health* (Feb. 1972), 223. Joint training efforts are being made in the State University of New York and at the University of Illinois; see also "Core Concept in Allied Health." *J. Allied Health* 2 (Summer 1973), entire issue; F. Abdellah, "Nursing and Health Care in the USSR." *Amer. J. Nursing* 73:2096–99 (Dec. 1973).

146. Gilpatrick, op. cit.

147. "Highlights of an Educational Plan," op. cit.

148. See, for example, *Guidelines for Training Entry Level Personnel,* op. cit.; Kohnke, op. cit.; Department of Finance, State of California, op. cit.; *Interagency Conference on Nursing Statistics,* op. cit.

149. HEW, "Optimal Health Care for Mothers and Children: A Report of Five Conferences Held During 1967" (Washington, D.C.: National Institutes of Health, 1968).

150. Hubbard, op. cit.

151. J. Cooper, "USSR and US Health Policies." *N. Eng. J. Med.* 286:722–24 (Mar. 30, 1973).

152. National Center for Health Statistics, *International Comparison of Perinatal and Infant Mortality: U.S. and Six West European Countries* (Washington, D.C.: Department of Health, Education, and Welfare, 1967); Moriyama et al., *Infant Loss in The Netherlands* (Washington, D.C.: Department of Health, Education, and Welfare, 1968).

153. J. Orring, *School in Sweden* (Stockholm: Sö-forlaget, 1969). See also Chapters 3 and 5 of the text.

154. Israel has recently used new personnel patterns in the new immigrant towns [Y. Yodfat, "A New Method of Teamwork in Family Medicine in Israel with the Participation of Nurses as Physician's Assistants." *Amer. J. Public Health* 62:953–56 (July 1972)].

155. N. Milio, " 'Outcast' Clients and Human Services Workers: Questions of Access and Equity" (unpublished research report), Boston University, 1973.

156. V. Sidel, "Feldshers and 'Feldsherism'." *N. Eng. J. Med.* 278:934–39, 987–92 (Apr. 25 and May 2, 1968).

157. World Health Organization, "Report of the Travelling Seminar on Nursing in the USSR" (Geneva: WHO, 1970); E. Forgotson and J. Forgotson, "Innovations and Experiments in Uses of Health Manpower: A Study of Selected Programs and Problems in the U.K. and Soviet Union." *Med. Care* 8:3–14 (Jan.–Feb. 1970).

158. J. Muller et al., "The Soviet Health System—Aspects of Relevance for

Medicine in the United States." *N. Eng. J. Med.* 286:693–702 (Mar. 30, 1972).

159. National Swedish Board of Education, "Training of Auxiliary Nursing Personnel" (Stockholm, Nov. 1968); *Internat. Nursing Rev.* 20 (May–June 1973).

160. R. Roemer, "Legal Systems Regulating Health Personnel: A Comparative Analysis." *Milbank Mem. Fund Quart.* 46:431–71 (Oct. 1968); International Congress of Nurses, *National Reports of Member Associations 1969* (Basel: Karger, 1969).

161. British Information Service, *Health Services in Britain* (London: Her Majesty's Stationery Office, 1968), 47–51.

162. "Report of the Community Health Centers Project to the Conference of Health Ministers." *Can. Med. Assoc. J.* 107:361–378 (Aug. 19, 1972), 377–78.

163. "Hospital Service Enquiry into the Deployment of Nursing and Midwifery Staff" (London: Department of Health and Social Security, 1966).

164. P. Hawthorne, *The Nurse Working with the General Practitioner—An Evaluation of Research and a Review of the Literature* (London: Department of Health and Social Security, July 1971); "Use of Ancillary Help in the Local Authority Nursing Services" (unpublished memo) (London: Department of Health and Social Security, Sept. 3, 1968).

165. *Greater Medical Profession,* op. cit., 184–88.

166. *Evidence to the Commission on Nursing (Briggs) by the Council for the Training of Health Visitors* (London: CTHV, Dec. 1970), 63.

167. *Greater Medical Profession,* op. cit., 192; *Internat. Nursing Rev.* 20 (May–June 1973).

168. *Greater Medical Profession,* op. cit., 148, 193.

169. International Council of Nurses, op. cit.; Great Britain Review Body on Doctors' and Dentists' Remuneration, *Twelfth Report* (London: Her Majesty's Stationery Office, 1970).

170. R. Klein, "The Political Economy of National Health," in Congressional Research Service, *Resolved: That the Federal Government Should Enact a Program of Comprehensive Medical Care for All United States Citizens* (Washington, D.C.: Government Printing Office, 1972), 377–388.

171. *Internat. Nursing Rev.* 20:69 (Sept.–Oct. 1973).

172. *International Nursing Review* 20:99 (Sept.–Oct. 1973); *International Nursing Review* 20 (May–June 1973); *International Nursing Review* 20:133, op. cit.; "Consultation on Multi-professional Training of Health Personnel," op. cit.; "Some Education and Training Activities Carried Out by WHO during the International Education Year, 1970" (Geneva: World Health Organization, Aug. 1970), 3; "Organizational Study of Methods of Promoting the Development of Basic Health Services: Report of the Working Group" (Geneva: World Health Organization, Jan. 16, 1973), 4.

173. W. Latham, *Community Medicine* (Bangkok, 1969).

174. B. Abel-Smith et al., "Can We Reduce the Cost of Medical Education?" *WHO Chronicle* 29:441–50 (Oct. 1972); C. Taylor, "Training Health Auxiliaries." East-West Center for Cultural and Technical Interchange, Conference on Public Health Training in Asian Countries, Honolulu, June 22, 1965 (mimeo); D. Shrivastar, "Nursing Around the World: India." *Internat. Nursing Rev.* 19:308 (1972).

175. WHO Medical School Survey, *World Health* (Nov. 1971).

176. Abel-Smith, op. cit.

177. Bryant, op. cit., 201; Abel-Smith, op. cit.; *The Use and Training of Auxiliary Personnel in Medicine, Nursing, Midwifery, and Sanitation* (Geneva: World Health Organization, 1961).

178. R. Fendall, *Auxiliaries in Health Care: Programs in Developing Countries* (Baltimore, Md.: Johns Hopkins Press, 1972), 44–47; P. Pene, "Health Auxiliaries in Francophone Africa." *Lancet* 1047–48 (May 12, 1973); F. Rosa, "Impact of New Family Planning Approaches on Rural Maternal and Child Health Coverage in Developing Countries: India's Example." *Amer. J. Public Health* 57:1327–32 (Aug. 1967); Bryant, op. cit., 248.

179. C. Flato, "China's Health Care." *Nation's Health* (Oct.–Nov. 1972); see also V. Sidel, "The Barefoot Doctors of the People's Republic of China." *N. Eng. J. Med.* 1292–1300 (June 15, 1972); J. Quinn (ed.), *Medicine and Public Health in the People's Republic of China* (Washington, D.C.: Department of Health, Education, and Welfare, 1972), Publ. NIH 72–67; "A Bibliography of Chinese Sources on Medicine and Public Health in the People's Republic of China: 1960–70" (Washington, D.C.: Department of Health, Education, and Welfare, 1973), Publ. NIH 73–439.

Images of Access iv, v

1. Based on a field visit to Mahsudpur with Miss Chahil, Rural Community Extension Program, Lady Irwin College, Feb. 21, 1971, and interviews with Dr. A. Lakshmy, Chairwoman, Child Development Program, Lady Irwin College, University of Delhi, Feb. 12, 1971; Dr. C. Nayar, Indian Council for Child Welfare, New Delhi, Feb. 23, 1971; Mrs. V. T. Lakshmi, Supervisor, Madras State Child Welfare Council Bala Sevika Training Centre, Madras, Mar. 25, 1971; Dr. G. Joseph, Head, Department of Preventive and Social Medicine, All-India Institute of Medical Science, New Delhi, Feb. 4, 1971. For well-documented studies of these programs, see A. Berg, *The Nutrition Factor: Its Role in National Development* (Washington, D.C.: The Brookings Institution, 1973).

2. Based on a field visit to Soíjin Community Center, and interviews with the Director and the Supervisor of the *hobo-san;* with Mrs. Kojima, Superintendent of the Kyoto City Child Welfare Section, and Miss

Umeoka, translator, June 9, 1971, Kyoto; also, Mr. Yamaguchi, head of the Foreign Affairs Department, Kyoto City Government, June 5, 1971, and written reports from the national Ministry of Health and Welfare, Children and Families Bureau; discussions with Dr. Nakazawa and Shirata-san, Director of Nursing, Kyoto City Department of Health, May 5 and June 12; Seiwa College President Miss Yamakawa, and Miss Sakai, head of the Early Childhood Development Program, June 22, Nishinomiya; and Dr. Suzuki, Childrens and Families Bureau, Ministry of Health and Welfare, Tokoyo, May 11, 1971; at the University of Tokyo, School of Health Sciences, Miss Shigeko Hayashi, Dr. H.Sc., May 6, 21; and Dr. Tadao Miyasaka, Chairman, Department of Health Sociology, May 24.

Chapter 8—Making and Implementing Decisions

1. N. Milio, "Health Care Organizations and Innovation." *J. Health Soc. Behav.* 12:163–173 (June 1971).
2. Congressional Quarterly Service, *Legislators and the Lobbyists* (Washington, D.C., 1965); see also A. Carr-Saunders and P. Wilson, "The Rise and Aims of Professional Associations" in *The Professions* (Oxford: Clarendon Press, 1933), 298–304; E. Rayack, *Professional Power and American Medicine* (New York: World, 1967).
3. V. Navarro, "National Health Insurance and the Strategy for Change" (unpublished paper). Johns Hopkins University, School of Hygiene and Public Health, Nov. 1972; see also Chapters 4 and 5 of the text.
4. S. Wolfe and R. Badgley, "The Family Doctor 1960 to 2000 A.D." *Med. Care* 11:363–72 (Sept.–Oct. 1973); Common Cause data, reported by Associated Press, Sept. 1973, *Boston Globe*.
5. For example, AMA's AMPAC; the Committee for National Health Security; the new ANA political arm [*Amer. J. Nursing* 73:1849 (Nov. 1973)]; the Coalition for Human Needs and Budget Priorities.
6. The Editors, "The American Medical Association: Power, Purpose and Politics in Organized Medicine." *The Yale Law Journal* 63:938–47 (May 1954); see also R. Steven, *American Medicine and the Public Interest* (New Haven: Yale University Press, 1971); J. and B. Ehrenreich, *The American Health Empire: Power, Profits, and Politics* (New York: Random House, 1970).
7. B. Myers, "Health Services Research and Health Policy Interactions." *Med. Care* 11:352–58 (July–Aug. 1973); see also W. Williams, *Social Policy Research and Analysis* (New York: American Elsevier, 1971); A. Rivlin, *Systematic Thinking for Social Action* (Washington, D.C.: The Brookings Institution, 1970).
8. E. Krause, "Health and the Politics of Technology." *Inquiry* 8:51–59 (Sept. 1971); see also S. Strickland, *Politics, Science and Dread Disease*

(Cambridge, Mass.: Harvard University Press, 1972); R. Elling, "The Shifting Power Structure in Health." *Milbank Mem. Fund Quart.* 46: 119–43 (Jan. 1968); A Chase, *The Biological Imperatives: Health, Politics, and Survival* (New York: Holt, Rinehart and Winston, 1971), 70, 71.

9. Hospital Research and Educational Trust, *Annual Report 1972* (Chicago: American Hospital Assoc. 1973), 1–2; see also Chapter 4 of the text.

10. M. Pitel and J. Vian, "Private Philanthropy and Nursing Research." *Nursing Res. Rept.* 8:1 (Oct. 1973); E. Flook and P. Sanazaro, *Health Services Research and R&D in Perspective* (Ann Arbor: Health Admin. Press, Univ. of Mich. 1973) 82–108.

11. *Health Planning Memorandum* 48 (Aug. 16, 1973).

12. H. Somers and A. Somers, *Medicare and the Hospitals* (Washington, D.C.: The Brookings Institution, 1967), 87; *AMA Legislative Roundup* 14 (Oct. 12, 1973), regarding regulations for skilled nursing facilities under the Social Security Amendments of 1972; ibid., Nov. 9, 1973, regarding definition of Professional Standards Review Organizations (PSROs). See also text later in this chapter.

13. Hearings on S. 3716, "Health Facilities, Manpower, and Community Mental Health Center Act of 1972," Rept. 92–1064, U.S. Senate Committee on Labor and Public Welfare (Aug. 16, 1972); *Med. Care Rev.* 29:973–77 (Oct. 1972).

14. *Drug Res. Rept.* (Sept. 30, 1972); *Washington Report on Medicine and Health* (Oct. 6, 1972); see also Carnegie Commission on Higher Education, *Higher Education and the Nation's Health,* Oct. 1970.

15. W. Pearse, "The Maternal and Infant Program." *Obstetrics and Gynecology* 35:114–119 (Jan. 1970); see also J. Wysong and R. Eichhorn, "The Health Services Complex: Inter-agency Relations in the Delivery of Health Services," in R. Elling (ed.), *National Health Care* (Chicago: Aldine, 1971), 229–44.

16. Comptroller General of the United States, *Study of Health Facilities Construction Costs* (Washington, D.C.: Government Printing Office, 1972), 857, 862, and many other examples.

17. Milio, op. cit.

18. See also Social Security Administration, *The Size and Shape of the Medical Care Dollar: Chartbook/1972* (Washington, D.C.: Government Printing Office, 1973).

19. I. S. Falk, "Medical Care in the U.S.A., 1932–72." *Health and Society* issue of *Milbank Mem. Fund Quart.* 51:1–40 (Winter 1973); B. Bullough, "The Medicare–Medicaid Amendments." *Amer. J. Nursing* 73: 1826–29 (Nov. 1973); see Sec. 1801, Social Security Amendments Act of 1965.

20. "A Survey of CHP Councils and Their Relation to Local United Funds" (unpublished) (Richmond, Va.: United Givers Fund, Apr. 30, 1970); "Funding Sources of Selected CHP Agencies," Nov. 5, 1970, and "Survey

of Funding Sources, 108 CHPs," Community Health, Inc. (memo), Mar. 1971; *Health Is a Community Affair—Revisited* (prepublication draft) (New York: Community Health, Inc., Sept. 1973).

21. Comptroller General of the United States, op. cit., 867–880.

22. W. Curran, *National Survey and Analysis of Certificate-of-Need Laws: Health Planning and Regulation in State Legislatures 1972* (Chicago: American Hospital Association, 1973); W. Curran, "Certificate of Need Legislation." *Amer. J. Public Health* 62:1549 (Nov. 1972).

23. Comptroller General of the United States, op. cit.; Curran, AHA, 1973, op. cit.

24. Ibid.

25. Ibid.

26. L. Olson and J. Daley, "Comprehensive Health Planning: The Drift Toward Federal Control." *Health Planning Memorandum* 10 (June 1973).

27. W. Curran, "A Severe Blow to Hospital Planning. 'Certification-of-Need' Declared Unconstitutional." *N. Eng. J. Med.* 288:723–4 (Apr. 5, 1973). The state was North Carolina.

28. Curran, AHA, 1973, op. cit.

29. R. Van Hoek, "Health Care and the Role of Health Services Research," 1973 Michael Davis Lecture (Chicago: University of Chicago Center for Health Administration Studies, 1973).

30. Comptroller General of the United States, op. cit., 869.

31. Olson and Daley, op. cit.; "Analysis of Guidelines for Improvement of Certificate-of-Need for Health Care Facilities and Services and Model Legislation" (mimeo) (Chicago: American Hospital Association, Nov. 1972).

32. *Health Planning Memorandum,* Oct. 12, 1973.

33. Curran, AHA, 1973, op. cit.

34. O'Donoghue, op. cit., 79.

35. C. Havighurst, "Government's Increasing Involvement in the Health Care Sector: The Hazards of Regulation and Less Hazardous Alternatives" (prospectus; mimeo, for National Health Forum, Mar. 20, 1973) and "Health Maintenance Organizations and the Market for Health Services" (mimeo) (Minneapolis: Institute for Interdisciplinary Studies, Health Services Research Center, Sept. 1971).

36. P. Ellwood et al., *Assuring the Quality of Health Care* (Minneapolis: InterStudy, 1973), 85. See also A. Wolfson and P. P. Wolfson, "The Food and Drug Administration and the Pill." *Social Policy* 52–56 (Sept.–Oct. 1970); J. Turner, *The Chemical Feast* (New York: Grossman, 1970); J. Esposito, *Vanishing Air* (New York: Grossman, 1970).

37. Ellwood, op. cit., 29–33.

38. Social Security Administration, *Hospital Utilization Review and Medicare: A Survey* (Washington, D.C.: Department of Health, Education,

and Welfare, Apr. 1971), Staff Paper 8; Comptroller General of the United States, op. cit., 827–29.

39. *Report of the U.S. Senate Committee on Finance,* No. 92-1230, Sept. 26, 1972, 254–69; Social Security Administration, op. cit.; Ellwood, op. cit.

40. *Report of the U.S. Senate Committee on Finance,* No. 92-1230, op. cit.

41. Ellwood, op. cit.

42. *Report of the U.S. Senate Committee on Finance,* op. cit.

43. "Health Components of H.R. 1." *Perspective* (Fourth Quarter 1972).

44. 92nd Congress, Social Security Amendments of 1972 (P.L. 92-603), Sec. 249F.

45. R. Egdahl, "Foundations for Medical Care." *N. Eng. J. Med.* 288:491–99 (Mar. 8, 1973), see also Chapter 4 of the text, and Flook and Sanazaro, op. cit., 150–184.

46. P. Sanazaro et al., "Research and Development in Quality Assurance." *N. Eng. J. Med.* 287:1125–31 (Nov. 30, 1972).

47. Myers, op. cit.

48. *U.S. Congressional Record* 118:S 1611–12.

49. The AMA initially introduced the PSRO as a statutory measure in its first Medicredit (national health insurance) bill, 1970; it called for Professional Review Organizations, statewide and equivalent to medical societies; this was dropped in its 1972 bill. The concept was picked up by Sen. Bennett (Utah) and became part of the Nixon Administration NHI bill, 1970–1971 [Association of American Physicians and Surgeons, *Newsletter* 27 (Feb. 1973)]; U.S. Joint House–Senate Conference Report, No. 92-1605, Oct. 14, 1972, pp. 19–20; Navarro, op. cit.; H.R. 4960, "Medicredit," AMA-sponsored bill, 1971.

50. *AMA Legislative Round-up* 14 (Nov. 9, 1973); AMA resolution reported in *Amer. J. Nursing* 73 (Sept., 1973).

51. *AMA News,* July 1973.

52. Van Hoek, op. cit.; Havighurst, op. cit.

53. American Hospital Association, *A Quality Assurance Program for Medical Care in Hospitals* (Chicago: AHA, 1972).

54. Egdahl, op. cit.; see also Chapter 4 of the text.

55. Health Insurance Council, "Professional Standards Review Organizations —The Role of the Private Sector: The Insurance Industry's Perspective." *Viewpoint* (July 1973).

56. Ibid.

57. Ibid.

58. *Health Planning Memorandum* 48 (Aug. 16, 1973).

59. *Health Planning Memorandum* 48 (Oct. 12, 1973).

60. Part of the proposed 1973 revision of the Public Health Service Act by the House Subcommittee on Public Health and Environment; and of an

HEW "Forward Plan for Fiscal 1975," Office of the Secretary, July 1973 [*Health Planning Memorandum* 48 (Oct. 12, 1973)].

61. Ibid.

62. Hearings Before the House Subcommittee on Public Health and the Environment "Health Maintenance Organizations—1973," Rept. 93-26, Mar. 6–7, 1973. See testimony by the Association of American Physicians and Surgeons; American Council of Medical Staffs, 258–361; "HMOs: A Growing Threat to Local Pharmacists." *Drug Topics* (July 3, 1972)—see also "Controlling Drug Costs." *Amer. J. Public Health* 62:755–56 (June 1972); M. Mintz, *By Prescription Only* (Boston: Houghton Mifflin, 1967).

63. House Hearings, Mar. 1973, op. cit., see testimony by the American Association of Dental Schools, American Society for Medical Technology, National League for Nursing, 341–61.

64. Ibid., see testimony by the American Association of Medical Colleges, or Association of University Programs in Hospital Administration, 362–64.

65. Ibid., see National Association of Insurance Commissioners testimony.

66. Ibid., see testimony of the Nixon Administration, 80–84, and of the Group Health Association of America; *Health Planning Memorandum* 48 (Aug. 16, 1973); "Health Maintenance Organizations," *U.S. Congressional Record,* Senate, Sen. Kennedy, Aug. 8, 1972; the AMA took credit for the change of position on HMOs by the Nixon Administration. The AMA claimed that its lobbying efforts were responsible for the change (*Amer. Med. News,* Nov. 19, 1973).

67. N. Hicks, "Insurers' Role Grows in Medical Plans." *New York Times* 31 (July 14, 1973); S. Kalman, "Toward the Political Economy of Medical Care." *Inquiry* 8:30–38 (Sept. 1971). For background see D. Clark, "A Cameo Study of Policy in the Health Services in the 1930's," in Flook and Sanazaro, op. cit., 109–125.

68. H.R. 2222, "Health Care Insurance Act of 1973" (Medicredit), Rep. Fulton; also S. 444, Sen. Hartke.

69. H.R. 1, "National Health Care Services Reorganization and Financing Act," Rep. Ullman.

70. H.R. 5200, "National Healthcare Act of 1973," Rep. Burleson; also S. 1100, Sen. McIntyre.

71. H.R. 22, "Health Security Act," Rep. Griffiths; also S. 3, Sen. Kennedy.

72. Personal communication, National Health Council official, May 1973.

73. Committee for Economic Development includes the wealthiest manufacturing corporations (automobile, communications equipment, oil, and steel) and the wealthiest (ranked by assets) of the financial corporations, having four of the top six: Prudential, Metropolitan, Equitable, and Aetna [see *Fortune* magazine (June and October 1973)].

74. Committee for Economic Development, *Building a National Health Care System* (New York: CED, 1973).

75. For example, The Committee for National Health Insurance, Washington, D.C.

76. G. Hodgson, "The Politics of American Health Care." *Atlantic Monthly* 232:45–61 (Oct. 1973); "Life, Death, and Medicine." *Scientific American* 229 (Sept. 1973), 160–66. For the potential benefit of insurance coverage of prescribed drugs, see also Social Security Administration, "Medical Insurance Sample: Prescription Drugs, 1967–71." *Health Insur. Stat.* (Oct. 12, 1973).

77. Legislation was under the Economic Opportunity Act in 1965; maternal–child funds under Social Security Amendments of 1963 and 1965; Model Cities and comprehensive health planning programs also provided funds. See N. Milio, "Dimensions of Consumer Participation and National Health Legislation." Fred T. Foard, Jr., Memorial Lecture, University of North Carolina School of Public Health, Chapel Hill, Apr. 16, 1973, *Amer. J. Public Health* (forthcoming); also R. Ulrich, "Tribal Community Health Representatives of the Indian Health Service." *Public Health Rept.* 84:11 (Nov. 1969); L. Reeder, "The Patient-Client As a Consumer: Some Observations on the Changing Professional–Client Relationship." *J. Health Soc. Behav.* 13:406–12 (Dec. 1972).

78. A. Colin and Waitzkin, "Prepaid Health Care: A Critique of Harvard's New Plan" (unpublished study). Harvard Medical School and Department of Sociology, 1971; Krause, op. cit.

79. Sheps, op. cit., 47–48.

80. These were comprehensive health planning funds, PL 89-749, Sec. 314(e), under which neighborhood health centers and HMOs were funded. Colin, op. cit.; Hicks, op. cit.; P. O'Donaghue et al., *A Descriptive Analysis of CHP "B" Agencies* (Minnesota: InterStudy: Feb. 1973); Milio, *J. Health Soc. Behav.*, op. cit.

81. L. Bellin et al., "Phase One of Consumer Participation in Policies of 22 Voluntary Hospitals in New York City." *Amer. J. Public Health* 62: 1370–75 (Oct. 1972).

82. Ibid.

83. Sheps, op. cit., 56.

84. *Study to Evaluate the OEO Neighborhood Health Center Program at Selected Centers, Final Report* (Washington, D.C.: Office of Economic Opportunity, Jan. 1972).

85. H. Tilson, "Stability of Physician Employment in Neighborhood Health Centers." *Med. Care* 11:384–400 (Sept.–Oct. 1973).

86. G. Gordon and S. Marquis, "Freedom, Visibility of Consequences, and Scientific Innovation." *Amer. J. Sociol.* 72:195–202 (Sept. 1966); N. Milio, *9226 Kercheval: The Storefront That Did Not Burn* (Ann Arbor, Mich.: University of Michigan Press, 1970).

87. *Amer. J. Nursing* 73:1867 (Nov. 1973); see also Chapter 6 of the text.

88. R. Bradbury, "A CHP Board of Directors." *Health Serv. Rept.* 87:905–908 (Dec. 1972); Sheps, op. cit., 50.

89. Bellin, op. cit.; Colin and Waitzkin, op. cit.

90. A Stokes et al., "The Columbia Point Health Association: Evolution of a Community Health Board." *Amer. J. Public Health* 62:1229–34 (Sept. 1972); J. Gordon, "Politics of Community Medicine Projects: A Conflict Analysis." *Med. Care* 7:419–28 (Nov.–Dec. 1969); E. Feingold, "A Political-Scientist's View of Neighborhood Health Centers As a New Social Institution." *Med. Care* 8:108 (Mar.–Apr. 1970).

91. Stokes, op. cit.; see also J. and B. Ehrenreich, *The American Health Empire* (New York: Random House, 1971).

92. *Health Law Newsletter* 31 (Nov. 1973).

93. O'Donaghue et al., 9; K. Parkum and V. Parkum, *Voluntary Participation in Health Planning* (Philadelphia: Pennsylvania Department of Health, Nov. 1973).

94. Ibid., 77–84.

95. New York City, *Health Planning Memorandum* 48 (Aug. 16, 1973).

96. "HIACA Revisited" (New York: Community Health, Inc., Aug. 1973); M. Creditor and D. Nelson, "Regional Medical Programs and the Office of Management and Budget." *N. Eng. J. Med.* 289:239–42 (Aug. 2, 1973).

97. D. Gossert and A. Miller, "State Boards of Health, Their Members and Commitments." *Amer. J. Public Health* 63:486–93 (June 1973).

98. P.L. 92-603, Sec. 249F, op. cit.

99. Health Insurance Council, op. cit.; *Health Planning Memorandum* 48 (Aug. 16, 1973); *Amer. J. Nursing* 73 (Oct. 1973).

100. *Health Law Newsletter* 25 (May 1973).

101. *Health Planning Memorandum* 44 (Apr. 25, 1973); Industrial Health and Safety Group, *Survival Kit* (Cambridge, Mass.: IHSG, 1973).

102. For examples of what happens to patients in circumstances where others limit their choices, see E. Goffman, *Asylums* (New York: Doubleday, 1961); R. D. Laing, *The Politics of Experience* (New York: Ballantine Books, 1967); T. Szasz, *The Manufacture of Madness* (New York: Harper & Row, 1970); R. Duff and A. B. Hollingshead, *Sickness and Society* (New York: Harper & Row, 1968).

103. A. Guttmacher, "Family Planning Need and the Future of the Family Planning Program." *Family Planning Perspectives* 5:175–76 (Summer 1973); J. Eliot, "Fertility Control and Coercion." Ibid., 132.

104. S. Levit, "Sterilization Associated with Induced Abortion: JPSA Findings." Ibid., 177–82; H. Rodman, Merrill–Palmer Institute, Detroit, in *Boston Globe* 21 (Aug. 19, 1973).

105. For example, in the Hearings on HMOs, 1973, op. cit., psychiatric professionals testified: "If given a choice, the consumer might pick a program of dental or drug benefits rather than mental health benefits. This does not indicate that the introduction of the consumer in shaping health care systems is a bad thing. Unfortunately, however, the consumer has

seldom been an effective force in improving our system of mental health services. Most people deny the possibility that they may develop a mental illness. And many who have experienced a psychiatric difficulty fail to speak out in favor of mental health benefits because of guilt and shame."

106. S. Strickland, *U.S. Health Care: What's Wrong and What's Right* (New York: Universe Books, 1971).

107. M. Olendzki, "Concerns of the Consumer" Paper, Conference on Redesigning Nursing Education for Public Health, Washington, D.C., May 22–25, 1973, Division of Nursing, Health, Education, and Welfare, National Center for Family Planning Services, "Non-physician Professionals Being Trained to Provide Family Planning Care." *Family Planning Digest* 2:1–6 (July 1973).

108. Olendzki, op. cit.

109. L. Harris, "American Favor 'Right to Die.' " *Boston Globe* 25 (Apr. 23, 1973).

110. For example, "Patient's Bill of Rights" (Chicago: American Hospital Association); H. Denenberg, "Citizens Bill of Hospital Rights" (Harrisburg, Pa.: Pennsylvania State Insurance Department, Apr. 1973).

111. W. Gaylin, "The Patient's Bill of Rights." *Saturday Rev.* 1:22 (Mar. 1973).

112. "Informed Consent Litigation." *APHA Med. Care Sec. Newsletter* 2 (Oct. 18, 1973); *Health Law News* 28 (Aug. 1973).

113. Rep. J. Symington, H.R. 11339, 92nd Congress. *PMA Newsletter* (Nov. 9, 1973).

114. S. 2360, 92nd Congress. *Legis. Roundup* 14 (Oct. 26, 1973).

115. *PMA Newsletter*, Nov. 16, 1973.

116. B. Shenkin and D. Warner, "Giving the Patient His Medical Record: A Proposal to Improve the System." *N. Eng. J. Med.* 289:688–92 (Sept. 27, 1973).

117. D. Hussar, "Drug Interactions." *Amer. J. Pharm.* 65–111 (May–June 1973).

118. Rodman, op. cit.

119. For example, from the Pennsylvania Insurance Department, Harrisburg, Pa.: "A Shoppers Guide to Surgery: 14 Rules on How To Avoid Unnecessary Surgery" (July 1972); "A Shoppers Guide to Dentistry" (Feb. 1973); "A Shoppers Guide to Hospitals in the Philadelphia Area" (Nov. 1971). Paperback books include *Go To Health* (New York: Dell, 1972); A. Frank and S. Frank, *The People's Handbook of Medical Care* (New York: Random House, 1973); M. Samuels and H. Bennett, *The Well Baby Book* (New York: Random House, 1973); T. McGuire, *The Tooth Trip* (New York: Random House, 1972); Boston–Cambridge Women's Book Collective, *Our Bodies, Our Selves* (New York: Simon and Schuster, 1973); R. Fisher and G. Christie, *A Dictionary of Drugs: The Medicines You Use* (New York: Schoken Books, 1972); ℞: *Consumers*

Guide to Prescription Prices (Syracuse, N.Y.: Consumer Age Press, 1973). See also H. Lewis and M. Lewis, *The Medical Offenders* (New York: Simon and Schuster, 1970).

120. E. Freidson (ed.), *The Hospital in Modern Society* (London: Collier-Macmillan Ltd., 1963); R. Bucher and J. Stelling, "Characteristics of Professional Organizations." *J. Health Human Behav.* 10:3–15 (Mar. 1969).

121. C. Perrow, "Hospitals, Technology, Structure, and Goals" in *Handbook of Modern Sociology* (Chicago: Rand McNally, 1964), 910–71.

122. M. Goodfellow, "Checklist on Susceptibility to Union: How Organizer Rates Your Hospital." *Hospital Topics* (Jan. 1973).

123. Council of Teaching Hospitals, *COTH Survey of House Staff Policy 1973* (Washington, D.C.: Association of American Medical Colleges, 1973).

124. AMA resolution, reported in *Amer. J. Nursing* 73:1614 (Sept. 1973).

125. Women's Bureau, *Child Care Services Provided by Hospitals* (Washington, D.C.: Department of Labor, 1970).

126. *Amer. J. Nursing* 73:1671 (Sept. 1973); B. Schutt, "Collective Action for Professional Security." *Amer. J. Nursing* 73:1946–51 (Nov. 1973); Goodfellow, op. cit.

127. Schutt, op. cit.; and, for example, "Agreement Between the Drug and Hospital Union, AFL-CIO, and the Albert Einstein College of Medicine of Yeshiva University, July 1, 1970 to June 30, 1972," Bronx, N.Y.

128. For another example, see R. Badgley and S. Wolfe, *Doctors' Strike: Medical Care and Conflict in Saskatchewan* (New York: Atherton Press, 1967).

129. K. Parkum, *Consumer Participation in Denmark's Health Insurance System: A Study of the Danish Sygekasse* (Harrisburg, Pa.: Pennsylvania Department of Health, 1972); E. Johnson, "Modern Implementation of Denmark's Tradition of Health Care Delivery." *Health Serv. Rept.* 88: 624–31 (Aug.–Sept. 1973).

130. B. Shenkin, "Politics and Medical Care in Sweden: The 7 Crowns Reform." *N. Eng. J. Med.* 288:555–59 (Mar. 15, 1973); The Swedish Institute, "Organization of Medical Care in Sweden" (Stockholm: The Institute, Dec. 1971).

131. "The National Health Service." *Med. Care Rev.* 29:1041–47 (Oct. 1972); R. Battistella and T. Chester, "The 1974 Reorganization of the British National Health Service—Aims and Issues." *N. Eng. J. Med.* 289:610–15 (Sept. 20, 1973).

132. J. Lister, "Reorganization of the NHS 1974—For Better or for Worse?" *N. Eng. J. Med.* 672–74 (Mar. 29, 1973).

133. For examples of this, see J. Christoph, "Great Britain: Advent of the National Health Service," in J. Christoph (ed.), *Cases in Comparative Politics* (Boston: Little, Brown, 1965), 3–43; G. Maddox, "Muddling Through: Planning for Health Care in England." *Med. Care* 9:439–448

(Sept.–Oct. 1971); D. Mechanic and R. Faich, "Doctors in Revolt: The Crisis in the English National Health Service." *Med. Care* 8 (Nov.–Dec. 1970); R. Klein, "The Political Economy of National Health," in Congressional Research Service, *Resolved: That the Federal Government Should Enact a Program of Comprehensive Medical Care for All United States Citizens* (Washington, D.C.: Government Printing Office, 1972), 377–88; R. Badgley et al., "Medical Power in Health Manpower Planning" World Congress of Sociology, 1970, Varna, Bulgaria (mimeo); W. Steslicke, "The Japan Medical Association and the Liberal Democratic Party: A Case Study of Interest Group Politics in Japan," *Studies on Asia.* 1965, 143–61.

134. Battistella and Chester, op. cit.; M. Joselow, "Occupational Health in the U.S.—The Next Decades." *Amer. J. Public Health* 63:929–30 (Nov. 1973).

135. Department of Health and Social Security, *Annual Report 1972* (London: Her Majesty's Stationery Office, 1973); Johnson, op. cit.; see also Chapter 7 of the text.

136. "Hospital Workers and Pay Policy." *Lancet* 730–31 (Mar. 31, 1973). Certain types of unionizing can lead to divisiveness, see J. Ben-David, "Professionals and Unions in Israel," in E. Friedson and J. Lorber (eds.), *Medical Men and Their Work* (Chicago: Aldine, 1972), 20–38.

137. "Organizational Study on Methods of Promoting the Development of Basic Health Services: Report of the Working Group" (Geneva: World Health Organization, Jan. 16, 1973).

138. Reported in *Lancet,* 730 (Mar. 31, 1973).

139. Johnson, op. cit.

140. Editorial *Can. Med. Assoc. J.* 108:1349 (June 2, 1973).

141. Shenkin, op. cit.; see Image of Access, iii in the text.

Chapter 9—Evaluating Health Care

1. P. Ellwood et al., *Assuring the Quality of Health Care* (Minneapolis: InterStudy, 1973). For an extensive summary of research, see E. Flook and P. Sanazaro, *Health Services Research and R&D in Perspective* (Ann Arbor: Health Admin. Press, Univ. Mich., 1973).

2. Ibid.; P. Sanazaro, "Research and Development in Quality Assurance." *N. Eng. J. Med.* 287:1125–31 (Nov. 30, 1972).

3. *Evaluation* 1:69 (Feb. 1973).

4. Social Security Administration, "Medicare: Inpatient Hospital Services by Region, 1967 and 1968." *Health Insur. Stat.* (May 30, 1973).

5. Social Security Administration, "Utilization and Reimbursements Under Medicare for Persons Who Died in 1967 and 1968." *Health Insur. Stat.* 51 (Oct. 17, 1973).

6. Social Security Administration, *Medicare: Health Insurance for the Aged 1971, Sec. 2: Enrollment* (Washington, D.C.: Government Printing Office, 1973), Table L.

7. "Witnesses Cite Continued Discrimination by Hospitals Against Medicare Recipients." *Nation's Health* (Oct. 1973).

8. Social Security Administration, *Medicare: Health Insurance for the Aged, 1969: Length of Stay by Diagnosis* (Washington, D.C.: Government Printing Office, 1973), Table A.

9. This was in spite of federal price controls imposed in August 1971. Social Security Administration, "Health Insurance for the Aged: Monthly Reimbursements per Person by State: 1971." *Health Insur. Stat.* 52 (Dec. 5, 1973).

10. U.S. Senate Special Committee on Aging, *Home Health Services in the United States, Current Status* (Washington, D.C.: Government Printing Office, July 1973), 54.

11. "The Cost of Standard Medical Services Under Alternative Delivery Systems" (Washington, D.C.: Department of Health, Education, and Welfare, Oct. 1972).

12. S. Berki, "The Economics of New Types of Health Personnel." Macy Conference on Intermediate-Level Health Personnel, Williamsburg, Va., Nov. 12–14, 1972 (mimeo).

13. House Committee on Ways and Means, "Cost Study of Health Insurance Proposals Introduced in the 92nd Congress," in Congressional Service, op. cit., 183–92; I. S. Falk, "Costs of National Health Security and Their Financing." Prepared for the Commission for National Health Insurance, Washington, D.C., Sept. 1971.

14. Ellwood, op. cit., 33–34; H. Freeman, "Outcome Measures and Social Action Experiments: An Immodest Proposal for Redirecting Research Efforts." *Amer. Sociol.* 17–19 (Nov. 1972).

15. Ellwood, op. cit.; A. Twaddle and R. Sweet, "Factors Leading to Preventable Hospital Admissions." *Med. Care* 8:200–207 (May–June 1970).

16. N. Anderson, "Services to Older Persons." *Evaluation* 1:02:4–6 (1973); L. Breslow, "Quality and Cost Control—Medicare and Beyond." *Med. Care* 12:95–114 (Feb. 1974).

17. A. Donabedian, "An Evaluation of Prepaid Group Practice." *Inquiry* 6:3–27 (Sept. 1969); G. Landsberg, "Consumers Appraise Storefront Mental Health Services." *Evaluation* 1, No. 2:66–68 (1973); see also A. Kisch and L. Reeder, "Client Evaluation of Physician Performance." *J. Health Soc. Behav.* 10:51–58 (Mar. 1969); N. Hershey and S. Bushkoff, *Informed Consent Study: The Surgeon's Responsibility for Disclosure to Patients* (Pittsburgh: Aspen Systems Corp., 1969).

18. C. Dean, "Staffing Patterns and Clinic Efficiency." *Family Planning Perspectives* 2:35–40 (Oct. 1970).

19. H. Chase (ed.), *A Study of Risks, Medical Care, and Infant Mortality*, Part II (Washington, D.C.: American Public Health Association, Sept.

1973); also published by the Institute of Medicine, National Academy of Science.

20. National Center for Health Statistics, Infant Mortality Rates: Socioeconomic Factors U.S. (Washington, D.C.: Department of Health, Education, and Welfare, Mar. 1972); other U.S. and international studies also conclude the prime importance of socioeconomic conditions (e.g., R. Lewis et al., "Relationships Between Birth Weight and Selected Social, Environmental and Medical Care Factors." *Amer. J. Public Health* 63: 973–81 (Nov. 1973; R. Puffer and C. Serrano, *Patterns of Mortality in Childhood* (Washington, D.C.: Pan American Health Organization, 1973); see also Chapter 2, Note 117.

21. For example, the National Academy of Sciences reported that it was difficult or impossible to evaluate the federally funded Maternity and Infant Care Programs (*Infant Death: An Analysis by Maternal Risk and Health Care*, Vol. 1 (Washington, D.C.: Institute of Medicine, National Academy of Sciences, 1973).

22. See Chapters 4 and 5 of the text.

23. "Life and Death and Medicine." *Scientific American* 229 (Sept. 1973), 24–32.

24. National Center for Health Statistics, "Annual Summary for the United States, 1972." *Monthly Vital Stat. Rept.* 21, June 27, 1973 (provisional).

25. Ellwood, op. cit., Chap. 5; for a method of assessing community health, see G. Christakis (ed.) *Nutritional Assessment in Health Programs, Amer. J. Public Health* 63 (Suppl.), Nov. 1973.

26. *Health Statistics Today and Tomorrow: Report of the Committee to Evaluate the National Center for Health Statistics* (Washington, D.C.: Department of Health, Education, and Welfare, Sept. 1972).

27. See, for example, R. Klein, "The Political Economy of National Health," in Congressional Research Service, op. cit., 377–88; H. Somers, "Profile of Health Care in America." *Perspective* 33–34 (Second Quarter 1973); "Epidemiological Considerations Underlying the Allocation of Health and Disease Care Resources." *Internat. J. Epid.* 1:69–74 (Spring 1972); R. Elling (ed.), *National Health Care* (Chicago: Aldine-Atherton, 1971, 250–260); D. Mechanic, *Medical Sociology: A Selective View* (New York: Free Press, 1968) 236–57; see also Chapter 1 of the text. For further discussion and approaches to evaluation, see: O. Deniston and I. Rosenstock, "Evaluating Health Programs." *Public Health Reports* 85:835–40 (Sept. 1970); D. Barr and C. Gaus, "A Population-Based Approach to Quality Assessment in HMOs." *Med. Care* 11:523–28 (Nov.–Dec. 1973); J. Williamson, "Evaluating Quality of Patient Care: A Strategy Relating Outcome and Process Assessment." *J. Amer. Med. Assoc.* 218:564–569 (Oct. 25, 1971); D. Smith and C. Metzner, "Differential Perceptions of Health Care Quality in a Prepaid Group Practice." *Med. Care* 8:264–75 (July–Aug. 1970); E. Sellers, "The Influences of Group and Independent General Practice on Patient Care: A Comparative Study in Ontario." *Can. Med. Assoc. J.* 93 (July 24, 1965);

M. Ingbar et al., "Differences in the Costs of Nursing Service: A Statistical Study of Community Hospitals in Massachusetts." *Amer. J. Public Health* 55:1699–1715 (Oct. 1966); R. Bailey, "Economics of Scale in Medical Practice," in H. Klarman (ed.), *Empirical Studies In Health Economics* (Baltimore, Md.: Johns Hopkins Press, 1970), 255–73; M. Feldstein, *Economic Analysis for Health Service Efficiency* (Chicago: Center for Health Administration Studies, 1968); M. Pauly, *Medical Care at Public Expense: A Study in Applied Welfare Economics* (New York: Praeger, 1971).

28. Major national environmental protection legislation includes: Water Quality Improvement Act of 1969 and subsequent amendments; Federal Clean Air Act Amendments of 1970; Solid Waste Disposal Act of 1965 as amended by Resource Recovery Act of 1970; Occupational Safety and Health Act of 1970; Port and Waterways Safety Act of 1971; Toxic Wastes Disposal Act of 1972; Noise Control Act of 1972; Safe Drinking Water Act of 1973.

29. E. Richter et al., "Housing and Health: A New Approach." *Amer. J. Public Health* 63:878–83 (Oct. 1973).

30. *Environmental Quality, 1973—The Fourth Annual Report of The Council on Environmental Quality* (Washington, D.C.: Government Printing Office, 1973).

31. U.S. Department of Commerce, *Statistical Abstract of the United States, 1972* (Washington, D.C.: Government Printing Office, 1972).

32. Reported in *Boston Sunday Globe,* A-17 (Dec. 16, 1973); A Chase, *Biological Imperatives* (New York: Holt, Rinehart and Winston, 1971), 168.

33. See Chapters 4 and 5, International Comparisons sections; also "The Cost and Financing of the Social Services in Sweden 1970" (Stockholm: National Central Bureau of Statistics, 1971).

34. See Chapter 2, text and citation by Fraser; also O. Anderson, *Health Care: Can There Be Equity?* (New York: Wiley-Interscience, 1972).

35. J. Lister, *N. Eng. J. Med.* 289:1184 (Nov. 29, 1973).

36. Reported in *Family Planning Digest* 2:10 (July 1973).

37. W. Steward and P. Enterline, "Effects of NHS on Physician Utilization and Health in England and Wales." *N. Eng. J. Med.* 265:1187–94 (1961); S. Greenhill and D. Haythorne, "Health Care Utilization Patterns of Albertans 1968 and 1970" (Edmonton, Canada: Department of Community Medicine, University of Alberta, 1972).

38. P. Enterline et al., "Effects of 'Free' Medical Care on Medical Practice— The Quebec Experience." *N. Eng. J. Med.* 288:1152–55 (May 31, 1973); P. Enterline, "Distribution of Medical Services Before and After 'Free' Medical Care—The Quebec Experience." *N. Eng. J. Med.* 289:1174–78 (1973).

39. See, for example, Shenkin and Maddox, cited in Chapter 8.

40. For example, National Center for Health Statistics, *Report of the Inter-*

national Conference on the Perinatal and Infant Mortality Problem of the United States (Washington, D.C.: Department of Health, Education, and Welfare, June 1966); "Organizational Study on Methods of Promoting the Development of Basic Health Services" (Geneva: World Health Organization, Jan. 16, 1973); Freeman, op. cit.

41. Lister, op. cit.
42. E. Vayda, "A Comparison of Surgical Rates in Canada and in England and Wales." *N. Eng. J. Med.* 289:1224–29 (1973).
43. For example, J. Schenken, "Infant Mortality Statistics" (Oak Brook, Ill.: Association of American Physicians and Surgeons, 1971), with rebuttal by H. Chase, op. cit. in Chapter 2 of the text.
44. For example, National Center for Health Statistics, *International Comparisons of Medical Care Utilization: A Feasibility Study* (Washington, D.C.: Department of Health, Education, and Welfare, June 1969); Freeman, op. cit.; for a bibliographic summary, see "International Health Services Research," in Flook and Sanazaro, op. cit., 184–191.

Chapter 10—Reshaping the Alternatives for Health Care

1. I. S. Falk, "Medical Care in the U.S.A., 1932–72." (*Health and Society*) *Milbank Mem. Fund Quart.* 51:1–40 (Winter 1973).
2. Copies of legislation are available on request to either the House (or Senate) Documents Room, U.S. Capitol, Washington, D.C. 20515 (or 20510 for the Senate). Requests should include the number of the bill, the Congressional representative's name, and title (e.g. H.R. 6, Rep. Brown, Health Care Act of 1973 or S. 10, Sen. White, Health Training Act of 1973) and a self-addressed mailing label.
3. *Washington Report on Medicine and Health* 1380 (Dec. 10, 1973).
4. This analytic summary concerns the following proposed Congressional legislative bills, which are representative of the scope of national health insurance bills introduced in the early 1970s: (1) S. 3, Sen. Kennedy, (H.R. 22, Rep. Griffiths) "Health Security, 1973"; (2) S. 1100, Sen. McIntyre, (H.R. 5200, Rep. Burleson) "National Health Care, 1973"; (3) H.R. 1, Rep. Ullman, "National Health Care Services Reorganization and Financing, 1973"; (4) S. 1623, Sen. Bennett, "National Health Insurance Standards, 1971"; (5) S. 2756, Sen. Scott, "Health Rights, 1973"; (6) S. 444, Sen. Hansen (H.R. 2222, Reps. Broyhill and Fulton), "National Health Care Insurance (Medicredit), 1973"; (7) S. 2513, Sens. Long and Ribicoff, "Catastrophic Health Insurance and Medical Assistance Reform, 1973."
5. See U.S. Senate Committee on Finance Report No. 92-1230 (Sept. 26, 1972), 254–69, and other references in Chapter 2, Notes 105 and 106.
6. The Institute of Medicine has recently recommended that coverage of catastrophic illnesses *not* be used as the approach to developing a national

health insurance [*Disease by Disease Toward National Health Insurance? Report of a Panel: Implications of a Categorical Catastrophic Disease Approach to National Health Insurance* (Washington, D.C.: National Academy of Sciences, June, 1973)].

7. "Cost Study of Health Insurance Proposals Introduced in the 92nd Congress," in Congressional Research Service, *Resolved: That the Federal Government Should Enact a Program of Comprehensive Medical Care for All United States Citizens* (Washington, D.C.: Government Printing Office, 1972) House Document 92-375, pp. 183–92.

Images of Access vi, vii, viii

1. Based on field visits to Konarak Subcentre and 20 other rural health programs between Apr. 4 and 18, 1971, with Miss Rama Rani Ray, Deputy Superintendent of Nursing for the State of Orissa. These visits included interviews with program directors, particularly, Dr. Pradon, State Director of Health and Family Planning, Bhubaneswar, and Mrs. Mohandi, Senior Tutor, ANM Training Centre, Puri; in addition, Miss Verghese, Lady Reading School for Health Visitors, New Delhi, Feb. 2 and 3, 1971. Other related field visits in March included 20 local community health programs, as well as discussions with many people at the Christian Medical College in Tamil Nadu, principally Mrs. Achyamma John, Chairwoman, Department of Community Health Nursing; Mrs. K. Sunder Rao; Miss A. Kuruvilla, Dean, College of Nursing; Dr. V. Benjamin, Chairman, Dept. of Community Health; Mr. Sunder Rao, head, Dept. of Biostatistics, College of Medicine, Mar. 11–23, 1971; Mr. Amor El Atki, Chief, Health Section, UNICEF, New Delhi, Feb. 2, 1971; Dr. J. Goddard, Program Adviser for Family Planning, Ford Foundation, New Delhi, Feb. 20; Dr. D. Bhattia, Family Planning Consultant, Ford Foundation, New Delhi, Feb. 26, 1971; Miss A. Cherian, Chief Nursing Advisor, Ministry of Health, New Delhi, Feb. 1, 1971; Dr. (Mrs.) S. Krishnan, Principal, College of Nursing, New Delhi, Feb. 19, 1971.

2. Based on a field visit to Bijlmer Meer, Oct. 21, 1971, and interviews with Marijke Mol, Oct. 21 and 23; a discussion with social workers and visiting nurses at Blankenberg Stiehling, Oct. 23; interview with Dr. J. Weijel, Board of Directors, Social Security System and Professor, Rehabilitation Center, University of Amsterdam, Oct. 22, Amsterdam.

3. Based on a field visit to Craigmillar, Dec. 10 and 12, 1971, and discussion with the Craigmillar Festival Society leaders; also with the staff of the Richmont Church of Scotland, and with Ian Reid, Director, the Iona Community, Dec. 7, 1971, Edinburgh; L. Hockey, Dept. of Nursing Studies, University of Edinburgh, Edinburgh, Dec. 8, 1971. "A Community on the Move: The Report of the Craigmillar Festival Society, 1970–1971." Other related field visits included the Daisy Bank Road Day Nursery and interviews with Miss Heeney, Matron and Miss Pickford,

Superintendent Deputy Matron, Nov. 25, 1971, Manchester; also Mr. Baker, Training Officer, Social Services Department, Borough of Camden Day Care Services, Nov. 3, London; staff at the Nursery School Association, Nov. 11, London; Isabel Menzies, psychoanalyst, Tavistock Institute of Human Relations, Centre for Applied Social Research, Nov. 12, London; Child Minders Registration personnel, City of Southampton, Nov. 19; Southampton Central Health Clinic Maternity Services midwives, Nov. 19; Mrs. Dickinson, Superintendent of Nursing, Manchester Health Authority, Nov. 22; Brunswick Health Center, Health Visitor staff and Miss Cannon, Group Advisor, Nov. 22, Manchester; Miss J. McFarlane, Department of Preventive and Community Medicine, University of Manchester, Nov. 23; a field visit to the Home Help Service and interview with Mrs. Taylor, Supervisor, Nov. 19, 1971, Southampton; also with Miss Vergebovsky and Miss Rule, Head, Department of Higher Education, Royal College of Nursing, Nov. 2, London; Miss Brooks, Head, Department of Community Nursing, RCN, Nov. 8, London; Miss Bussby, Chief Nursing Officer, Queen's Institute for District Nursing, Nov. 10, London; Miss King, Midwifery Advisor, Department of Health and Social Security, Nov. 10, London; Miss P. O'Connell, Lecturer in Health Visiting, University of Southampton, Nov. 15 and 16; in the Southampton City Council Central Health Clinic, Miss Clarke, Head of Health Visiting; Miss Ames, Head of District Nursing, Nov. 19, Southampton; and the following official papers, Department of Health and Social Security, "The National Health Service: the Future Structure" ("Green Paper") (London: Her Majesty's Stationery Office, 1970); "The Organization of Group Practice: Excerpts from a Report of a Sub-committee" Oct. 1971, Central Health Services U.K.; "The Mayston Report," Oct. 1969, Department of Health and Social Security, London.

Appendix Tables

Appendix Table 1 Distribution of Resources Within Underdeveloped Countries

Urban–Rural Differences in Latin America, Environmental Security

Data Years		Urban Areas	Rural Areas
1967	Water supplies (% having)	69	20
	Sewerage systems (% having)	45	2–3
1961–1967	Construction funds invested (%)		
	for water/sewerage service	100	100
	National government sources	57	80
	International sources	43	20
	U.S. Agency for International Development	16	2
	Inter-American Development Bank	73	98

Source: Pan American Health Organization, *Goals in the Charter of Punta del Este: Facts on Health Progress* (Washington, D.C.: PAHO, July 1969).

Appendix Table 2 Distribution of Resources Within Affluent Countries

Differences in Access to Higher Education,
by Socioeconomic Status, Sex, and Ability, United States

	Enrollment (%) at Senior and Junior Colleges of 1968 High School Graduates			
	Poorest Quartile		Wealthiest Quartile	
Ability Level	Male	Female	Male	Female
Least able quartile	14	17	40	55
Most able quartile	75	67	88	88

Source: Educational Testing Service, adapted from Report of CSS Panel on Financing Poor and Minority Students (Princeton, N.J., 1968).

Appendix Table 3   Distribution of Resoures Within Underdeveloped Countries

Urban–Rural Differences in Latin America, Basic Education

	Urban Areas	Rural Areas	Data Years
Facilities (5-year schools, % having)	66	6	1966
Literacy (% of area pop.)			
Argentina	90.5	81.0	Early 1960s
Brazil	73.5	32.5	
Colombia	84.5	64.5	
Venezuela	93.2	75.0	
(Men only)			

Sources: Pan American Health Organization, *Goals in the Charter of Punta del Este: Facts on Health Progress* (Washington, D.C.: PAHO, July 1969).

International Committee for the Development of Education, *Learning To Be* (Paris: UNESCO, 1972).

Appendix Table 4   Distribution of Resources Within Underdeveloped Countries

Access to Education by Females Compared to Total[a] Students, 1960–68

	Annual Rate of Increase in Enrollment (%)							
	Primary Level		Secondary Level		Higher Education		Total	
	Total	Female	Total	Female	Total	Female	Total	Female
Africa	5.6	6.6	9.7	10.8	7.4	11.3	5.4	7.1
Latin America	5.4	5.3	10.2	11.2	11.4	10.9	6.3	6.2
Asia[b]	5.2	5.7	4.5	6.1	10.2	13.7	5.2	5.9

	Female Enrollment, 1968			
	Primary	Secondary	Higher	Total
Asia[b]				
% of total students	38.6	33.9	28.5	37.0
% increase, 1967–1968				
Total students	4.5	3.8	6.9	4.4
Females	4.6	3.7	7.8	4.5

[a] 1965–1968.

[b] Not including China, North Korea, or North Viet Nam.

Source: International Committee for the Development of Education, *Learning To Be* (Paris: UNESCO, 1972).

Appendix Table 5   Population Characteristics, United States

Age, Race, and Sex, 1971

	%
Age (yr)	100.0[a]
—17	33.5
17–44	36.2
45–64	20.4
65 and over	9.9
Race	100.0
White	87.7
65 and over[b]	(10.3)
Other races	12.3
Black	(11.0)
65 and over	(6.8)
Sex	100.0
Male	48.7
65 and over[b]	(8.5)
Female	51.3
65 and over[b]	(11.3)

[a] $N = 207$ million.

[b] 1970.

Source: U.S. Bureau of Census, *Statistical Abstract of the United States 1972* (Washington, D.C.: Government Printing Office, 1972).

Appendix Table 6   Distribution of Population, United States

Blacks, by Region, 1971

	Total (%)
United States	100.0
Northeast	19.0
North Central	20.0
South	53.0
West	8.0

Source: U.S. Bureau of Census, *Statistical Abstract of the United States 1972* (Washington, D.C.: Government Printing Office, 1972).

Appendix Table 7   Distribution of Population, United States

Urban–Rural Residence, White and Black Races, 1970

	Total Population (%)	Whites (%)	Blacks (%)
Urban areas			
Central cities	31.5	27.9	56.5
City fringe	26.8	28.9	12.2
Outside urbanized areas	15.2	15.7	12.0
Rural areas	26.5	27.5	19.3
	100.0	100.0	100.0

Source: U.S. Bureau of Census, *Statistical Abstract of the United States 1972.* (Washington, D.C.: Government Printing Office, 1972).

Appendix Table 8   Distribution of Population, United States

High- and Low-Income Groups, Race and Region, 1970

	Family Income (%)			
	White		Black	
	$—5,000	$10,000 or more	$—5,000	$10,000 or more
Northeast	14.2	56.5	37.6	34.7
North Central	15.9	53.5	30.9	36.0
South	20.7	44.9	47.8	17.3
West	17.0	52.4	28.7	39.1

Source: U.S. Bureau of Census, *Statistical Abstracts of the United States 1972* (Washington, D.C.: Government Printing Office, 1972).

Appendix Table 9 **Population Characteristics of More Affluent and Less Affluent States**

Birth, Death, and Infant Mortality Rates, 1972

	More Affluent States			Region	Less Affluent States		
	Birth Rate	Death Rate	Infant Mortality Rate		Birth Rate	Death Rate	Infant Mortality Rate
United States	15.6	9.4	18.0				
				Northeast			
Conn.	12.7	8.6	16.3	Me.	15.4	10.9	16.7
				North Central			
Ill.	15.6	9.7	20.0	S.Da.	15.8	10.4	21.3
				South			
Tex.	18.9	8.6	19.4	W.V.a.	16.7	11.6	20.8
				West			
Cal.	14.8	8.2	15.8	Mont.	15.8	9.5	18.3

Source: National Center for Health Statistics, "Annual Summary for the United States, 1972." *Monthly Vital Stat. Rept. 21,* July 27, 1973 (provisional).

Appendix Table 10 Distribution of Health Care Resources, United States

Physicians, Dentists, and Registered Nurses in More Affluent and Less Affluent States, 1970

	More Affluent States			Region	Less Affluent States		
	M.D. and D.O. (per 100,000 population)	D.D.S.[b]	R.N.[a]		M.D. and D.O. (per 100,000 population)	D.D.S.[b]	R.N.[a]
United States	171	47	313[c]				
				Northeast			
Conn.	193	59	536	Me.	131	36	414
				North Central			
Ill.	140	48	330	S.Da.	86	36	308
				South			
Tex.	123	37	188	W.Va.	111	32	260
				West			
Cal.	192	58	312	Mont.	109	46	354

[a] 1966, active.
[b] Nonfederal.
[c] 1970 estimate is 345.

Source: National Center for Health Statistics, *Health Resources Statistics 1971* (Washington, D.C.: Department of Health, Education, and Welfare, 1972).

Appendix Table 11 Distribution of Health Care Resources, United States

Physicians in Primary Care and Group Practice in More Affluent and Less Affluent States

	More Affluent States						Region	Less Affluent States					
	Nonfederal M.D.s[a]				M.D.s in Medical Groups[b]			Nonfederal M.D.s[a]				M.D.s in Medical Groups[b]	
	Total	General Practice	Internal Medicine	Pediatrics	Total	General Practice Groups		Total	General Practice	Internal Medicine	Pedi-atrics	Total	General Practice Groups
United States	298,745	54,376	36,755	16,349	40,028	2,681							
Conn.	5,800	664	832	361	601	41	Northeast Me.	1,100	267	102	43	55	0
Ill.	15,300	3,058	1,932	827	1,726	95	North Central S.Da.	534	203	37	17	187	47
Tex.	13,000	2,936	1,314	716	2,293	223	South W.Va.	1,823	442	204	80	298	4
Cal.	38,031	7,040	4,545	2,000	6,543	312	West Mont.	722	245	62	30	212	30
Totals	72,131	13,698	8,623	3,914	11,163	671		4,179	1,157	405	170	752	81
% of U.S. total	24	25	20	24	28	25		1.4	2.1	1.1	6.3	1.9	3.0

a 1970.

b 1969.

Source: National Center for Health Statistics, *Health Resources Statistics 1971* (Washington, D.C.: Department of Health, Education, and Welfare, 1972).

Appendix Table 12   Distribution of Health Care Resources, United States

Nursing Personnel Ratios to Inpatient Beds in More Affluent and Less Affluent States

| | More Affluent States | | | | Region | Less Affluent States | | | |
| | R.N.s (per 1,000 beds) in | | LPNs (per 1,000 beds) in | | | R.N.s (per 1,000 beds) | | LPNs (per 1,000 beds) | |
	Hospital[b]	Skilled Nursing Facilities[a]	Hospital[b]	Skilled Nursing Facilities[a]		Hospital[b]	Skilled Nursing Facilities[a]	Hospital[b]	Skilled Nursing Facilities[a]
United States	268	36.6	111.5	49.7					
					Northeast				
Conn.	336	73.6	84.8	49.6	Me.	257	43.5	62.0	64.4
					North Central				
Ill.	269	29.5	77.2	47.1	S.Da.	267	34.6	64.9	27.0
					South				
Tex.	218	20.9	213.7	71.7	W.Va.	252	39.0	115.4	58.6
					West				
Cal.	330	35.4	111.8	40.8	Mont.	425	48.4	130.3	52.1

[a] 1969.
[b] 1968.

Source: National Center for Health Statistics, *Health Resources Statistics 1971* (Washington, D.C.: Department of Health, Education, and Welfare, 1972).

Appendix Table 13 Distribution of Health Care Resources, United States

Inpatient Facilities in More Affluent and Less Affluent States

	More Affluent States				Less Affluent States		
	Total Hospital Beds (per 1,000 pop.)[a]	General Medical–Surgical Beds (per 1,000 pop.)[a]	Skilled Nursing Facilities Beds (per 1,000 Medicare enrollees)[b]	Region	Total Hospital Beds (per 1,000 pop.)[a]	General Medical–Surgical Beds (per 1,000 pop.)[a]	Skilled Nursing Facilities Beds (per 1,000 Medicare enrollees)[b]
United States	7.6	5.0	14.3				
Conn.	6.8	4.0	35.7	Northeast Me.	9.2	5.9	6.2
Ill.	7.9	5.2	7.2	North Central S.Da.	10.1	6.9	6.1
Tex.	6.9	5.1	4.1	South W. Va.	9.5	6.1	5.8
Cal.	6.2	4.6	43.0	West Mont.	7.0	6.4	10.4

[a] 1970.
[b] 1972.

Sources: National Center for Health Statistics, *Health Resources Statistics 1971* (Washington, D.C.: Department of Health, Education, and Welfare, 1972).
Social Security Administration, "Medicare: Participating Health Facilities, July, 1972." *Health Insur. Stat.* 48 (July 20, 1973).

Appendix Table 14 Distribution of Health Care Resources, United States

Outpatient Facilities (N) in More Affluent and Less Affluent States

	More Affluent States						Less Affluent States				
	Hospital with Outpatient General Medical–Surgical Services (1970)	Medical Groups 1969 Total	General Practice	Community Mental Health Centers[a]	Home Health Agencies[b]	Region	Hospital with Outpatient General Medical–Surgical Services (1970)	Medical Groups 1969 Total	General Practice	Community Mental Health Centers[a]	Home Health Agencies[b]
United States	6,495	6,357	783	609	2,217						
Conn.	48	104	13	5	89	Northeast Me.	60	14	0	8	23
Ill.	261	293	30	14	81	North Central S.Da.	69	36	13	1	22
Tex.	534	408	67	28	46	South W.Va.	81	34	1	7	19
Cal.	569	81	15	66	83	West Mont.	67	36	9	4	10
Totals	1,412	886	125	115	299		277	120	23	20	74
% U.S. total	22	14	16	19	13.5		4.2	1.9	2.9	3.3	3.3

[a] Funded, 1971.

[b] Participating in Medicare, 1972.

Source: National Center for Health Statistics, *Health Resources Statistics 1971* (Washington, D.C.: Department of Health, Education, and Welfare, 1972). Social Security Administration, "Medicare: Participating Health Facilities, July, 1972." *Health Insur. Stat.* 48, July 20, 1973.

Appendix Table 15   Distribution of Health Care Resources, United States

Nursing Personnel, Schools, and Students in More Affluent and Less Affluent States, 1970

	U.S. Population (%)	R.N.		LPN	
		Schools % (N)	Students % (N)	Schools % (N)	Students % (N)
United States	100.0	100.0 (1,330)	100.0 (165,000)	100.0 (1,233)	100.0 (55,000)
More affluent states	22.3	17.1 (228)	20.0 (32,900)	22.4 (277)	22.2 (12,250)
Less affluent states	2.0	2.7 (36)	2.5 (4,180)	2.7 (34)	2.1 (1,190)

Source: National Center for Health Statistics, *Health Resources Statistics 1971* (Washington, D.C.: Department of Health, Education, and Welfare, 1972).

Appendix Table 16 Distribution of Health Care Resources, United States

Medical and Nursing Personnel Training Facilities in More Affluent and Less Affluent States, 1970

	More Affluent States Schools (No.)			Region	Less Affluent States Schools (No.)		
	M.D.ᵃ	R.N.	LPNᵇ		M.D.ᵃ	R.N.	LPNᵇ
United States	107	1,330	1,233				
				Northeast			
Conn.	1	24	10	Me.	0	6	5
				North Central			
Ill.	5	78	40	S.Da.	1	9	5
				South			
Tex.	4	44	145	W.Va.	1	16	16
				West			
Cal.	6	82	82	Mont.	0	5	8
Total	16	228	277		2	36	34
% U.S. total	14.9	17.1	22.4		1.4	2.7	2.7

ᵃ Includes six 4-yr schools of osteopathic medicine.

ᵇ Licensed practical nurse.

Source: National Center for Health Statistics, *Health Resources Statistics 1971* (Washington, D.C.: Department of Health, Education and Welfare, 1972).

Appendix Table 17   Distribution of Health Care Resources, United States

Medical Schools[a] and Medical Students[b] in More Affluent and Less Affluent States

	Medical Schools (No.)		Students	Region	Medical Schools (No.)		Students
	Public	Private	(per 100,000 population)		Public	Private	(per 100,000 population)
United States	55	52	5.8				
				Northeast			
Conn.	0	1	4.9	Me.	0	0	2.0
				North Central			
Ill.	1	4	6.7	S.Da.	1	0	7.5
				South			
Tex.	3	1	4.1	W.Va.	1	0	5.0
				West			
Cal.	3	3	4.2	Mont.	0	0	4.1

[a] 1969–1970.

[b] 1971–1972.

Sources: National Center for Health Statistics, *Health Resources Statistics 1971* (Washington, D.C.: Department of Health, Education, and Welfare, 1972).
Council on Medical Education, *J. Amer. Med. Assoc.* 222 (Nov. 20, 1972).

Appendix Table 18a Summary of Population Characteristics and Distribution of Some Health Care Resources in Certain Countries

	United States	Canada	United Kingdom	Sweden	Denmark	Federal Republic of Germany	Nether- lands	Japan	U.S.S.R.	India	Argentina	Brazil
Population characteristics[1]												
Total population (millions) 1970	205	21.5	49	8	4.9	59.5	13	103.7	243	550	24	95.3
Life expectancy (male years)	66.6	68.7	68.7	71.8	70.7	67.5	71	69.1	70	41.9	64	60.7[a]
Gross domestic product[2] (per person)	$4,734	$3,676	$2,128	$4,055	$3,141	$3,034	$2,353	1,911	$1,110[b]	$94	$974	$362
Density (km.²)[3]	22	2	270	18	114	240	377	280	11	167	9	11
Urban (%)[3]	73	74	79	77	75	79	78	72	56	20	41	56
Minority (%)[1,3,4]	12	n.a.	2.4	−1	n.a.	5.5	3.8	n.a.	46.7[c]	n.a.	n.a.	n.a.
Aged (% 65 and over)[3]	9.9	7.8	12.8	13.7	12.8	12.9	10.1	6.9	n.a.	3	n.a.	n.a.
Infant death rate (per 1,000 live births)	19.8	19.3	18.0	11.7	14.8	23.6	12.7	13.1	24.4	139	58.3	170[b]
Distribution of health care resources[1,5]												
Physicians M.D.s per 100,000 population	170	138	113	120	134	155	125	109	228	20	164	44
Persons per M.D.	670	700	810	768	600	568	832	898	433	5,800	500	1,953

Appendix Table 18a   Summary of Population Characteristics and Distribution of Some Health Care Resources in Certain Countries (continued)

	United States	Canada	United Kingdom	Sweden	Denmark	Federal Republic of Germany	Netherlands	Japan	U.S.S.R.	India	Argentina	Brazil
Urban M.D.s/ rural M.D.s (per 100,000 population)	132/81	n.a.	110/96	n.a.	277/120[d]	n.a.	n.a.	127/70	230/35[e]	14/2	337/110	71/28
Dentists (per 100,000 population)	56.7	32	26	83	67	52	23	35	35	n.a.	53	27
Nurses (per 100,000 population)	361	605	504	290	220	287	443	258	400	11	104	10
Midwives (per 100,000 population)	2.4	n.a.	36	25	12	12	6	28	117	12	12	2
Nursing auxiliaries (per 100,000 population)	479	123	103	15	n.a.	13.6	1.4	n.a.	n.a.	3	34	73
Hospital beds (per 1,000 population)	7.4	14.5	9.2	16	8.8	11.6	5.1	12.5	9.6	0.5	6	2.9
Urban–rural	6.2/10.1	n.a.	9–13/9–10	n.a.	n.a.	n.a.	n.a.	n.a.	n.a.	n.a.	8.2/5	7.1/2.6
Persons per bed	137	98	106	67	112	87	192	79	9.4	1700	160	325
Medical schools (N):[G] Before 1960	86	12	27	5	2	19	6	46	76	55	9	20
New 1960–1970	21	4	0	1	1	7	1	0	7	40	0	53
Population (million) per medical school	1.9	1.3	2.1	1.3	1.6	2.3	1.9	2.2	2.8	5.7	2.7	1.2

Appendix Table 18a   Summary of Population Characteristics and Distribution of Some Health Care Resources in Certain Countries (*continued*)

	Chile	Colombia	Venezuela	Guate-mala	Mexico	Israel	Egypt	Senegal	Nigeria	Kenya	Li-beria	Tan-zania[f]	South Africa
Population characteristics[1]													
Total population (million) 1970	9.8	21.1	10.4	5.2	49.1	2.9	33.3	3.9	55.1	11.2	1.2	13.3	20.1
Life expectancy (male years)	54.4	44.1	63.8[a]	48.2	61	69.5	51.6	41[a]	37	47.5[a]	36.1	40[a]	49[a]
Gross domestic product[2] (per person)	$681	$401	$979	$363	$663	$1,836	$170[b]	$170[b]	$70[b]	$140	$210[b]	$97	$864
Density (km.[2])	13	19	11	48	25	141	33	20	60	19	11	14	16
Urban (%)[3]	76	53	75	34	59	82	42	n.a.	16	9.9	26.2	5.5	48
Minority (%)[1,3,4]	na.a	n.a.	n.a.	35	6.3	n.a.	6	n.a.	0.1	1.8	n.a.	0.5	31
Aged (% 65 and over)[3]	5.4	2.6	n.a.	2	3.6	n.a.	n.a.	n.a.	2	3.5	3.4	2.1	n.a.
Infant death rate (per 1,000 live births)	91.6	70.4	46.9	88.4	68.5	22.9	118	92.9	n.a.	55	137	162	n.a.
Distribution of health care resources[1,5]													
Physicians													
M.D.s per 100,000 population	58	44	84	22	55	251	49	6.6	4	11	10	4.4	62.5
Persons per M.D.	2,443	2,220	1,100	4,030	1,850	400	2,000	15,150	50,000	8,720	9,240	23,200	1,500[g]
Urban M.D.s/ rural M.D.s (per 100,000 population)	103/33	49/23	93/57	60/8	223/3	n.a.	n.a.	45/1.7	n.a./0.7	n.a.	n.a.	n.a.	n.a.

Appendix Table 18a Summary of Population Characteristics and Distribution of Some Health Care Resources in Certain Countries (continued)

	Chile	Colombia	Venezuela	Guate-mala	Mexico	Israel	Egypt	Senegal	Nigeria	Kenya	Li-beria	Tan-zania[t]	South Africa
Dentists (per 100,000 population)	10	15	21	4.6	7	50	n.a.	n.a.	n.a.	n.a.	n.a.	n.a.	n.a.
Nurses (per 100,000 population)	21	7	49	13	19	381	27	42	22	70	n.a.	29	207
Midwives (per 100,000 population)	9	n.a.	1.3	3.6	n.a.	17.7	36	7.7	22.5	28	n.a.	5	150
Nursing auxiliaries (per 100,000 population)	154	60	141	52	94	n.a.	n.a.	n.a.	n.a.	n.a.	n.a.	n.a.	n.a.
Hospital beds (per 1,000 population)	4.2	2.5	3.2	2.3	2	5.8	2.1	1.3	0.5	1.2	1.8	1.4	4.4
Urban–rural	4.5/3.2	2.9/2.2	6.2/2.6	7.3/1.4	n.a.	n.a.	n.a.	n.a.	n.a.	n.a.	3.3	n.a.	n.a.
Persons per bed	284	420	315	420	550	130	472	740	1,870	750	509	47	189
Medical schools (N)[6]													
Before 1960	4	7	4	1	22	1	3	1	1	0	0	0	5
New 1960–1970	1	2	3	0	3	2	4	0	3	1	1	1	0
Population (million) per medical school	2	2.3	1.4	5	2	1	4.7	4	16	11	1	15	4

ᵃ Average for men and women.

ᵇ GNP, 1969 (U.S. Gross National Product per capita = $3,980). Population Reference Bureau, "1971 World Population Data Sheet." GNP is about $200–500 more than the GDP per capita in most affluent countries [see J. Kasun, "U.S. Poverty in World Perspective" *Current History* 64:247–52 (June 1973)]; "OECD Member Countries, 1973 Edition." *OECD Observer* 63 (Apr. 1973).

ᶜ Russians (53.4%) are the largest of 92 nationality groups in U.S.S.R.

ᵈ For Copenhagen compared with all other areas.

ᵉ Working in ambulatory services only.

ᶠ Most figures are for Tanganyika.

ᵍ Because of apartheid policies, this translates into one M.D. per 400 whites, and one M.D. per 44,000 Africans ("Health Care in South Africa." *Lancet*, Sep. 15, 1973).

Sources: ¹ United Nations, *Statistical Yearbook 1971* (New York: UN, 1972). UN figures are estimates for 1970 or latest available; "urban" designations in Latin America vary, and in Columbia and Venezuela include populations of 1,500 and 1,000 persons, respectively. In Latin America, minorities are mainly Indian; in Africa, mainly nonblack or non-Muslim groups.

² GDP is the total value of goods and services produced within a country. U.S. Bureau of Census, *Statistical Abstract of the United States 1972* (1970 data).

³ United Nations, *Demographic Yearbook 1971* (New York: UN, 1972).

⁴ J. Power, *The New Proletarians* (London: British Council of Churches, 1972).

⁵ Most figures for the United Kingdom are from Great Britain Department of Health and Social Security, *Social Trends 1972* (London: Her Majesty's Stationery Office, 1973); for Latin America, from Pan American Health Organization, *Facts on Health Progress* (Washington, D.C.: Pan American Health Organization, 1969) (1966 data) ("urban" in Latin American countries refers to capital cities). Some U.S.S.R. figures are from G. Popov, *Principles of Health Planning in the USSR* (Geneva: World Health Organization, 1971). Data bases for computing ratios varied with sources. U.S. data from National Center for Health Statistics, *Health Resources Statistics 1972–73* (Washington, D.C.: Department of Health, Education, and Welfare, 1973). (Nursing auxiliaries are practical nurses, aides, orderlies); urban–rural hospital beds are for contrasting urban and rural states. Most other nurse auxiliary data are from International Council of Nurses National Reports of Member Associations 1969 (Basel, Switz.: ICN, 1969).

⁶ World Health Organization Survey, *World Health* (Nov. 1971).

Appendix Table 18b   Summary of Health Care Financing in Certain Countries

	Canada	Great Britain
National Programs for Health Care Financing		
Type[a]	Social insurance Direct revenues	Social insurance Direct revenues
Sources of funds	50% national government; remainder determined by province	85% government revenues; 15% social insurance taxes and direct consumer cost
Population coverage	99%	100%
Benefits[b]	Cash; comprehensive in- and output services (except dental)	Cash; comprehensive services
Payment method to: Specialists GPs	Arranged by provinces; alternative to fee-for-service being proposed (1973)	Salary Capitation
Administration National level	Health and Welfare Department	Department of Health and Social Security
Local level	Provincial departments of health	Regional and area health authorities
Other social insurance programs[c]	Old age; work injury; unemployment; family allowance	Old age; work injury; unemployment; family allowance

Appendix Table 18b Summary of Health Care Financing in Certain Countries (*continued*)

Sweden	Denmark	Federal Republic of Germany
Social insurance Direct revenues	Direct revenues	Social insurance Direct revenues
55% national government revenues; employer/employee payroll tax; direct consumer cost	Governmental general revenues; direct consumer costs	Small government contribution for poor and for maternity grants; 5% employee payroll tax; employer tax 5%
100%	100%	90% (compulsory for most workers)
Cash; comprehensive services	Cash; comprehensive services	Cash; medical, dental, midwifery, drugs
Salary	Salary; fee-for-service contract for primary care	Fee-for-service
Salary	(All salaried in Copenhagen)	Fee-for-service
Social Insurance Board	Ministry for Social Affairs	Ministry of Labor and Social Affairs
County government council	Local government council	State insurance office and sick funds (non-government)
Old age; work injury; unemployment; family allowance	Old age; work injury; unemployment; family allowance	Old age; work injury; unemployment; family allowance

	Netherlands	Japan
National Programs for Health Care Financing		
Type[a]	Social insurance Direct revenues	2 programs: social insurance direct revenues
Sources of funds	Government subsidy for poor; 4–6% employee payroll tax; employer tax	1. Govt. subsidy to employer–employee program 2. 40% government for those not in (1)
Population coverage	Over 70% (compulsory for most workers); 100% for catastrophic care	98%
Benefits[b]	Cash; comprehensive services	1. Cash; comprehensive services 2. Comprehensive services
Payment method to: Specialists	Salary; fee	Fee-for-service
GPs	Capitation	Fee-for-service
Administration National level	Ministry of Social Affairs and Public Health	Ministry Health and Welfare
Local level	Sick funds (nongovernment)	1. Prefectural government and insurance societies (nongovernment) 2. Local government health insurance funds
Other social insurance programs[c]	Old age; work injury; unemployment; family allowance	Old age; work injury; unemployment; family allowance

U.S.S.R.	India	Argentina
Social insurance (for cash benefits) Direct revenues	Social insurance Direct revenues	Social insurance
Employee tax for cash benefits; 100% government revenues for service benefits	Employer/employee taxes; 12% government revenues	Employer–employee taxes
100%	Lower-paid workers in larger urban firms	Workers and dependents
Cash; comprehensive services	Cash; medical and maternity	Cash; comprehensive services
Salary	Capitation	n.a.
Salary	Capitation	n.a.
Ministry of Health	Ministry of Labor	Ministry of Social Welfare; National Institute of Social Services
Republic ministries of health	State insurance corporations	
Old age; work injury; family allowance	Old age; work injury; unemployment	Old age; work injury; unemployment; family allowance

	Brazil	Chile
National Programs for Health Care Financing		
Type[a]	Social insurance Direct revenues	Social insurance Direct revenues
Sources of funds	Employer–employee taxes; government pays administrative costs	Employer–employee taxes; government pays at 5.5% of earnings, plus grants for given programs
Population coverage	Workers	Workers
Benefits[b]	Cash; comprehensive services in National Social Insurance Institute facilities	Cash; comprehensive services, in National Health Service facilities (owns 88% of hospital beds and most outpatient facilities)
Payment method to: Specialists	Salary	Salary
GPs	Salary	Salary
Administration National level	Ministry of Labor and Social Insurance; National Social Insurance Institute	Ministry of Health; National Health Service
Local level		13 health zones
Other social insurance programs[c]	Old age; work injury; unemployment; family allowance	Old age; work injury; unemployment; family allowance

Appendix Table 18b   Summary of Health Care Financing in Certain Countries (*continued*)

Colombia	Venezuela	Guatemala
Social insurance Direct revenues	Social insurance Direct revenues	Social insurance Direct revenues
Employer–employee taxes; government pays at 2.5% of earnings	Employer–employee taxes; government pays at 1.5% of earnings	Employer–employee taxes; government pays 25%
Farm and industrial workers	Full-time workers	Workers in capitol area (10% of population; 29% of workers)
Cash; comprehensive services in Colombia Social Insurance Institute hospitals	Cash; comprehensive services in Venezuela Social Insurance Institute facilities	Cash; comprehensive medical services in Guatemala Social Security Institute facilities
Salary	Salary	Salary
Salary	Salary	Salary
Colombia Social Insurance Institute	Ministry of Labor; Venezuela Social Insurance Institute	Ministry of Labor and Social Welfare; Guatemala Social Security Institute
Old age; work injury; unemployment; family allowance	Old age; work injury	Old age; work injury

	Mexico	Israel
National Programs for Health Care Financing		
Type[a]	Social insurance Direct revenues	Two programs: (1) mandatory; (2) voluntary Social insurance
Sources of funds	Employer–employee taxes; government pays at 1.6% of earnings	1. Employer–employee taxes 2. Enrollee and government subsidy
Population coverage	Nondomestic workers (23% of population)	1. Working women 2. 80% of population
Benefits[b]	Cash; comprehensive services in Mexico Social Insurance Institute hospitals	1. Maternity, cash, and medical services 2. Comprehensive medical care
Payment method to: Specialists	Salary	Salary
GPs	Salary	Salary
Administration National level	Ministry of Labor and Social Welfare; Mexico Social Insurance Institute	1. Ministry of Labor and National Insurance Institute
Local level		2. Kupat Holim and kibbutzim sick funds
Other social insurance programs[c]	Old age; work injury	Old age; work injury; unemployment; family allowance

Egypt	Senegal	Nigeria
Social insurance	Social insurance Direct revenues	Provident fund
Employer and employee taxes	Employer–employee taxes; government pays 33%	Employer 5%; employee 95%
Industrial workers	Working women	Workers in firms of over 10 employees
Cash; medical (no dental) care in facilities under contract with Social Insurance Organization	Cash for maternity; maternity	Cash, as contributed prior to need
Salary	Salary	Salary
Salary	Salary	Salary
Ministry of Labor and Social Insurance Organization	Ministry of Public Services and Labor	Ministry Labor and Social Welfare; National Provident Fund
Unemployment	Work injury; family allowance	Old age; work injury

	Kenya	Liberia
National Programs for Health Care Financing		
Type[a]	Hospital insurance	None
Sources of funds	Employees	
Population coverage	Workers earning $140 or more monthly	
Benefits[b]	Hospital care	
Payment method to: Specialists	Cash reimbursement to hospital	
GPs		
Administration National level	Ministry Health; National Hospital	
Local level	Insurance Fund	
Other social insurance programs[c]	Old age; work injury	Work injury

Appendix Table 18b   Summary of Health Care Financing in Certain Countries
(concluded)

Tanzania	South Africa
Provident Fund	None (see below)
Employers 5%; employees 95%	
Workers in firms of 4 and over	
Cash for sickness as contributed prior to need	
Salary	
Salary	
Ministry Communications, Transport and Labor; National Provident Fund	
Old age; work injury	Old age; work injury; unemployment (includes some health benefits); family allowance

[a] All are statutory and mandatory unless noted otherwise.

[b] Varying time limits for maternity and sickness benefits.

[c] Limited to certain groups, especially in poorer countries.

Sources: Social Security Administration, *Social Security Programs Throughout the World 1971* (Washington, D.C.: Government Office, 1971).

W. Glazer, *Paying the Doctor: Systems of Remuneration and Their Effects* (Baltimore, Md.: Johns Hopkins University Press, 1970).

E. Long and A. Vian, "Health Care Extension Using Medical Auxiliaries in Guatemala." *Lancet* 127–130 (Jan. 26, 1974).

	Canada	Great Britain	Sweden	Denmark
National health service[a]	No	Yes	Yes	Yes
Hospital ownership and support	Mixed private–public; government controls 90% of beds.	All national government; 50% of health services expenditures.	All county government; 47% of health expenditures (plus 24% for M.D., dental care in OPDs).	Government decreasing support for inpatient facilities; hospitals publicly owned.
Ambulatory care alternatives	Integration proposed (1972) of hospital and ambulatory care facilities, with increased outpatient options and home care.	Maternal Child Health–birth control care integrated through health centers in which GPs practice. Emphasis on health centers, which increased from 31 (1965) to 341 (1971); from 300 GPs (1966) to 1800 (1971). GP maternity homes (1–7-day delivery facilities run by midwives with GP and hospital backup). Home health and personal care services. ECFs. Child and adult day care.	50% of services rendered in hospital outpatient departments; 23% in county health centers (90% without referral); 26% private M.D.s. Maternal Child Health–birth control integrated as above. Emergency medical service and ambulance network. Integrated industrial health services. Home health and personal care services. ECFs. Child and adult day care.	Maternal Child Health–abortion–family planning integrated. Independent M.D.s salaried in Copenhagen area. Home health and personal care services. ECFs. Child and adult day care.

Federal Republic of Germany	Netherlands	Japan	U.S.S.R.
No	No	No	Yes
62% federal; 38% voluntary.	Majority private with government subsidy.	Mixed.	100% government.
Predominance of nonintegrated clinics and independent private medical practitioners. Infant and pre-school centers.	Regional maternity centers with home help services. Home delivery (55% of births) by midwives (49%) or M.D.s (51%).	Regional health centers for public health services. Maternal Child Health centers (543 in 1968). Family planning supplies distributed through nongovernment channels with government subsidy. Predominance of private independent medical care.	General medical primary care units (uchastoks) per 10,000–15,000 population. Emergency medical network, including first aid stations. Dispensaries for close follow-up on certain groups. Gynecological–women's comprehensive social services clinics. Extensive primary home medical care services. Industrial worker health services.

395

	Canada	Great Britain	Sweden	Denmark
Physicians and other health personnel	49% of M.D.s in Quebec in general practice.	49% (¾ in group or health center settings) in general practice. 51% of M.D.s employed in hospital as specialists; virtually all other personnel employed by government National Health Service.	35% GPs, 56% specialists ⎬ 14% private practice. 9% of all M.D.s in administration (5% foreign origin) Virtually all other personnel employed by government health service.	36% GPs, 14% specialists ⎬ Nonhospital practice (49% women). 41% hospital-based; 8% administration. Most personnel employed by government.
Controls	National Health Insurance fiscal controls. National personnel policy making. National and provincial planning and policy making with consumer input.	National Health Insurance fiscal controls. National planning and policy, standard setting. Regional allocations and coordination. Local administration and consumer input.	National Health Insurance fiscal controls. National planning: standards, physician posts, construction. Regionalized services with graded care. Local government administration through elected council.	National Health Insurance controls. National planning and standards.

ᵃ Most of the countries of Asia, Africa, and Latin America have some system of national health service, usually not extensive, and most often concentrated in capital areas; roughly one half to two thirds of their physicians are salaried under these systems.

Sources: "Report of the Commission of the Health Center Project." *Can. Med. J.* (Aug. 19, 1972).

O. Anderson, *Health Care: Can There Be Equity?* (New York: Wiley, 1972).

K. Parkum, *Consumer Participation in Denmark's Health Insurance System* (Harrisburg, Pa.: Department of Health, 1972).

A Brief Report on Public Health Administration in Japan 1968 (Tokyo: Ministry of Health and Welfare, 1968).

M. Field, *Soviet Socialized Medicine* (New York: Free Press, 1967).

(Government of Canada *Statistics Canada 1971* (Ottawa: Government of Canada, 1973))

See references in Appendix Tables 18a and 18b.

Field research in these countries by author, 1967, 1971, 1973.

Federal Republic of Germany	Netherlands	Japan	U.S.S.R.
85% of M.D.s have some insurance patients.	Majority of M.D.s are in private practice and treat sick fund members.	Govt. employs 7.5% of M.D.s, dentists; 21% of nurses; midwives are in private practice.	50% of M.D.s make home calls; all personnel employed by government.
National Health Insurance fiscal controls.	National Health Insurance, fiscal controls (e.g., full capitation for up to 1,400 patients per M.D.; lesser thereafter to 2,800 patients). Some regional training.	Ministry of Health and Welfare sets standards for public health services and conditions for compulsory insurance funds.	Ministry of Health. All personnel employed by government. National planning and policy. Regional coordinating and grading of services. National education system and payment for training of personnel in return for limited service.

Index

Italic page numbers refer to figures.

Health status, 15–19, 39–48
  economic development and, *21*
  environment and, 49–53
  family planning and, *21*
  health services and, 53–57
  population growth and, *21*
  See also Disability; Disease; Growth
    and development; Life expectancy;
    Mental health; Mortality
Health visitors, 82t, 163t
Home Services, 70t, 91–93, 107, 117,
  260–61, 285
Hospitals, 68, 82t, 85–90, 93, 235, 240,
  379–83t, 394–97t

Illiteracy, 7, 10
India, 18, 23, 29–30, 33, 53
  health services in, 108, 128–31, 162,
    207–11, 299–302, 343n, 379–80t,
    387t
Integrated health training, 195–201
Israel
  health services in, 381–82t, 390t

Japan, 25, 28, 29t, 34, 49
  health services in, 81, 83, 108, 162,
    203, 379–80t, 386t, 394–97t

Kenya
  health services in, 381–82t, 392t

Labor unions, 186, 250, 252
Latin America, 8, 14, 17–18, 24–25, 30,
  45, 83, 108, 127, 365–66t
Legislation, health, 360n. *See also* Decision making, Congressional; Education, Health professions; Medicaid;
  Medicare; Controls; National health
  insurance; Organization, health services
Liberia
  health services in, 381–82t, 392t
Licensure, 181, 182, 184–85, 203, 256.
  See also Credentialing
Life expectancy, 16t, 17, 46, 379–83t
Low income, 10, 23, 26t, 27, 36t, 41t,
  66t, 67t, 264, 368t
  health occupations and, 145, 153t, 182,
    186, 202
  health services and, 80t, 116t, 129,
    173, 247, 259, 274–85t

Medicaid, 97, 118–19, 122, 189, 227,
  232, 246, 328n
Medical care assistants, 166–76
Medical schools, 73, 122, 156t, 174, 190,
  203, 206, 377t, 379–83t

Medicare, 70t, 87, 90–93, 97, 98, 101,
  117–18, 122, 189, 227, 232, 246, 256–
  58, 260, 328n
Mental health, 49–51, 103
Mexico
  health services in, 381–82t, 390t
Midwives, 82t, 163t, 202, 379–83t
Minorities, 37, 41t, 42t, 46, 379–83t
  health occupations and, 156t, 163t,
    182, 202
  health services and, 80t, 82t, 116t, 259,
    274–85t
Mortality, 49t, 49–50
  infant, 39–45, 82t, 259, 379–83t
  See also Health status

National health insurance, 125–27, 132,
  189, 239–41, 268, 271–94, 302–305,
  361–62n
Netherlands, 15, 34, 83, 126, 131–34,
  162, 202, 379–80t, 386t, 394–397t
New minorities, 34–35
Nigeria
  health services in, 81, 108, 127, 162,
    381–82t, 391t
North America, 8, 17
Nurse practitioners (NP), 172, 175–76,
  183–85, 201
Nurses, 72t, 82t, 151–53, 163t, 181, 379–
  83t
Nursing homes, 70t, 90–91, 120

Occupational Safety and Health Act, 246
Organization, health services, 85–109,
  104t, 284–88
Outcasts, 32–49, 83–84, 201, 260, 271,
  276–82t, 287, 292. *See also* American
  Indians; Blacks; Elders; Low income;
  Minorities; Spanish-speaking; Rural
  areas; Women

Patients' rights, 248–49. *See also* Con-
  sumers-as-patients
Pharmacists, 156t
Physician assistants (PA), 167, 169–77,
  183–85, 201
Physicians, 72t, 96t, 125, 149–50, 156–
  57t, 163t, 268. *See also* General prac-
  titioner; Specialists
Planning, 108. *See also* Comprehensive
  Health Planning Agency
Population, 8, 19, 46, 66t, 379–83t
  economic development and, 20
  family planning and, 9
  health and, 21t
Poverty, 27, 39t. *See also* Low income;
  Outcasts